Atlas of
External diseases of the eye

Volume IV
Anterior chamber, iris, and ciliary body

Atlas of
External diseases of the eye

VOLUME IV Anterior chamber, iris, and ciliary body

DAVID D. DONALDSON, M.D.

*Associate Professor of Ophthalmology, Massachusetts Eye and Ear
Infirmary and Howe Laboratory of Ophthalmology, Harvard University
Medical School; Associate Surgeon, Massachusetts Eye and Ear Infirmary;
Consultant in Ophthalmology, Massachusetts General Hospital,
Boston, Massachusetts*

*With 328 illustrations
112 stereoscopic views in full color on 16 View-Master® reels
and a View-Master® compact viewer*

THE C. V. MOSBY COMPANY

Saint Louis   1973

Volume IV

Copyright © 1973 by The C. V. Mosby Company

All rights reserved. No part of this book may be reproduced in any manner without written permission of the publisher.

Volume I copyrighted 1966, volume II copyrighted 1968, volume III copyrighted 1971

Printed in the United States of America

Distributed in Great Britain by Henry Kimpton, London

Library of Congress Cataloging in Publication Data

Donaldson, David D
  Atlas of external diseases of the eye.

  Stereoscopic color views on View-Master® reels with a compact viewer in pockets.
    Includes bibliography.
    CONTENTS. v. 1. Congenital anomalies and systemic diseases.—v. 2. Orbit, lacrimal apparatus, eyelids, and conjunctiva.—v. 3. Cornea and sclera. [etc.]
    1. Ophthalmology—Atlases. I. Title.
[DNLM: 1. Ophthalmology—Atlases. WW17 D676ae 1966]
RE71.D59   617.71   66-26959
ISBN 0-8016-1429-5 (v. 4)

To David Glendenning Cogan,
my constant friend through the years, whose personal integrity
and devotion to scientific research inspire and support all of us
who have had the good fortune to know and work with him.

Foreword from volume I

This volume, the [fourth] of a series to be published, has a solid foundation. Dr. Donaldson has had a background uniquely suited for such an undertaking. Brought up in Dearborn, Michigan, under the shadow of the Ford Motor Company and under the particular patronage of the elder Henry Ford himself, Dr. Donaldson learned machine shop technique at an early age. In high school he developed a more than average interest in photography, an interest which was to be applied to problems in publication when he later became editor of the campus magazine at the University of Michigan.

The importance of stereoscopic photography for medical purposes struck Dr. Donaldson as a hitherto unexplored field while he was a student at the University of Michigan Medical School in the early 1940's. Accordingly, he set about to take stereoscopic photographs of neuroanatomic specimens in the laboratory of Dr. Elizabeth Crosby. This was accomplished by taking two separate photographs with a single camera mounted on an arc frame and then viewing the pictures in a stereoscope. However, in order to take clinical photographs, it was necessary to have two cameras operating simultaneously. Calling on his early machine shop training, Dr. Donaldson made the first double camera combination while serving in the armed forces in Panama.

While subsequently attending a postgraduate course at the Harvard Medical School and, still later, while spending what was planned to be only a few months in the Howe Laboratory of Ophthalmology, Dr. Donaldson developed his technique of taking three-dimensional photographs of the eye. This involved the design of a camera that would permit appropriate magnifications, adjustable inter-lens distances, and avoidance of keystone optical aberrations, as well as methods for individual and group viewing. The original few months extended to years and to a career that is now well advanced in its second decade.

I have had the privilege of intimate association with Dr. Donaldson during his years at the Howe Laboratory of Ophthalmology and the Massachusetts Eye and

Ear Infirmary. I have seen Donaldson cameras designed, constructed, and varied while a steady stream of patients were referred to him or to his assistants for ocular photography. The result is an impressive collection of more than ten thousand photographs, a storehouse of sixteen years' documentation, illustrating a vast array of common and uncommon clinical conditions.

This volume and the others to follow are a tribute to Dr. Donaldson's ingenuity and industry. They will expand a service which has already proved to be of inestimable value to students, practitioners, and others concerned with ocular disease.

David G. Cogan

Director of Howe Laboratory of Ophthalmology,
Harvard University Medical School, and Chief of Ophthalmology,
Massachusetts Eye and Ear Infirmary

Preface

This volume, *Anterior Chamber, Iris, and Ciliary Body,* is the fourth in a series entitled *Atlas of External Diseases of the Eye* and represents a companion text to the three preceding atlases: *Congenital Anomalies and Systemic Diseases* (Vol. I), the *Orbit, Lacrimal Apparatus, Eyelids, and Conjunctiva* (Vol. II), and *Cornea and Sclera* (Vol. III). All of these atlases have been received with unanticipated enthusiasm; the last, on cornea and sclera, apparently has filled a void in the literature, and the response to it has been unusually gratifying.

In this volume the term external disease is used in the broadest sense; that is, any condition that can be visualized by means of slit-lamp biomicroscopy.

The format of this volume follows that of the previous ones with brief descriptions of the various disease entities followed by selected cases that are illustrated by stereoscopic photographs and/or text figures. The main parts of the book are subdivided on an etiologic basis. Because of the complexity of the anterior chamber angle, the presentation of the material in this atlas deviates from the previous volumes in that a number of labeled text figures are presented which have been reproduced from the stereoscopic photographs in the reels. Since the text figures are merely for the purpose of identifying structures within the chamber angle, the corresponding stereoscopic photograph on the reel must be utilized in conjunction with these labeled figures, in order that the reader may grasp the significance of the condition being illustrated. In fact, some of the labeled figures are almost meaningless without simultaneous viewing of the stereoscopic photograph. Although viewing of the reel photographs can be accomplished with the stereoviewer included in the book, a more substantial battery-operated stereoviewer is readily available and should be obtained.

In reading the abstracts of the histories in this volume, the reader must realize that some of these cases were seen and treated more than 25 years ago. Therefore, the treatment utilized, such as intravenous typhoid therapy, may have long since been superceded by other, newer therapeutic methods and agents.

During the 23 years of my tenure as a member of the Howe Laboratory of Ophthalmology at the Massachusetts Eye and Ear Infirmary, some 20,000 stereophotographs have been collected from which the illustrations for this volume were selected. During these many years, Dr. David G. Cogan, Director of the Laboratory, has taken an active and personal interest in the development of the photographic techniques and has been a constant encouragement as well as a source of important clinical material. Particularly in my earlier years, his willingness to assist me with all phases of my work made my years of clinical research and these volumes possible. Miss Inez M. Berry, who has been my chief assistant since I joined the Laboratory, has not only kept the photographic collection intact but has also been important in every phase of the production of this present volume. Her role in photographing the patients, organizing and keeping the collection intact, and selecting the photographs for this present volume has been invaluable. Also I am indebted to my secretary, Miss Agnes Love, for the many tedious hours she has spent typing and retyping the manuscript. As with previous volumes, Dr. Irving L. Pavlo has made a most valuable contribution by his constructive criticism and the proofreading of the entire manuscript. In addition, I had the good fortune of having Dr. Dennis Waltman work with me as a fellow during the major work on this volume. Not only was he involved in selecting photographs and in reviewing the literature, he was also primarily involved in the microscopic sections of tumors. I greatly appreciate the many hours spent by Dr. Waltman in the collection of microscopic slides and the production of photomicrographs to illustrate the important aspects of iris and ciliary body tumors.

It is impossible to mention all of the individuals directly and indirectly involved in the production of this volume, and I am indebted to the cooperation of innumerable fellows, residents, and staff members at the Massachusetts Eye and Ear Infirmary. Their referral for consultation and photographic recording of unusual cases has made possible the extensive collection. Funding for the development of the collection has been from the National Institute for Neurological Diseases and Blindness (Grants NB 5424, NB 3017, and NB 05691).

Following are the physicians who referred to me patients whose valuable case material is used in this volume: Dr. Lloyd M. Aiello, Reel XII–5 and Fig. 146; Dr. D. Robert Alpert, Fig. 53; Dr. William P. Beetham, Reel XIV–1 and Figs. 171 and 201; Dr. Frederic B. Breed, Fig. 141; Dr. Virgil G. Casten, Fig. 145; Dr. Paul A. Chandler, Reel III–1 and Figs. 16, 71, 100, and 189; Dr. David L. Clarke, Reel IX–2; Dr. David G. Cogan, Reels XII–2 and XIV–4 and Figs. 80, 88, 149, and 177; Dr. George B. Corcoran, Jr., Fig. 74; Dr. Thomas P. Cronin, Reel XI–5; Dr. Francis A. D'Ambrosio, Reel VII–2; Dr. William F. Donoghue, Fig. 61; Dr. Edwin B. Dunphy, Fig. 160; Dr. H. MacKenzie Freeman, Fig. 51; Dr. Carl G. Freese, Fig. 178; Dr. Edwin B. Goodall, Reel XVI–4 and Fig. 202; Dr. Edward F. Goodman, Reel XIII–1; Dr. Trygve Gundersen, Fig. 54; Dr. B. Thomas Hutchinson, Reels V–3 and V–4 and Fig. 124; Dr. Carl C. Johnson, Reel XV–6 and Fig. 194; Dr. Onni C. Kangas, Reel VI–3; Dr. Dewey Katz, Reel IX–4; Dr. Aaron H. Levin, Fig. 144; Dr. Sumner D. Liebman, Fig. 137; Dr. Bernard McGowan, Fig. 122; Dr. John M. McIver, Reel IX–5 and Figs. 34 and 81; Dr. J. Wallace McMeel, Reel III–6; Dr. Stanislaw A. Milewski, Fig. 142;

Dr. Irving L. Pavlo, Reel XII–6 and Figs. 77, 105, and 148; Dr. Arnold R. Perlman, Reel XIV–3 and Fig. 176; Dr. Charles D. J. Regan, Fig. 52; Dr. Francesco Ronchese, Fig. 89; Dr. Herbert S. Rubin, Fig. 119; Dr. Baruch J. Sachs, Figs. 151 and 154; Dr. Alfred W. Scott, Reel X–1; Dr. David H. Scott, Reels VII–6 and VII–7; Dr. Elmer A. Shaw, Fig. 35; Dr. Jules H. Shaw, Reel XV–4; Dr. Richard J. Simmons, Reels VIII–7 and IX–3; Dr. Albert E. Sloane, Figs. 12 and 150; Dr. Taylor R. Smith, Reels XV–3 and XVI–2 and Figs. 130 and 191; Dr. Julius C. Sozanski, Reel XII–3 and Fig. 140; Dr. Garrett L. Sullivan, Figs. 44, 155, 161, 179, and 193; Dr. H. Frederick Stephens, Fig. 123; Dr. Richard A. P. Thoft, Reel III–2; Dr. Robert R. Trotter, Reel XV–5 and Figs. 32 and 192; Dr. Ora H. Wagman, Fig. 31; Dr. David S. Walton, Fig. 64; Dr. Michael S. Wiedman, Reel VII–4; University of California, San Francisco Medical Center (Dr. Robert N. Shaffer), Reel VI–2 and Fig. 190; Estelle Doheny Eye Foundation (Dr. Otto Jungshaffer and Mr. Zolton Yuhasz), Reel V–7 and Fig. 62; University of Miami, Bascom Palmer Eye Institute (Drs. Richard K. Forster, Norman S. Jaffe, and Edward W. D. Norton), Reel II–3 and Figs. 56, 57, 86, and 200.

David D. Donaldson

Contents

Contents

Part three Ciliary body, 325

Part one

ANTERIOR CHAMBER

The function of the anterior chamber is a most important one. It is filled with aqueous, which is in constant production by the ciliary body. The relation between the rate of aqueous production and the resistance to aqueous outflow at the anterior chamber angle determines the intraocular pressure. When the intraocular pressure is elevated, the eye becomes glaucomatous and a number of structures within the eye can be permanently damaged. The complex embryonic and fetal development of the anterior chamber particularly of its angle, is responsible for the frequency of congenital anomalies. Moreover, it is vulnerable to various exogenous insults; corneal penetrations, foreign bodies in the anterior chamber, and bleeding (hyphema) may commonly result even from trauma of too mild a degree to affect more posteriorly located tissues. The majority of intraocular surgical procedures involve the anterior chamber; for example, cataracts are removed through the anterior chamber, and glaucoma surgery is performed to modify it.

Anatomically, the anterior chamber is bounded in front by the cornea, laterally by the sclera and ciliary body, and posteriorly by the iris and that portion of the lens within the pupillary opening. A most important portion of the anterior chamber is the so-called angle, which is visible ordinarily only through a gonioscopic device. The structures of the angle are important in considering abnormalities primarily associated with glaucoma but also in considering inflammatory processes, foreign bodies, and various congenital anomalies. These structures may be difficult to differentiate, particularly in the blue-eyed and in the young patient. They especially stand out when excessive pigment deposition has taken place, as in pigmentary glaucoma (Reel I-1 and Fig. 1). Posteriorly, the angle REEL I-1 recess begins just beyond the final iris roll. The floor of the recess is formed by FIG. 1 the ciliary body, which extends anteriorly to the scleral spur. On gonioscopic examination the ciliary body is seen as a light brown structure—the ciliary body band. At the anterior termination of the ciliary body band is another, narrower

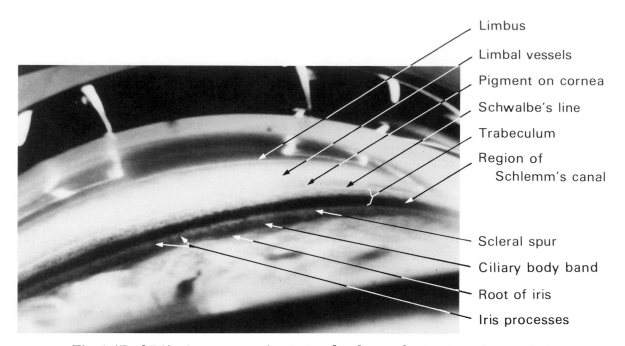

Limbus
Limbal vessels
Pigment on cornea
Schwalbe's line
Trabeculum
Region of
  Schlemm's canal

Scleral spur
Ciliary body band
Root of iris
Iris processes

Fig. 1 (Reel I-1). *Appearance of anterior chamber angle structures in a patient with pigmentary glaucoma.* The structures of the angle seen gonioscopically are accentuated by the presence of the excessive pigmentation selectively deposited on various portions of the angle. The meshwork overlying Schlemm's canal is black with pigmentation, while the portion of the meshwork just above it is covered with granules of pigment. Schwalbe's line is easily visible due to its being outlined by pigment on the cornea anteriorly and pigment granules on the trabecular meshwork posteriorly. The scleral spur is visible as a light gray line just below the trabecular meshwork, and the ciliary body is only lightly pigmented.

band, gray-white in color—the scleral spur or posterior border ring. This also represents the posterior boundary of the trabecular meshwork. The latter is contained in the scleral groove and represents the anterior wall of the angle. The posterior portion of the trabecular meshwork overlies Schlemm's canal and is the functional filtering portion of the meshwork. Ordinarily it has an irregular, roughened surface, composed of trabecular bands and intratrabecular spaces. In the brown-eyed older individual this portion of the trabecular meshwork is brown due to collections of melanin pigmentation. In the patient with pigmentary glaucoma it is most prominent, being almost black. The relatively nonfunctional portion of the trabecular meshwork occupies the anterior portion of the groove and finally ends at Schwalbe's line or the anterior border ring, the termination of Descemet's membrane. Schwalbe's line is generally considered the internal limbus; the external limbus, along with the limbal vessels, is frequently visible gonioscopically through the cornea. Schlemm's canal is deep in the scleral sulcus at about the junction of the middle and posterior thirds of the trabecular meshwork. Ordinarily it is not visible gonioscopically; but in congested or

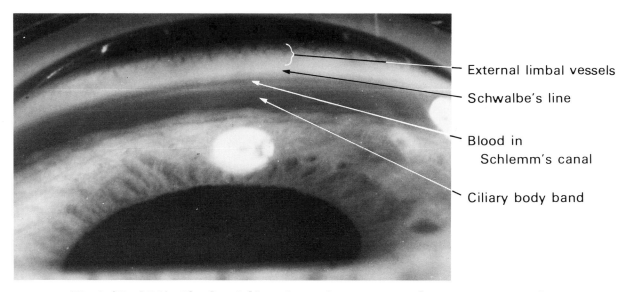

— External limbal vessels

— Schwalbe's line

— Blood in
    Schlemm's canal

— Ciliary body band

Fig. 2 (Reel I-2). *Blood in Schlemm's canal in a patient whose eye was recently subjected to blunt trauma.* The posterior portion of the trabecular meshwork has a distinct pink color due to reflux of blood into Schlemm's canal. Associated with the trauma is a recession of the iris root, which gives the impression of a wider ciliary body band than is usually seen.

recently traumatized eyes, particularly when the intraocular pressure is low, blood can reflux back into the canal, producing a prominent pink line (Reel I-2 and Fig. 2).

REEL I-2
FIG. 2

The corneoscleral meshwork constitutes the major portion of the trabecular meshwork and inserts on the scleral sulcus, the scleral spur, and the anterior ciliary body. The uveal meshwork, which arises at the periphery of the iris, bridges the angle recess and usually terminates near the scleral spur. However, some of the uveal meshwork may extend onto the inner surface of the corneoscleral meshwork to end near or at Schwalbe's line. When viewed gonioscopically, the single fibers of the uveal meshwork are called iris processes. They are seen as fine, delicate, vertically oriented fibers disappearing in the region of the scleral spur (Reel I-3 and Fig. 3). In the brown-eyed patient they are brown and show up against the lighter background of the ciliary body band and especially the scleral spur (Fig. 1 and Reel I-1). In the blue-eyed patient they are light gray or white and may be easily missed unless numerous (Fig. 3 and Reel I-3). Iris processes are sometimes referred to as pectinate ligaments because they are somewhat similar in appearance to and may be vestigial remains of the pectinate ligament of lower animals. Iris processes should not be confused with synechias and ordinarily do not have any effect on the outflow of aqueous. When abundantly present, particularly when they insert beyond the scleral spur, they may represent a true congenital anomaly of the angle involving incomplete cleavage and may predispose to chronic open angle glaucoma.

REEL I-3
FIG. 3

Determination of the width of the angle of the anterior chamber is one of the most important objectives of gonioscopy. While it may not be possible to deter-

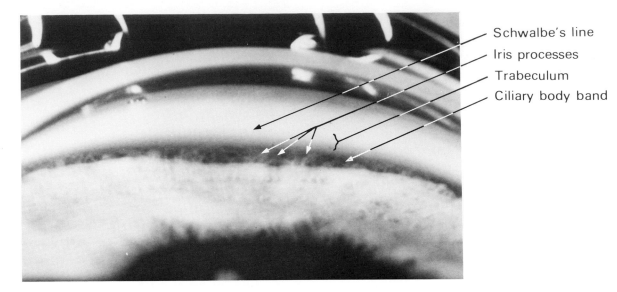

Schwalbe's line
Iris processes
Trabeculum
Ciliary body band

Fig. 3 (Reel I-3). *Prominent iris processes in a young myopic woman.* In the angle recess there is no ciliary body band visible due to the large amount of iris processes (uveal meshwork) that extend up to the scleral spur. The trabecular meshwork is lightly pigmented, and Schwalbe's line can be identified due to a number of pigment granules that have been deposited on it. The angle is very wide, typical of a myopic eye.

mine with absolute certainty whether an angle can be or is actually closed, functional provocative tests are not necessary in the presence of an obviously open angle. Thus the finding of an open angle during periods of elevated tension indicates that the glaucoma is not due to angle closure. However, if the angle appears to be closed when the tension is elevated or if the angle is extremely narrow and predisposed to closure, with a typical history suggestive of acute angle closure glaucoma (halos, redness, pain, and so on), further testing is mandatory to determine the exact cause. The fact that a simple peripheral iridectomy in uncomplicated cases of angle closure is curative requires that this differential diagnosis be made with maximum deliberation and accuracy. It must be constantly kept in mind that the corneoscleral meshwork is normal in angle closure glaucoma, but the aqueous humor is prevented from reaching the meshwork by apposition of the peripheral iris to the meshwork. In open angle glaucoma the aqueous has direct and unimpeded access to a defective filtering meshwork, which is the cause of increased resistance to outflow.

The width of the angle must be interpreted by the gonioscopist and a determination made about whether closure is possible. If the angle is slitlike and only a portion of the trabecular meshwork is visible, it is potentially a case of angle REEL I-4 closure (Reel I-4). If in at least some areas no trabecular meshwork is visible and in other areas only a small portion is visible, this is possibly a case of angle closure, or it may be some time in the immediate future. If no angle is visible, either the tension should be elevated, or there is a technical error in the gonioscopic examination.

Limbal vessels
Ciliary synechias
Scleral spur
Schwalbe's line

Trabeculum
Ciliary body band
Root of iris

Fig. 4 (Reel I-5). *Ciliary synechias and clumped pigmentation in the angle of a man with recurrent fibrinous iritis.* The ciliary body band is almost totally obscured by multiple tentlike synechias that extend only to the scleral spur. The trabecular meshwork is partially covered by pigment clumps, along with some pigment deposition on the peripheral cornea.

Gonioscopic evaluation of the angle of the anterior chamber involves the determination of the presence or absence of peripheral anterior synechias (P.A.S.) and, if present, their type and extent. Peripheral anterior synechias are abnormal adhesions of the iris to a portion of the anterior chamber angle. In some instances these adhesions may extend only onto the ciliary body band, while in other cases they may extend even beyond Schwalbe's line onto the cornea. The most common cause of peripheral anterior synechia formation in the open angle is inflammation, particularly of the chronic type. Less commonly they result from a flat anterior chamber following intraocular surgery. They are also common in the presence of iris bombé, both phakic and aphakic. In essential iris atrophy, both of the progressive type and in Chandler's syndrome, they frequently extend onto the cornea. Various types of trauma, such as perforating corneal wounds, also produce anterior synechias.

In the absence of inflammatory disease of the anterior chamber or other obvious causes, neovascular hemorrhagic glaucoma associated with occlusion of the central retinal vein or diabetic retinopathy must be seriously considered in explaining the presence of synechias. Even before the synechias develop, glaucoma is usually present due to the fibrovascular membrane commonly found in this condition.

In angle closure glaucoma, synechia formation is the rule, especially if the eye is congested and the attack lasts for more than 2 days. Subacute angle closure glaucoma without inflammation, when present for a prolonged period of time, also will produce peripheral anterior synechias. Often in an eye with acute

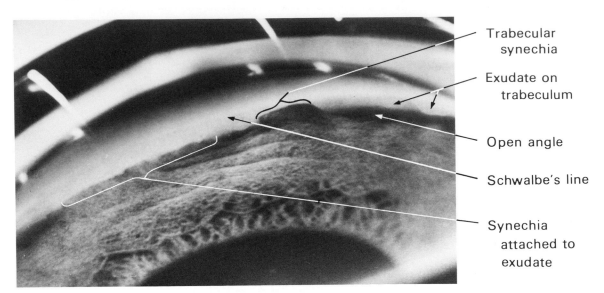

Trabecular
synechia

Exudate on
trabeculum

Open angle

Schwalbe's line

Synechia
attached to
exudate

Fig. 5 (Reel I-6). *Trabecular synechias and exudates on the trabecular meshwork in a woman with tuberculous iritis.* One peripheral anterior synechia extends to Schwalbe's line, while another broad synechia is attached to an exudate on the trabeculum. Elsewhere exudates project downward from the meshwork but have not yet come into contact with the iris to form synechias.

angle closure glaucoma it is very difficult to determine whether there is peripheral anterior synechia formation, and chamber deepening prior to the actual surgery may be necessary.

The importance of peripheral anterior synechias lies in the interference they may cause with aqueous outflow by obstruction of the filtering meshwork. Narrow and relatively tenuous peripheral anterior synechias that are not too numerous usually cause no difficulty. So-called ciliary synechias do not extend beyond the scleral spur; even though extensive, they produce no REEL I-5 obstruction to outflow (Reel I-5 and Fig. 4). This type of synechia involving only FIG. 4 the ciliary body is commonly associated with chronic iritis and is generally the precursor to trabecular synechias, which involves the trabecular meshwork as REEL I-6 well (Reel I-6 and Fig. 5). The trabecular synechia is particularly prone to de- FIG. 5 velop when exudates form on the trabecular meshwork. When such exudates become sufficiently large, they touch the iris, resulting in organization and a permanent and strongly adherent band involving variable amounts of the trabecular meshwork. In the presence of active iritis, there may be little or no development of glaucoma due to the relatively open blood-aqueous barrier. However, when the inflammation has subsided, secondary glaucoma, sometimes intractable, may result. In certain instances, particularly in progressive essential iris atrophy, extensive iridocorneal adhesions are frequently found, despite which the intraocular pressure and facility of outflow are normal. This is explained by the fact that the synechias bridge the meshwork and do not come into contact with the functioning trabecular tissue.

6

Chapter 1

Congenital and systemic conditions involving the anterior chamber

MEGALOCORNEA

Congenital enlargement of the cornea, which is stationary, characterizes megalocornea. In this condition the diameter of the cornea must exceed 13 mm. and is often as large as 16 mm. The congenital and stationary aspects, in the absence of increased intraocular pressure and glaucomatous cupping of the disc, eliminate the possibility of congenital glaucoma. Megalocornea is frequently familial, is usually bilateral, and is almost entirely restricted to males. It is commonly transmitted as a sex-linked recessive trait, and the pathogenesis is thought to be associated with development during embryologic life, where the rate of growth of the ectoderm of the optic cup slows but the ciliary ring continues to enlarge. This results in an increased size of the entire anterior segment.

The typical findings associated with megalocornea are a normal or increased curvature of the cornea, a well-marked limbus, and frequently an arcus juvenilis (anterior embryotoxon). The anterior chamber is very deep, and iridodonesis is frequent because there is no corresponding enlargement of the crystalline lens; therefore, the iris floats freely. Visual acuity is usually good, but astigmatism is not uncommon. The posterior segment of the eye is normal except for the enlarged ciliary ring. The latter is particularly evident by gonioscopy, where the ciliary body band is seen to be wider than the entire trabecular meshwork and scleral spur. Unlike buphthalmos (infantile glaucoma), the angle contains no grossly abnormal tissue.

Megalocornea is sometimes complicated by subluxation of the lens, which can then produce glaucoma. Also, in persons between the ages of 40 and 50 years it is not uncommon for cataracts to develop, and these may be associated with dislocation of the lens.

Megalocornea

History. Recently this 20-year-old man was rejected by the Army because of "glaucoma." The patient had no visual complaints and had never had his eyes examined previously.

Findings. The vision in both eyes is 20/20. Both corneas have a diameter of 14 mm., and the anterior chambers are very deep. The irides are normal except for a marked iridodonesis. The media are clear; and fundi, including the discs, are normal. Gonioscopy reveals that the angle is very wide, with a flat iris. The ciliary body band is unusually wide, and there are a number of iris processes REEL I-7 reaching up to the scleral spur (Reel I-7 and Fig. 6). A few abnormal vessels FIG. 6 run longitudinally around the angle. Intraocular tension in both eyes is 8 mm. Hg (Schiøtz).

Megalocornea

History. Two years ago this 46-year-old man noted painless loss of vision in the right eye and was discovered to have a posterior subcapsular cataract. About a year ago he was found to have inferior peripheral retinal holes, with minimal detachment in both eyes. The larger holes in the right eye were treated with cryopexy, and the postoperative reaction was good. The lens opacity in the right eye was slowly progressive, and recently the left eye was also found to have a cataract. The patient's older brother had eyes with a very similar appearance.

Findings. Vision in the right eye is counting fingers at 3 feet and in the left FIG. 7 20/40. Both eyes appear to be large and prominent (Fig. 7, A). The corneal diameter of the right eye is 13.5 mm., and there is a minimal arcus senilis. The

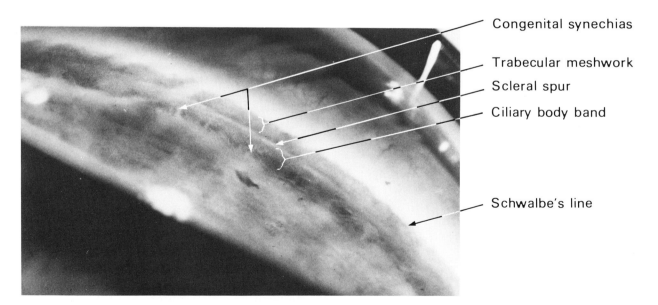

Congenital synechias

Trabecular meshwork

Scleral spur

Ciliary body band

Schwalbe's line

Fig. 6 (Reel I-7). *Unusually wide anterior chamber angle in a 20-year-old man with megalocornea.* The ciliary body band is wider than the trabecular meshwork, and a number of iris processes reach the scleral spur. The patient has normal vision and has no ocular complaints.

anterior chamber is extremely deep and contains minimal cells and no flare (Reel II-1). The iris is concave, transilluminates around its periphery, and REEL II-1 exhibits iridodonesis. In the lens there is a moderate nuclear sclerosis and a dense posterior subcapsular opacification. Through the lens opacity the posterior pole appears to be normal. Gonioscopy reveals the extremely deep anterior chamber, with a concave iris and wide ciliary body band (Fig. 7, *B*). The trabecular meshwork is heavily pigmented, and there are no peripheral anterior synechias or neovascularization. The left eye is identical to the right except that in the left eye the lens opacity is confined to the posterior subcapsular region and is much less dense. Tension revealed by applanation tonometry is 12 mm. Hg in the right eye and 14 mm. Hg in the left.

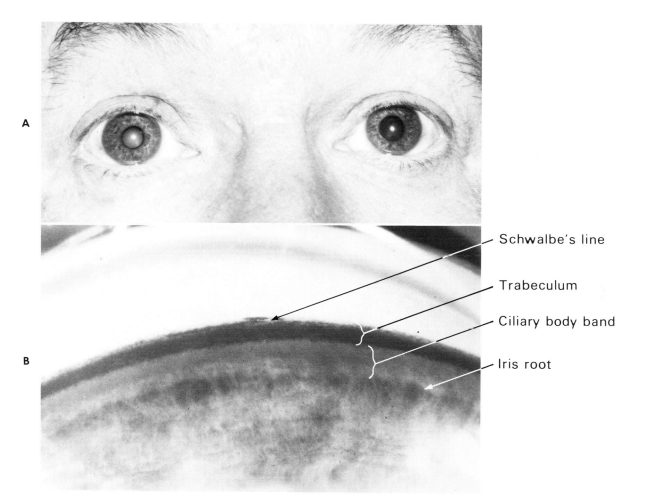

Schwalbe's line

Trabeculum

Ciliary body band

Iris root

Fig. 7. *Enlarged corneas (13.5 mm. in diameter) in a 46-year-old man with bilateral megalocornea.* **A,** The eyes are very prominent due to the megalocornea, and the right eye recently developed a posterior subcapsular cataract. **B,** Gonioscopy shows that the anterior chamber angle is very wide due to the exceptional width of the ciliary body band. The iris is concave and the trabecular meshwork heavily pigmented. The patient's older brother also has megalocornea.

Course. Cataract extraction was performed without complications, and the postoperative course was uneventful. Two months later with aphakic correction the patient had 20/20 vision in the right eye and was fitted with a contact lens. Fundus examination showed cystoid degeneration with many pars plana cysts and some lattice degeneration near the equator. The areas of the cryopexy were also visible. Two years later he was doing well and was still wearing his contact lens.

FAULTY CLEAVAGE ANOMALIES AND SYNDROMES

Congenital maldevelopment of the iridocorneal angle results in a number of anomalies and when associated predominantly with the cleavage process is often referred to as the faulty cleavage syndrome. Formation of the iridocorneal angle is a complex process, and many names have been applied to various anomalies of the angle. It is not surprising, therefore, that much confusion exists regarding the pathogenesis of these anomalies. It seems quite clear that during the earlier stages of development of the anterior chamber a gradual process of cell ingrowth and displacement takes place, with dissolution or atrophy of the mesodermal tissue. At about the fourth month a cleavage process begins as a part of the normal embryologic phenomenon, along with a decrease in the absorptive process of the mesodermal elements. Thus both processes play an important part in the pathogenesis of various developmental defects of the anterior chamber. The fact that these defects are primarily mesodermal in origin is undeniable, and the term dysgenesis mesodermalis of the iris and cornea is appropriate. Although some of the anomalies of the angle cannot be classified into a definite entity, others appear to have findings sufficiently distinct to classify them as a specific anomaly or syndrome. Posterior embryotoxon (Axenfeld's anomaly), Peters' anomaly, and Rieger's syndrome seem to be distinct entities.

A pathologically prominent Schwalbe's line with iris adhesions to the line represents posterior embryotoxon as described by Axenfeld and should be referred to as *Axenfeld's anomaly.* The condition is usually bilateral but may involve only a small segment of the angle in only one eye. A familial tendency is not uncommon. The condition may be an isolated finding and produce no symptoms, but many times it is associated with other, more extensive developmental defects of the anterior chamber. Clinically, a white line is seen concentric with and close to the limbus. Slit-lamp biomicroscopy shows this line to be on the posterior surface of the cornea, and frequently iris processes can be seen attached to it. Gonioscopic examination reveals the characteristic picture of a thickened white ring that is displaced centrally, with multiple strands of iris bridging the meshwork and attaching to it. The thickening of Schwalbe's line is of variable degree, but in some instances it has a ropelike appearance and in places is detached from the cornea. The trabecular zone appears widened, depending on the degree of anterior displacement of Schwalbe's line. The pathogenesis appears to be a defect in the cleavage process after the fourth month of embryologic development.

Histopathologically, in Axenfeld's anomaly the prominent Schwalbe's ring is related to mesodermal tissue of the uveal meshwork rather than to Descemet's

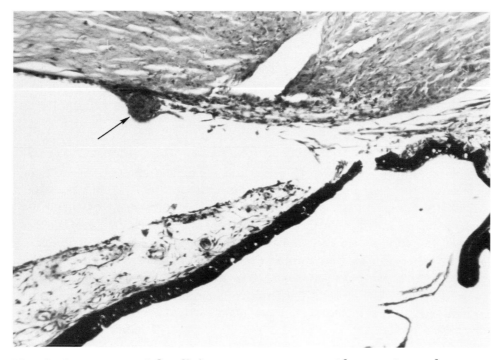

Fig. 8. *A prominent Schwalbe's ring in a patient with posterior embryotoxon (Axenfeld's anomaly).* A thickened anterior Schwalbe's ring (arrow) is a prominent finding, along with bits of uveal meshwork extending up on the angle recess and attaching to the ring. (Masson stain; ×400.)

membrane (Fig. 8). Iris tissue is attached to the ring, and in some cases there is FIG. 8 a meridional ciliary muscle that bypasses the scleral spur.

Congenital central corneal opacification, usually associated with iridocorneal adhesions to the edge of the opacity, characterizes *Peters' anomaly* (dysgenesis mesodermalis of the cornea). The condition is usually transmitted as a recessive trait. Clinically, the typical defect in Peters' anomaly consists of a central corneal opacity involving the deepest layers most extensively. The mildest degree of this anomaly is probably seen as nothing more than a central posterior kerato-conus. In more advanced stages there is a central leukoma, with distinct edges and a number of iridocorneal adhesions arising from the collarette and extending to its borders. Sometimes the lens is involved, showing anterior polar cataract formation. Microcornea is commonly present in Peters' anomaly, as opposed to its rather infrequent occurrence in Rieger's syndrome. The opposite is true of glau-coma, which occurs less frequently in Peters' anomaly. The pathogenesis appears to occur very early in the development of the anterior chamber, with a dis-turbance in separation of the primary lens vesicle from the superficial ectoderm. The condition is usually bilateral but occasionally unilateral. When associated with other developmental defects of the anterior segment or congenital anomalies other organ systems, it should be referred to as secondary dysgenesis mesoder-malis of the cornea. A number of such cases have been reported. Maternal rubella may give rise to a secondary type of Peters' anomaly.

Hypoplasia of the iris stroma, anomalies of the iridocorneal angle, bilaterality of the ocular defects, and dental defects comprise the findings now generally referred to as *Rieger's syndrome* (dysgenesis mesodermalis of the iris). Because of the prominent findings in the iris associated with this syndrome, detailed discussion of it is given in Chapter 5. However, it too must be considered to be a congenital maldevelopment of the iridocorneal angle associated with incomplete or disturbed cleavage.

Faulty cleavage syndrome

History. At birth this 16-year-old boy was noted to have abnormal eyes. During the past few years various drops and pills were given, presumably for glaucoma.

Findings. Vision in the right eye is 20/80 with correction and in the left counting fingers at 1 foot. In the right eye there is moderate conjunctival injection, and the corneal diameter is 11 mm. The central cornea and a portion of the nasal cornea are clear, but most of the peripheral cornea is densely opacified REEL II-2 (Reel II-2). To the opacified cornea are attached numerous strands of iris stroma, some of which arise at the pupillary margin. Some areas of the iris are markedly atrophic, and the pupil is irregular, miotic, and displaced temporally

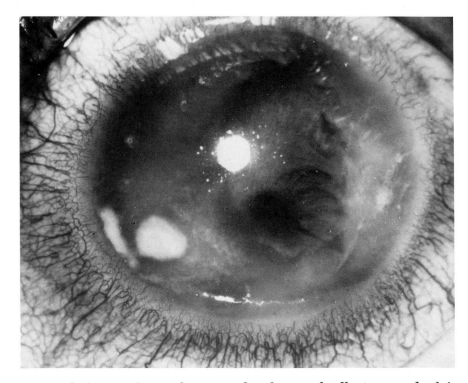

Fig. 9. *Marked corneal opacification and iridocorneal adhesions in the left eye of a 16-year-old boy with a faulty cleavage syndrome.* The right eye (Reel II-2) is similarly involved but to a lesser extent, having only peripheral corneal opacification, with useful vision. Intraocular pressure, however, is markedly elevated. The left eye has a normal intraocular pressure but progressively has become more edematous until the eye has become blind.

due to the iridocorneal adhesions. There are some opacities in the lens, and only a red reflex can be obtained from the fundus. In the left eye the conjunctiva is markedly injected, and the cornea is almost entirely opacified except for a small area centrally (Fig. 9). Again, there are numerous adhesions of iris to cornea FIG. 9 associated with the corneal opacification. The pupil is miotic and displaced downward. Only a red reflex can be obtained. The intraocular pressure revealed by applanation tonometry is 60 mm. Hg in the right eye and 20 mm. Hg in the left. Because of the corneal opacification, gonioscopy is difficult and does not reveal any additional information about either eye. Visual field examination of the right eye reveals symmetrical constriction and an enlarged blind spot.

Course. Echothiophate (Phospholine) iodide (1/4%) was used topically in the right eye and resulted in a gradual lowering of the intraocular pressure to normal levels. Despite consistent findings of normal intraocular pressures on a number of occasions, 6 months later there was an increase in the field defect, with a large upper Bjerrum scotoma. Epinephrine (1%) drops and acetazolamide (Diamox) were added to the regimen, but despite this in another 3 months there was a further increase in the field defect and a decrease in the visual acuity. At times the intraocular pressure was found to be in the low 30's, and more intensive medications were instituted. Three years later because of difficulty in control of the intraocular pressure, penetrating cyclodiathermy was performed, and this was repeated in another year. Two years later a corneal trephine procedure was performed, and a year later cyclocryotherapy was carried out. In another year a cataract had formed in the right eye, so a cataract extraction was performed. When the patient was last seen 2 years later, the intraocular pressure was 7 mm. Hg (Schiøtz), and his vision was 20/200. The central cornea in the right eye was still clear, but the left eye was blind and the entire cornea opacified.

Incomplete Peters' anomaly

History. At birth this 12-year-old boy was found to have corneal opacity in his right eye. During the next 6 months much of the opacity cleared, but a residual opacity remained stationary since then. When the boy was 4 years old, muscle surgery was performed for an exotropia of 30 prism diopters.

Findings. Vision in the right eye is 20/50 and in the left 20/20 with correction. The cornea of the right eye has a central diffuse opacity limited inferiorly by three anterior synechias, which arise from the collarette (Reel II-3). Else- REEL II-3 where there is evidence of other synechias that have become detached from the cornea, resulting in a scalloped, irregular collarette. The remainder of the anterior chamber and iris is normal, the pupil is round, and the media and fundus are normal. The left eye is normal.

Course. For the next 4 years the patient had no change in his ocular status, and his vision remained the same.

Congenital anterior synechia

History. This 62-year-old woman was seen because of tearing of her left eye and difficulty in reading. She gave a history of having had a splinter of wood removed from one of her eyes 2 years previously.

FIG. 10 *Findings.* Vision in both eyes is 20/40 with correction. The right eye is normal, but the left has a broad attachment of the iris to the cornea at the 3 o'clock position, causing an oval-shaped pupil (Fig. 10). Gonioscopy reveals that the angle structures on each side of the synechia are normal and that no abnormality of the iris is present except in the area of the iridocorneal adhesion, where the stroma is somewhat thinned. The anterior extent of the synechia is several millimeters beyond Schwalbe's line. Some incipient lens changes are evident in the cortex, and the fundus is normal.

Course. With careful refraction the patient's vision was corrected to 20/25 in each eye. A ^{32}P test showed no evidence of increased uptake in the region of the synechia. On several occasions intraocular tensions were found to be in the high teens. She was seen several times during the next 6 years, and there was no change in the appearance of the synechia formation. When she was last seen, her vision was reduced to 20/70 in each eye due to lens changes.

Severe posterior embryotoxon (Axenfeld's anomaly)

History. Early in life this 8-year-old girl was noted to have peculiar-appearing eyes. Recently her optometrist found the vision in both eyes, and particularly in the left, to be reduced. Her parents have normal eyes, and her two brothers are said to have ocular abnormalities similar to hers.

Findings. Vision in the right eye is 20/70 and in the left 20/50 with correction. In the right eye the entire nasal half of the cornea is involved by a prominent white ring, which is attached to the posterior surface of the cornea

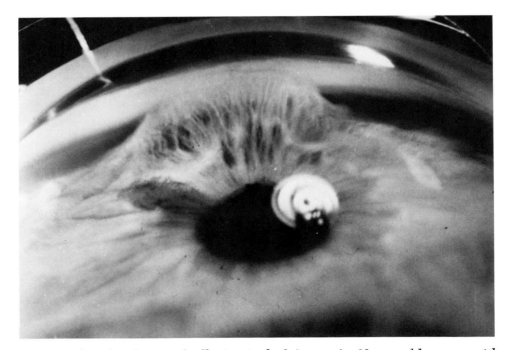

Fig. 10. *A broad iridocorneal adhesion in the left eye of a 62-year-old woman with a congenital anterior synechia. The patient's only complaint is difficulty in reading due to a refractive error, and the congenital defect is found incidentally.*

several millimeters in from the limbus. This ringlike structure extends temporally, but in some places disappears behind the external limbus. To the white ring are attached numerous strands of iris stroma arising from various portions of the iris as far in as the collarette. In the left eye there is a similar but more extensive process as the white ring extends around the entire cornea, with extensive iridocorneal adhesions (Fig. 11). Gonioscopy shows that all the iris stromal attach- FIG. 11 ments are inserted on a thickened and anteriorly displaced Schwalbe's line (Reel II-4). In some areas the angle structures can be visualized between the REEL II-4 numerous iris adhesions and appear to be normal. The anterior chambers are of normal depth, and the pupil is round and reactive. The media are clear, and the fundus is normal. Intraocular tension is 20 mm. Hg (Schiøtz) in both eyes.

Course. Tonography showed both eyes to have a low normal facility of outflow. Repeated intraocular tensions indicated that the right eye was consistently normal, but tension in the left was occasionally elevated. Four years later the

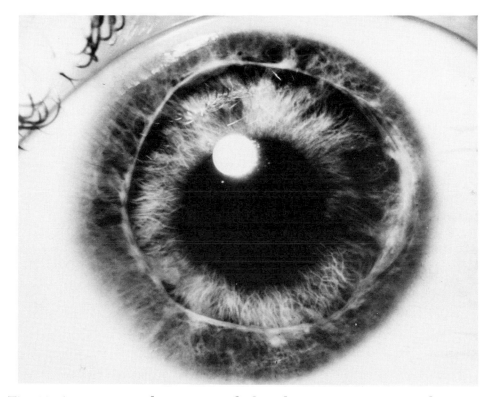

Fig. 11. *A prominent white ring attached to the posterior surface of the cornea in the left eye of an 8-year-old girl with severe posterior embryotoxon (Axenfeld's anomaly).* Since early life the patient had peculiar-appearing eyes. There is a similar appearance in both eyes, but in the left the process is more extensive, with a thickened and anteriorly displaced Schwalbe's line extending around the entire circumference of the cornea. To this are attached numerous iris adhesions, which are particularly well visualized gonioscopically (Reel II-4). Tonography shows a somewhat decreased facility of outflow in both eyes, but the intraocular pressure remains in the normal range most of the time.

girl developed an exotropia, with a reduction of vision in the right eye to 20/70 and improvement of her vision to 20/30 in the left. The left eye was occluded for 3 months, and the vision in the right eye improved to 20/50. With intermittent occlusion for the next year the vision remained at that level. When she was last seen 14 years later, her intraocular pressures were normal, and her vision with correction was 20/50 in the right eye and 20/30 in the left. The congenital abnormalities remained unchanged.

Posterior embryotoxon (Axenfeld's anomaly)

History. Two years ago this 53-year-old man cracked the right lens of his glasses. Immediately thereafter his right eye developed tearing and photophobia. The vision also became poorer, although admittedly this was an eye that had never had good vision. There was an almost constant sensation of foreign body in the eye, with some recent partial relief.

Findings. The vision in the right eye is 20/100 and in the left 20/15. In the right eye the lower one third of the cornea is edematous, with bedewing of the corneal epithelium and striate keratopathy. Encircling the entire cornea close to the limbus is a white irregular line, which by slit-lamp biomicroscopy can be seen to be on the posterior surface of the cornea (Fig. 12, *A*). The anterior chamber is clear and of normal depth, and the pupil is normal. There are no abnormalities of the posterior segment. Gonioscopy shows a ropelike structure extending around the entire periphery of the cornea just anterior to the normal location of Schwalbe's line. There are a number of attachments of the iris to this abnormal structure (Fig. 12, *B*). The edematous cornea inferiorly can be seen extending down into the angle, but no spicule of glass or other cause to explain the edematous cornea is visible. There are no deviations from normal in the left eye, including any that might be revealed by gonioscopic examination. Intraocular pressure is 20 mm. Hg (Schiøtz) in the right eye and 17 mm. Hg in the left.

FIG. 12

Course. Because of persistence of the corneal edema, a year later a conjunctival flap was performed to cover the lower half of the cornea. Six months later there was persistence of some edema above the flap, so hypertonic salt ointment was prescribed. A year later the flap was still in place, and there was no edema. The cause of the corneal edema remained a mystery.

Congenital glaucoma due to posterior embryotoxon

History. No reliable ocular history was obtainable on this 13-year-old boy, except that since the age of 4 he had very poor vision. In addition, he was almost deaf. About a month ago he was found to have an intraocular pressure of 50 mm. Hg (Schiøtz) in the right eye and 46 mm. Hg (Schiøtz) in the left. His corneas were markedly enlarged, and intensive medical therapy was instituted, using pilocarpine hydrochloride (4%) and epinephrine (1%) drops in both eyes at frequent intervals. At times the intraocular pressures were found to have been reduced to the low 30's, but on other occasions were found again to be markedly elevated.

Findings. Vision in the right eye is 20/70 and in the left 20/200 with correction. In both eyes the corneal diameters are 16 mm., and the corneas have a

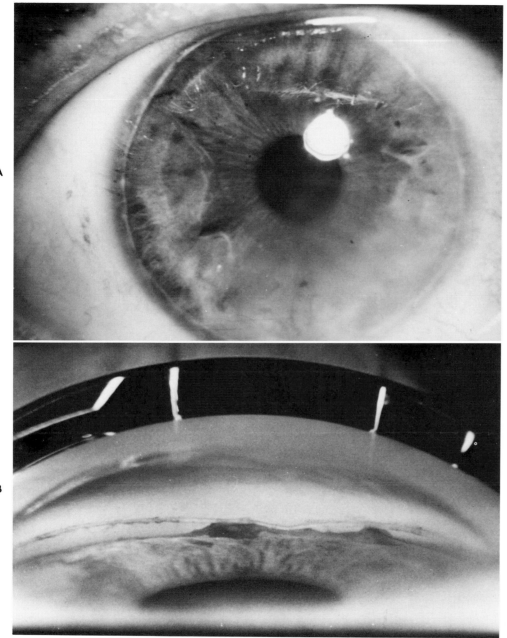

Fig. 12. *An anteriorly displaced, thickened Schwalbe's line in the right eye of a 53-year-old man with posterior embryotoxon (Axenfeld's anomaly).* **A,** In addition to the typical posterior embryotoxon, the inferior half of the cornea has been edematous since injury from a fragment of glass when his spectacles were accidentally shattered 2 years ago. **B,** Gonioscopy reveals the ropelike Schwalbe's line to which iris is attached in several places. Subsequently, a conjunctival flap was placed over the lower half of the cornea, and gradually the edema subsided.

slight diffuse opacification. The anterior chambers are deep and the iris planes flat. The pupils are miotic, and the optic nerve heads show deep glaucomatous cupping and atrophy in both eyes. Gonioscopy reveals that in the right eye there is a prominent thickened refractile Schwalbe's line, which is displaced an-

FIG. 13 teriorly onto the cornea (Fig. 13). In some places this is detached from the cornea and has iridocorneal attachments and dark pigment deposits on its surface. The trabecular meshwork is indistinct and is covered with a whitish membrane. In the left eye the abnormalities are similar but more extensive, with large pillar synechias attached to the anteriorly displaced and thickened Schwalbe's line

REEL II-5 (Reel II-5). Elsewhere there are anterior insertion of the iris and multiple anomalies of the angle, with excessive pigmented tissue and a filmy membrane on the trabecular meshwork. The intraocular pressure is 40 mm. Hg (Schiøtz) in both eyes. The field in the right eye is approximately 10° in size, using an 18-mm. test object; in the left eye the field is so constricted that no adequate examination can be performed.

Course. A goniopuncture was performed on the right eye and an iridencleisis on the left. Intraocular pressures were under better control for several years, although miotics and acetazolamide were necessary. Finally, 4 years later the intraocular tension became elevated in the right eye and a goniotomy was per-

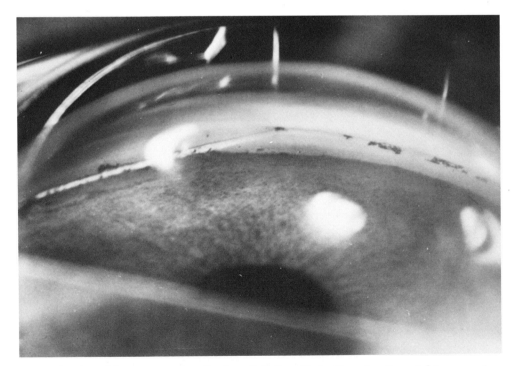

Fig. 13. *Ropelike anteriorly displaced Schwalbe's line in the right eye of a 13-year-old boy with congenital glaucoma due to posterior embryotoxon.* Clumps of pigment and iris attachments are seen on Schwalbe's line, which is actually detached from the cornea. In the left eye (Reel II-5) more extensive abnormalities are present, with large pillar synechias attached to the thickened Schwalbe's line. The patient has markedly enlarged corneas (16 mm. in diameter) and markedly constricted fields.

formed, and within the next 2 years two additional filtering procedures were necessary. Nine years after the patient had first been seen, the intraocular pressure was in the 20's when the patient was receiving maximal medications, and his vision was counting fingers at 2 feet in the right eye and light perception in the left.

CONGENITAL GLAUCOMA

A combination of corneal enlargement and edema and increased intraocular pressure within the first 6 months of life constitute congenital or infantile glaucoma (buphthalmos). Primary congenital glaucoma occurs in the absence of other congenital defects of the eye or systemic diseases. In contrast, secondary congenital glaucoma is usually associated with congenital anomalies such as aniridia, Sturge-Weber syndrome, Marfan's syndrome, Lowe's syndrome, and persistent hyperplastic primary vitreous. Juvenile glaucoma, developing after the first 6 months of life but usually before the patient is 20, is considered by some to be a delayed type of congenital glaucoma. Typical congenital glaucoma is usually transmitted as a recessive hereditary trait. It is bilateral about 75% of the time. The cardinal symptom is photophobia, but epiphora and blepharospasm are also seen frequently even before corneal cloudiness and enlargement become obvious. The increased intraocular pressure results in a markedly distended eyeball, giving rise to the term buphthalmos, or ox eye. If the cornea is more than 10 mm. in diameter, glaucoma should be suspected; 12 mm. is usually diagnostic, especially if accompanied by other signs, such as breaks in Descemet's membrane and diffuse corneal haziness. The anterior chamber becomes markedly deepened and the iris flattened and hypoplastic in appearance. Multiple breaks in Descemet's membrane occur concentric with the limbus peripherally; centrally the breaks are linear.

The appearance of the angle is still in dispute. The hypoplastic-appearing iris is flat and frequently has areas of marked hypoplasia at its base. Some ophthalmologists believe that it inserts into the trabecular meshwork, covering a portion of the trabeculum and causing a decrease in facility of outflow. All infants have a persistence of uveal meshwork in the angle that causes a hazy, unclear appearance in the angle structures and a decrease in the angle recess. Some increased opacification of the angle structures can be appreciated, but this abnormality is certainly not uniformly seen in all cases. Otto Barkan first described a fine gelatinous membrane that covers the trabecular meshwork, which may explain the marked decrease in facility of outflow seen in these patients, no matter what the appearance of the angle might be.

Successful treatment of congenital glaucoma depends on early diagnosis and prompt therapy. Medical treatment is only occasionally successful, but the surgical technique of goniotomy offers a high degree of success in those patients in which the disease becomes manifest after the second month of life. When the glaucoma is present earlier or at birth, the success rate is less than 50%.

Congenital glaucoma

History. Since birth this 13-year-old girl's right eye was larger than the left. When the girl was 2 years of age, the right cornea measured 15 mm. and the left

12 mm. With the patient under general anesthesia, the tension in the right eye was 48 mm. Hg and in the left 22 mm. Hg. A Reese type of sclerotomy was performed, and postoperatively a large cystoid staphyloma formed. Three months later the intraocular pressure was found to be 20 mm. Hg in the right eye but 30 mm. Hg (Schiøtz) in the left. Pilocarpine (2%) drops were used 4 times a day in both eyes. For the next 4 years the intraocular pressures were well controlled, but then the pressure in the right eye gradually became elevated. Cooperation was adequate to perform a visual field examination, which showed the nasal field of the right eye to be constricted. The right disc showed glaucomatous cupping, but the left disc was normal. Over the next 5 years there was gradual progression of the field defect, with moderately elevated tensions in the right eye despite medical treatment.

Findings. The vision in the right eye is 3/200 and in the left 20/15 with correction. The cornea of the right eye is markedly enlarged to about 17 mm., and FIG. 14 the anterior chamber is very deep (Fig. 14). The pupil is miotic and reacts slightly. The optic nerve head is pale and deeply saucerized, with an absence of the normal disc rim temporally. When viewed gonioscopically, the iris plane is flat, and at the periphery of the iris there is stromal thinning. The angle is wide open, but there is a hazy appearance to the structures, as if they are covered by a membrane. There are numerous dark, pigmented fibrils filling in REEL II-6 the angle and extending up onto the trabecular meshwork (Reel II-6). Neither the scleral spur nor Schwalbe's line can be identified. In the left eye the cornea is of normal size and the anterior chamber of normal depth. The pupil is miotic and the optic nerve head normal. Here, too, gonioscopy reveals structures in the

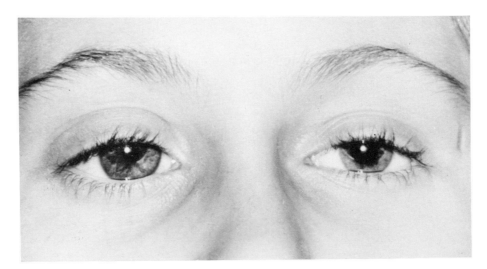

Fig. 14. *Enlarged right cornea in a 13-year-old girl with unilateral congenital glaucoma.* The right cornea is 17 mm. in diameter, and the intraocular pressure is 34 mm. Hg (Schiøtz). Gonioscopy (Reel II-6) shows that the iris plane is flat and that there is a hazy appearance to the angle structures, with numerous dark, pigmented fibrils filling in the angle and extending up onto the trabecular meshwork.

angle that are less visible than normal but with less fibrillar material in the angle and on the meshwork than in the right eye. Intraocular pressure in the right eye is 34 mm. Hg and in the left 23 mm. Hg (Schiøtz), and tonography shows the facility of outflow to be definitely in the glaucomatous range in the right eye and normal in the left. Visual fields are normal in the left eye but show moderate constriction, particularly nasally, in the right.

Course. With the patient receiving maximum medications in the right eye the tension still remained somewhat elevated, and 6 years later there was no appreciable change in her findings.

Congenital glaucoma

History. At birth this 13-year-old boy was noted to have large eyes, and at 1 year of age his left cornea developed a gray haze. Intraocular pressures were high normal in the right eye but markedly elevated in the left; a goniotomy, goniopuncture, and iridodialysis were performed on the left eye. Because of the continued elevation of tension in the left eye, additional goniotomies and a sclerectomy were necessary. A year later the intraocular tensions were normal in both eyes, but the left eye was found to be developing first a cataract and then a spontaneous hyphema with recurrent bleeding over the next 3 years. Paracenteses were to no avail, and finally the eye developed phthisis bulbi and was enucleated when the patient was 6 years old. For several years the intraocular pressure in the right eye was found to be normal when measured with the patient under

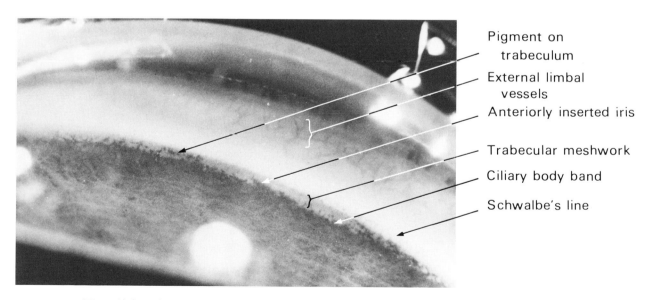

Pigment on
  trabeculum
External limbal
  vessels
Anteriorly inserted iris

Trabecular meshwork
Ciliary body band
Schwalbe's line

Fig. 15 (Reel II-7). *Insertion of the iris near the scleral spur in the right eye of a 13-year-old boy with congenital glaucoma.* By gonioscopy the iris can be seen to insert anteriorly just behind or at the scleral spur, with pigment clumps on the surface of the trabecular meshwork. The cornea is enlarged to 15 mm. in diameter. The intraocular pressure is moderately elevated but is controlled by medical therapy. The left eye has been enucleated following severe glaucoma and multiple operative procedures.

anesthesia, but when the boy reached age 10 the intraocular tensions were in the low 30's. However, the disc did not show glaucomatous cupping, and sometimes the intraocular tensions were in the mid 20's. About 3 months ago applanation tonometry indicated that the tension was elevated to 40 mm. Hg, and pilocarpine (2%) and epinephrine (1%) drops were instituted, with a return of the intraocular pressures to normal levels.

Findings. Vision in the right eye with a high myopic correction is 20/100, and the left eye is anophthalmic. There is a coarse nystagmus. The corneal diameter REEL II-7 is 15 mm. The anterior chamber is deep and the iris flat. When viewed gonio- FIG. 15 scopically, the iris inserts just behind or at the scleral spur (Reel II-7 and Fig. 15). Pigment clumps are on the surface of the trabecular meshwork, and Schwalbe's line is visible. There is an anterior polar cataract, and the disc is pink, with a moderate-sized physiologic cup. Intraocular pressure revealed by applanation tonometry is 20 mm. Hg.

Course. The intraocular pressure was generally well controlled but was occasionally elevated to the low 30's. With echothiophate (¼%) there seemed to be more consistent control. However, in another 18 months the tensions were again elevated, occasionally to the high 30's. A trephine procedure was performed, which resulted in a filtering bleb. Intraocular pressure was controlled over the next 5 years with the addition of epinephrine (1%) drops. Vision with a high myopic correction was 20/300.

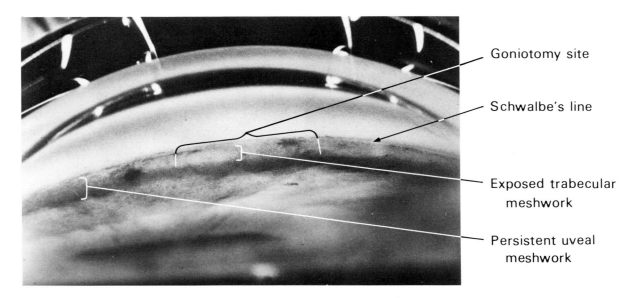

Goniotomy site

Schwalbe's line

Exposed trabecular meshwork

Persistent uveal meshwork

Fig. 16 (Reel III-1). *A wide open angle with visibility of the trabecular meshwork and ciliary body band in the right eye of a 38-year-old man following a goniotomy procedure for congenital glaucoma.* By gonioscopic examination there is a good visualization of the trabecular meshwork and ciliary body band in the area of a previous goniotomy; other portions of the angle contain a gray, thickened tissue covering the angle structures. There is total glaucomatous cupping of the disc, and the fields show marked glaucomatous changes. The previously elevated intraocular pressure is now normal following an iridencleisis procedure. The left eye has been enucleated due to severe glaucoma.

Goniotomy site in congenital glaucoma

History. At age 1 this 38-year-old man had his left eye enucleated because of glaucoma. About 20 years ago two glaucoma operations were performed on his right eye, and until the past year his intraocular pressures were normal, with no further field loss. Two months ago a goniotomy was performed, but within several months the intraocular tension again became elevated, requiring intensive medical treatment. Despite this, the intraocular pressure rose to the mid 30's.

Findings. Vision in the right eye is 20/20, and the left is anophthalmic. The cornea is enlarged, and there is a complete surgical iris coloboma superiorly. The anterior chamber is deep, the iris plane flat, and gonioscopy shows that there are several areas of broad synechias. From the 5 to 7 o'clock position the angle is wide open, with the trabecular meshwork and ciliary body band visible in the area of the previous goniotomy (Reel III-1 and Fig. 16). Elsewhere in the angle there REEL III-1 is a gray, thickened tissue, which covers the angle structures up to Schwalbe's FIG. 16 line. The optic nerve head is totally cupped, and fields show a double Bjerrum scotoma and an upper nasal step, with moderate peripheral constriction. The intraocular pressure is 35 mm. Hg (Schiøtz).

Course. An iridencleisis procedure was carried out, and the postoperative course was uneventful. Five years later the intraocular pressure again became elevated, and over the next 5 years multiple cyclodiathermy procedures were carried out to control the intraocular pressure. The patient then developed a posterior subcapsular cataract, with reduction of vision to 20/300, and cataract extraction was advised.

Juvenile glaucoma

History. Two months ago this 20-year-old man consulted an ophthalmologist because of frontal headaches. Applanation tonometry revealed elevated intraocular pressure in the left eye, 26 mm. Hg, while the tension in the right eye was only 23 mm. Hg. Tonography showed a decreased facility of outflow in both eyes. Epinephrine (1%) drops 3 times a day were initiated in the left eye. The patient's 27-year-old brother had almost identical findings.

Findings. Both anterior chambers are quite deep, and the irides are flat, with 4-mm. pupils. When viewed gonioscopically, the irides are flat with wide open angles, with a heavy, coarsely pigmented uveal meshwork obscuring most of the ciliary body band and scleral spur (Reel III-2). In some areas the pig- REEL III-2 ment on the meshwork is so heavy that it has the appearance of synechias. In addition, in some places there is also a more transparent membranous material that extends across the trabecular meshwork to reach Schwalbe's line. Visual fields are normal in both eyes.

Course. During the next year the introcular pressure was well controlled by the use of epinephrine drops. Then the intraocular pressure rose to borderline levels in the left eye, and echothiophate ($\frac{1}{16}$%) drops at bedtime were added to the treatment. In another 2 months the pressure was again elevated, and echothiophate administration was increased to twice a day. Two years later it was necessary to increase the echothiophate administration to $\frac{1}{8}$% twice a day in the left eye only. Four years later acetazolamide and pilocarpine (4%) were added, and the intraocular pressure in the left eye was only under borderline control. During the next 2 years control was fair in both eyes with continuation of the same treatment.

PERSISTENT HYPERPLASTIC PRIMARY VITREOUS

Retrolenticular vascularized membrane, spherophakia, hyperplastic ciliary processes, and a shallow anterior chamber characterize persistent hyperplastic primary vitreous. In this unilateral congenital defect there is usually some progression of the process during the first 5 years of life, with gradual increase in opacification of the lens and shallowing of the anterior chamber. The most prominent finding is that of the white pupil due to the retrolenticular membrane, which in turn is associated with the persistence of the hyaloid artery and hyperplastic primary vitreous. Commonly, ciliary processes can be seen around the periphery of the lens, which is smaller than normal. The pupil is difficult to dilate, and blood vessels are visible in the stroma of the iris. Sometimes it is possible to visualize the persistent hyaloid artery, which is always seen on microscopic sections. Frequently the cornea is smaller than normal, and the shallowing of the anterior chamber may precipitate subacute angle closure glaucoma. The shallowing may be secondary to swelling of the cataractous development of the lens but more commonly is probably associated with retraction of the retrolenticular tissue. Another complication that may occur is spontaneous vitreous hemorrhage as a result of bleeding of the persistent hyaloid artery.

Because persistent hyperplastic primary vitreous resembles retinoblastoma, the eyes are often enucleated. The most important differential point is the presence of a hyperplastic and elongated ciliary process around the periphery of the small lens. Until recently, the surgical treatment of these patients has been extremely poor, but several cases have been reported with good results in which a two-stage operation is done. Aspiration of the cataract is performed first, followed by an excision of the retrolenticular membrane. It is said that if the retrolenticular membrane extends to the ciliary processes, then early surgery is necessary to prevent loss of the eye.

Persistent hyperplastic primary vitreous

History. The right eye of this 3½-month-old female infant was noted to be abnormal at birth. Furthermore, it seemed to be photophobic and contained a mucoid exudate. Two weeks ago when the child was examined under anesthesia, the intraocular tension was found to be elevated, and a mass was observed behind the lens.

Findings. The right eye is slightly smaller than the left, the anterior chamber extremely shallow or possibly flat in places, and the pupil is small and nonreactive both directly and consensually. Behind the pupil is a yellow opaque mass seen through an apparently clear lens. In places the iris appears atrophic. Ultrasonography reveals an anteriorly displaced lens and a mass less than 2 mm. thick adherent to the posterior lens capsule. The globes are of equal and normal axial length, and there is no abnormality of the posterior segment.

Course. The eye was considered to be blind, and retinoblastoma could not be completely ruled out. An enucleation was performed. Histopathologic examination showed an atrophic iris, which was bowed forward and nearly flat against the cornea (Reel III-3). In turn, the lens was spherical and against the posterior REEL III-3 surface of the iris. On the posterior surface of the lens was a maze of slightly vascularized tissue, from the back of which arose the hyaloid artery, which extended back to the disc. Attached to the periphery of the retrolenticular mass were prominent hyperplastic ciliary processes.

Persistent hyperplastic primary vitreous

History. Shortly after birth this 1-year-old child was noted to have a "congenital cataract" and an enlarged cornea in the left eye.

Findings. The right eye is normal. The left cornea is larger than normal. There is nearly continuous peripheral iridocorneal adhesion extending several millimeters onto the cornea. A white mass extends up from the pupil and is adherent to the central cornea (Fig. 17). It appears that a pupillary block with FIG. 17 iris bombé is responsible for formation of the peripheral anterior synechias. Intraocular pressure is 26 mm. Hg (Schiøtz).

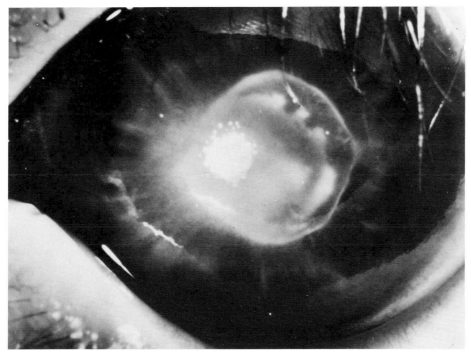

Fig. 17. *A white mass extending from the pupil and adherent to the central cornea in the left eye of a 1-year-old child with persistent hyperplastic primary vitreous.* A pupillary block appears to be present with iris bombé due to a continuous iridocorneal adhesion. The intraocular pressure was elevated, and a peripheral iridectomy was performed in an attempt to free the peripheral anterior synechias. Because the patient's intraocular tension remained elevated and the eye was apparently blind, it was enucleated. The gross pathologic specimen (Reel III-4) shows a persistent hyaloid artery containing blood, hyperplastic ciliary processes, and a tubular structure extending from a fibrotic pupillary membrane to the cornea.

Course. A peripheral iridectomy was performed, and the peripheral anterior synechias were freed. The cornea became clearer but gradually increased in size. Another tension measurement was 50 mm. Hg (Schiøtz). It became apparent that there was no light perception in the eye, and an enucleation was performed. The pathologic gross specimen showed a central corneal opacity attached to a tubular structure that was continuous with a dense fibrotic REEL III-4 pupillary membrane (Reel III-4). Attached to the posterior surface of the membrane was a persistent hyaloid artery containing blood. Throughout the periphery of the membrane were numerous hyperplastic ciliary processes. The peripheral iris was in contact with the cornea, and the retina was detached. Microscopic examination showed the persistence of the primary vitreous and a tunica vasculosa lentis. A year later the magnetic implant that had been used at the time of enucleation became exposed, and this was repaired. The right eye remained normal.

ARACHNODACTYLY

Long, slender bones, minimal subcutaneous fat, flaccid musculature, relaxed joints, and, frequently, subluxated lenses characterize arachnodactyly (Marfan's syndrome). Deformities of the chest and cardiovascular disease may be present. The dislocated lenses occur in approximately 60% of all patients with arachnodactyly, and bilateral involvement is the rule. Frequently the lenses are dislocated upward but may be dislocated into the vitreous or anterior chamber. When the latter occurs, pupillary block, glaucoma, and corneal edema are common complications and require immediate intervention. Glaucoma may also occur in patients with arachnodactyly due to angle anomalies such as abnormal persistence of the uveal meshwork and congenital peripheral anterior synechias. When these anomalies occur, the case is generally considered to be a secondary type of congenital glaucoma. Arachnodactyly is congenital and familial; it is generally transmitted as a dominant hereditary trait.

Dislocated lens in Marfan's syndrome

History. Early in life this 13-year-old boy was noted to be tall and thin, with long fingers and a high, arched palate. At 6 years of age he was discovered to have poor vision due to partially dislocated lenses. A congenital heart defect was also detected. During the past 2 months the size of his pupils varied, and yesterday the right pupil became dilated and remained so. This morning on examination he was found to have a partially anteriorly dislocated lens in the right eye. Treatment was instituted by maximally dilating the pupil while the boy was kept flat in bed.

Findings. Vision in both eyes is 20/400 with a high myopic correction. The cornea of the right eye has an area of stromal edema inferotemporally where the FIG. 18 partially dislocated lens touches the posterior surface of the cornea (Fig. 18, A). The pupil is well dilated, and the nasal half of the lens is behind the iris plane, while the temporal half is tilted outward well into the anterior chamber. No adequate view of the fundus can be obtained. The intraocular pressure is 25 mm. Hg (Schiøtz). In the left eye the lens is partially dislocated posteriorly. This fundus is also difficult to visualize.

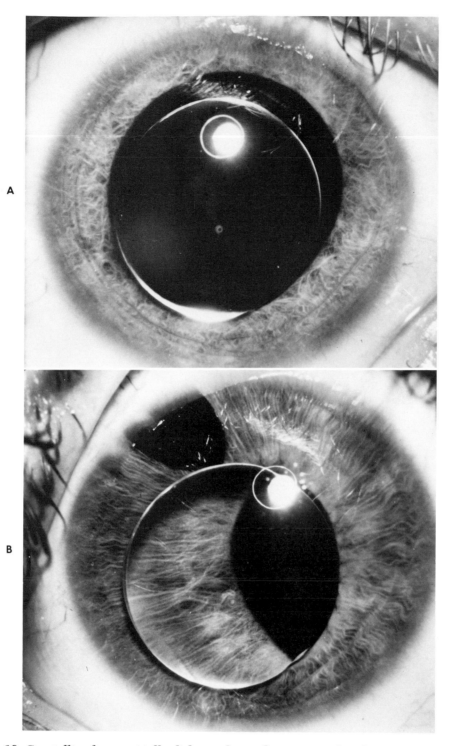

Fig. 18. *Crystalline lens partially dislocated into the anterior chamber in a 13-year-old boy with Marfan's syndrome.* **A,** In the right eye the lens is in contact with the cornea inferotemporally, producing an area of corneal edema. Following use of acetazolamide and glycerol the lens settled posteriorly. A peripheral iridectomy was performed and the patient kept on a regimen of miotics. **B,** Despite this treatment the lens has again prolapsed into the anterior chamber; but with pressure through the cornea it is displaced posteriorly, and echothiophate is used to keep it in place.

Course. Despite the widely dilated right pupil, the lens still remained dislocated anteriorly; therefore, acetazolamide and glycerol were given at frequent intervals in an attempt to decrease the size of the vitreous body. This treatment was continued for 24 hours, during which the lens gradually settled posteriorly and the pupil could be constricted with miotics. The next day a peripheral iridectomy was performed, and the convalescence was uneventful. The patient kept on a regimen of miotics; but when he was next seen in about 3 weeks, the lens had again dislocated into the anterior chamber except for a very small portion nasally (Fig. 18, *B*). By pressure through the cornea, the lens was again displaced posteriorly, and echothiophate drops kept it in place. A year later an aphakic correction gave 20/40 vision in each eye.

Congenitally dislocated lenses and glaucoma

History. Since birth this 37-year-old woman had dislocated lenses. Two years ago she was found to have elevated intraocular pressures and a very poor facility of outflow (C = 0.04). Moderate glaucomatous field changes were found in both eyes. Treatment with pilocarpine (4%) was initiated, and intraocular pressures remained in the normal range. Her two children also had congenitally dislocated lenses.

Findings. Vision in the right eye is 20/60 and in the left counting fingers at 10 feet. In both eyes the anterior chambers are deep, and there is a prominent iridodonesis. No lenses can be seen within the pupillary areas, and there is no vitreous in the anterior chamber. Fundus examination shows diffuse pigmentary changes and retinal degeneration at the posterior pole. Through dilated pupils

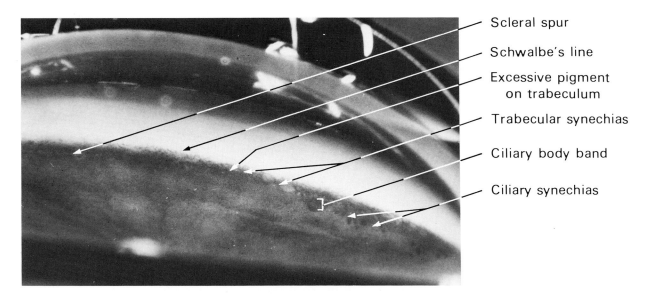

Scleral spur

Schwalbe's line

Excessive pigment on trabeculum

Trabecular synechias

Ciliary body band

Ciliary synechias

Fig. 19 (Reel III-5). *Multiple peripheral anterior synechias and heavy pigmentation in the angle of a 37-year-old woman with congenitally dislocated lenses.* In both eyes the patient has a markedly decreased facility of outflow and requires medical therapy to keep her intraocular pressure in the normal range. Two of her children also have congenitally dislocated lenses.

the lenses are found to be relatively opaque and are free floating inferiorly. Gonioscopy reveals an angle in which the ciliary body band and much of the trabecular meshwork are covered by multiple peripheral anterior synechias composed possibly of dense uveal meshwork (Reel III-5 and Fig. 19). Where a trabecular meshwork is visible, it is heavily pigmented. The iris plane is concave. Applanation tension is 20 mm. Hg in both eyes. There is almost complete loss of the upper field in the right eye and a dense double Bjerrum scotoma in the left.

REEL III-5
FIG. 19

Course. Seven years later the patient's intraocular tensions and visual fields remained essentially the same, although treatment with acetazolamide was added because of occasional borderline tensions.

INVOLVEMENT OF THE CHAMBER ANGLE IN SYSTEMIC DISEASES

Although many systemic diseases may involve the anterior chamber angle, several have important characteristic findings that deserve special attention. In long-standing chronic granulomatous disease such as tuberculosis or Boeck's sarcoid, classic mutton-fat keratic precipitates form; but in addition in these granulomatous uveitides the angle is frequently involved. In the angle large accumulations of yellowish white exudate occur, chiefly limited to the trabecular meshwork, projecting downward toward the iris until in many instances contact occurs. This results in the formation of permanent trabecular synechias, due to the organization of the exudate in contact with the cornea. In this manner the facility of outflow is reduced, and a secondary glaucoma occurs. On the other hand, the vascularized nodules that are commonly seen in Boeck's sarcoid usually do not involve the angle structures or, if they do, complete resorption is the rule, and no permanent defect occurs as with deposition of exudates on the trabecular meshwork.

Rubeosis iridis associated with diabetes may in addition involve the trabecular meshwork with the same neovascular process. Circumferential vessels from the iris are seen to extend to its root in instances of prominent neovascularization of the iris. Some of these vessels then extend across the ciliary body band up to the trabecular meshwork where numerous neovascular tufts occur, producing minute vessels that permeate the filtering meshwork and extend into Schlemm's canal. With further progression of the process, peripheral anterior synechias form, and an intractable glaucoma develops. As in the case of rubeosis iridis, recurrent hemorrhages from any of the areas of neovascularization are common, with development of a severe hyphema. The vessels may tend to disappear with the marked elevation of tension, but the glaucoma becomes absolute, with complete loss of vision.

Diabetic rubeosis iridis

History. Two years ago this 55-year-old man had blurring of vision and was found to have diabetes. Treatment with insulin was instituted. One week ago on awakening he had marked blurring of vision in the right eye and was found to have a retinal hemorrhage and glaucoma in that eye.

Findings. Vision in both eyes is 20/200. In the right eye there is a moderate

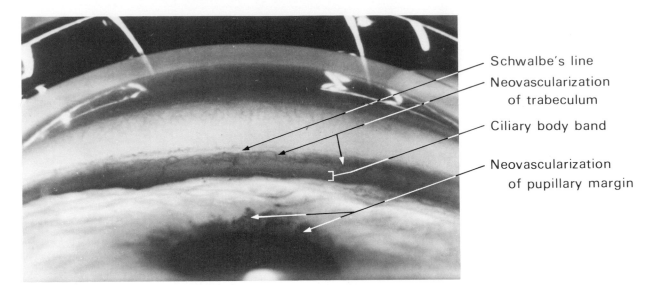

Schwalbe's line

Neovascularization
of trabeculum

Ciliary body band

Neovascularization
of pupillary margin

Fig. 20 (**Reel III-6**). *Neovascularization of the trabecular meshwork in the left eye of a 55-year-old man with diabetic rubeosis iridis.* The trabeculum is infiltrated with many fine blood vessels arising from the root of the iris. The patient is receiving insulin for the treatment of his diabetes; he has recently developed retinal hemorrhages and glaucoma in this eye.

conjunctival injection, and the sphincter region of the iris is red due to neovascularization. The media are clear, but in the fundus there are some scattered intraretinal hemorrhages and venous tortuosity and dilatation. Gonioscopy reveals that the peripheral iris has moderate neovascularization and that the trabecular meshwork is infiltrated with many fine vessels, with feeder vessels arising from the root of the iris. In the left eye there is no conjunctival injection, and the rubeosis iridis is less marked. The same is true of the vascularization of REEL III-6 the angle (Reel III-6 and Fig. 20). The fundus findings are about the same FIG. 20 except for a few strands of new vessel formation on the superior temporal vein. Intraocular pressure in the right eye is 32 mm. Hg (Schiøtz) and in the left 25 mm. Hg (Schiøtz).

Course. Despite intensive medical therapy, the intraocular pressure gradually became more elevated in the right eye, necessitating cyclodiathermy. Postoperatively, the intraocular pressure remained within normal limits. The patient was considered a good risk for hypophysectomy, so he underwent a stereotaxic radiofrequency hypophysectomy a week later. Six months later the vision remained the same, and fundus findings were constant.

Sarcoid uveitis

History. About 8 months ago this 23-year-old black man had a deep bilateral thrombophlebitis for which a bilateral femoral vein ligation was performed. At this time he also was found to have hyperglobulinemia, a negative tuberculin skin test, and x-ray findings of bilateral mottling of the lungs and hilar nodal enlargement typical of sarcoidosis. About 2 months ago he noted some difficulty

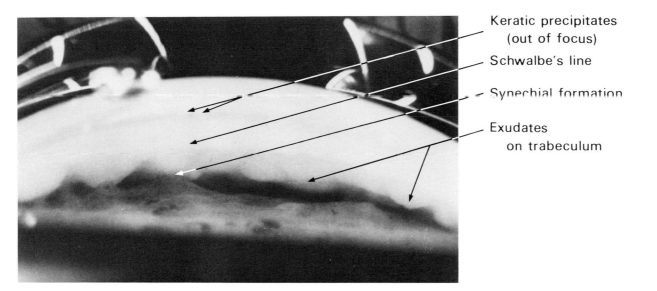

Keratic precipitates
(out of focus)

Schwalbe's line

Synechial formation

Exudates
on trabeculum

Fig. 21 (Reel III-7). *Massive collections of exudate on the trabecular meshwork of a 23-year-old man with sarcoid uveitis.* The exudates are so extensive that some extend down and touch the peripheral iris, forming peripheral anterior synechias. The patient also has hyperglobulinemia and chest x-ray findings typical of sarcoidosis.

with his eyes for which he was treated with eye drops twice a day. About 2 months ago keratic precipitates were noted, and the use of intensive topical corticosteroid drops and mydriatics was initiated. There were some exudates and hemorrhages in the fundi. Recently the patient also developed anorexia, vomiting, and peripheral neuropathy.

Findings. The vision in both eyes is 20/20. In both eyes there is a moderate circumcorneal injection, many keratic precipitates, particularly in the lower half of the cornea, and a moderate number of cells and a flare in the anterior chamber. Gonioscopy reveals massive collections of exudate on the trabecular meshwork, some of which extend down to touch the peripheral iris (Reel III-7 REEL III-7 and Fig. 21). Several of these appear to be undergoing organization and form- FIG. 21 ing extensive peripheral anterior synechias. Anteriorly, the exudates stop abruptly at Schwalbe's line.

Course. The topical corticosteroid administration was increased to every hour, and mydriatics were continued. The patient did not return for his follow-up visits.

Chapter 2

Degenerative conditions involving the anterior chamber

ANGLE CLOSURE AND MALIGNANT GLAUCOMA

Shallow anterior chambers are the common denominator for the two conditions angle closure glaucoma and malignant glaucoma. The mechanism and treatment for angle closure glaucoma are well understood; on the contrary, the pathogenesis of malignant glaucoma is not completely understood, and the treatment is still controversial.

Classical angle closure glaucoma is associated with a relative pupillary block and a narrow entrance to the anterior chamber angle. It is relatively common, usually inherited, and primarily due to anatomical factors in the anterior segment of the eye. With advancing age the lens thickens, and the anterior chamber becomes shallow. Hyperopia, with a small cornea and an already shallow anterior chamber, is contributory. The production of an attack of acute angle closure glaucoma is dependent on the differential of pressure between the posterior and anterior chambers. In predisposed eyes, the lens may be pushed against the iris, causing a relative pupillary block and trapping aqueous behind the iris. When the pupil is miotic (due either to bright light or the use of miotics), the relative pupillary block is maximum; but as the iris is also stretched out and thinned to its maximum, the tendency for the iris to come into contact with the trabecular meshwork is reduced. The pupillary block still exists as the pupil dilates, and in middilatation the thickened and lax peripheral iris is pushed forward against the trabecular meshwork, initiating the acute angle closure. Maximal dilatation of the pupil is not as dangerous, because the iris is no longer against the lens and therefore no pupillary block exists. However, the iris is markedly thickened due to the dilatation, and blocking of the angle structures may occur due to peripheral "bunching" against the filtering meshwork.

The classical signs and symptoms of angle closure glaucoma usually occur in

32

relative darkness, which causes the pupil to be semidilated; they do not occur in sleep, however, because the pupil is miotic during sleep. Elevation of intraocular pressure produces the phenomenon of colored halos around lights due to edema of the corneal epithelium. Mydriasis, venous congestion, aqueous flare, and a variable amount of pain during the early stages support the diagnosis. Later there is further shallowing of the anterior chamber, marked corneal edema, an irregular, dilated pupil, and an extremely congested eye, with excruciating pain, frequently radiating to other parts of the head. Nausea and vomiting may be misinterpreted as a gastrointestinal upset or infection.

Treatment is directed at breaking the attack by normalizing the intraocular pressure medically by the use of hyperosmotic agents such as oral glycerol and miotics to pull the iris out of the angle. Unfortunately, in a severe attack the latter is relatively ineffective. A peripheral iridectomy must be performed if there is reason to believe that the angle is not permanently closed with peripheral anterior synechias. In addition, it is equally important to perform a peripheral iridectomy for prophylactic reasons on the other eye, inasmuch as almost invariably this eye too has a narrow angle and is subject to closure and acute glaucoma. Permanent closure of the anterior chamber angle by peripheral anterior synechias following a prolonged attack of acute angle closure glaucoma usually necessitates a filtering procedure, with a markedly decreased chance of "cure." In the same vein, however, synechial closure in consequence of repeated overt or even subclinical episodes of angle closure (chronic angle closure) must not be overlooked, lest one fall into the error of performing a futile peripheral iridectomy in an eye that demands a filtering procedure.

As already mentioned, malignant glaucoma is poorly understood. There may be more than one mechanism involved in its production. Typically, patients who appear to have angle closure glaucoma, either the acute or chronic type, have an operative procedure performed, either a peripheral iridectomy or a filtering operation. Following this procedure, either immediately or after a period that may be as long as a number of months, the chamber will become extremely shallow, with an elevated intraocular pressure, despite the effectiveness of the operative procedure in producing an adequate peripheral opening in the iris. The lens appears to be actively pushed forward and is the primary cause for the marked shallowing of the anterior chamber. At least in some cases, aqueous collects in the vitreous body in the so-called aqueous diversion syndrome, and the swollen vitreous body in turn pushes the lens forward, producing a ciliovitreal block. More recently it has been proposed that a ciliovitreal block is the primary factor; but the absence of total overlapping of ciliary processes onto the lens in the presence of malignant glaucoma is against this hypothesis.

Medical therapy of malignant glaucoma is surprisingly effective in about half the cases and relieves the ophthalmologist of the necessity of surgical treatment. This effectiveness depends on the use of mydriatic-cycloplegic drops, which may have to be supplemented temporarily by carbonic anhydrase inhibitors and hyperosmotic agents. The mydriatic-cycloplegic treatment tightens the zonular ligament (due to the relaxed ciliary body) and pulls the lens-iris diaphragm slightly backward, thus deepening the anterior chamber. Some cases require intensive use of these drugs, even up to 5 days. It may be necessary to continue the mydriatic-cycloplegic treatment for a month or even indefinitely to avoid the development of another attack of malignant glaucoma. If the medical therapy fails, surgical intervention is required. There is no agreement on the optimum procedure, but pars plana vitreous puncture and aspiration with re-formation of the anterior chamber by air has given good results. Should a cataract already be present, lens extraction is also usually successful, but incision of the hyaloid membrane may also be required to avoid a shallow or flat chamber postoperatively. As a last resort in extremely stubborn cases some have suggested vitrectomy. Although much has yet to be understood in so-called malignant glaucoma, at one time most of these eyes were lost, whereas now the majority can be saved.

Acute angle closure glaucoma

History. For a year and a half this 60-year-old man, an alcoholic, noted rainbows and halos, particularly at night. Six months ago, after his tension in both eyes was found to be over 40 mm. Hg, he was told he should have peripheral iridectomies performed on both eyes. At that time he was given pilocarpine drops to use until he came in for surgery. Three days ago he developed severe pain in his left eye, and the vision rapidly became blurred. Yesterday the pain was less, but his vision did not improve.

Findings. Vision in the right eye is 20/20 and in the left counting fingers at 2 feet. Except for a shallow anterior chamber, the right eye is normal. The pupil is miotic due to the pilocarpine drops. The left eye has moderate conjunctival injection and marked ciliary injection. The central cornea is edematous, REEL IV-1 with prominent striate keratopathy (Reel IV-1). The anterior chamber is markedly shallow, the pupil moderately dilated and ovoid. Only a dull red reflex of the fundus can be obtained. Intraocular tension in the right eye is 14 mm. Hg (Schiøtz) and in the left 31 mm. Hg (Schiøtz).

Course. Peripheral iridectomy was performed on the left eye, and 4 days postoperatively the cornea was clearer, and the anterior chamber had deepened. The intraocular tension was 16 mm. Hg (Schiøtz). Two months later the patient returned and had a peripheral iridectomy, which was uneventful, performed on the right eye. The patient was then lost to follow-up.

Acute glaucoma and iridoschisis

History. Three years ago this 41-year-old man developed acute angle closure glaucoma in the left eye, which was treated as conjunctivitis for 5 days. By this time there was a bullous keratopathy and "iritis," with an intraocular tension of 72 mm. Hg (Schiøtz). A peripheral iridectomy was performed, followed by a prophylactic iridectomy in the uninvolved right eye. Postoperatively, some vision returned in the left eye. It was found necessary to use echothiophate (¼%) and acetazolamide in an attempt to control the tension in the left eye. In spite of maximum medication, the tensions remained somewhat elevated; so a year after his acute attack a scleral cautery filtration procedure as performed on the left eye. A good filtering bleb formed, and the intraocular pressures remained normal.

Findings. The vision in the right eye is 20/50 and in the left counting fingers at 15 feet. In the right eye the anterior chamber is somewhat shallow, and there is a large peripheral iridectomy at the 11 o'clock position. There is a moderate nuclear sclerosis, and the disc is normal. There is some pigment disturbance in the macular region. In the left eye there is a large filtering bleb at the 10 o'clock position and a peripheral iridectomy at the 2 o'clock position. The pupil is moderately dilated and fixed. The entire inner one third of the iris extending to the pupillary margin is fragmented, leaving strands of stroma floating up into the aqueous (Reel IV-2). This region is also prominently de- REEL IV-2 pigmented, in contrast to the dark brown of the remaining iris. There are several anterior subcapsular lens opacities, probably representing glaucoma flecken. There is glaucomatous cupping to the rim and abnormal pigmentation of the macular region. Gonioscopy of the right eye shows an open angle and a peripheral iridectomy. In the left, numerous anterior synechias are present, with only about one quarter of the angle remaining open. Both the filtering bleb and peripheral iridectomy appear functional. The intraocular pressures are 18 mm. Hg (Schiøtz) in the right and 20 mm. Hg (Schiøtz) in the left.

Course. Intermittently, the intraocular pressure was elevated in the left eye, and miotics were begun along with massage. The pressures remained controlled for 3 years, at which time the patient was lost to follow-up.

Malignant glaucoma

History. For about 10 years this 69-year-old woman has had intermittent attacks of frontal headaches and transient blurring of vision lasting 2 to 3 hours but without halos, colored lights, or redness of her eye. When first seen by an ophthalmologist 4 months ago, she was found to have somewhat elevated intraocular tension in her left eye but normal tension in her right. The angles in both eyes were found to be slitlike and actually closed superiorly in the left eye. Three months ago she underwent bilateral peripheral iridectomies, which were uneventful except for a small postoperative hyphema in the left eye, which cleared rapidly. The intraocular pressures remained normal until 3 weeks later when tension in the left eye was 30 mm. Hg (Schiøtz), while that in the right was only 18 mm. Hg (Schiøtz). Pilocarpine (1%) drops were started 4 times a day, and a week later she returned with an intraocular tension of 40 mm. Hg by applanation tonometry in the left eye. Examination now showed the anterior chamber to be very shallow in the left eye and the angle to be completely closed throughout 360°. In the right eye the angle was narrow but open and the anterior chamber deeper. Therapy was immediately instituted with mydriatics administered topically in the left eye and acetazolamide and glycerol administered systemically. Within a few hours the intraocular pressure was 18 mm. Hg (Schiøtz), and 2 days later all medications except the mydriatics were stopped, and the intraocular pressures remained in the teens. Although the iridectomy in the left eye was very peripheral and small, it was definitely open and the chamber was now approximately of the same depth as that of the right eye. She continued the use of scopolamine drops twice a day in the left eye. When she was seen 3 weeks later, her intraocular pressure in the left eye was 48 mm. Hg (Schiøtz), and the angle was again found to be completely closed. She was again intensively treated with mydriatics, acetazolamide, and glycerol, with return of a normal intraocular pressure. However, this time the angle did not entirely open, and a small amount of acetazolamide along with 2% atropine twice a day was required to keep the intraocular pressure within normal limits. For the past week more intensive mydriatics (phenylephrine [Neo-Synephrine] hydrochloride, cyclopentolate [Cyclogyl] hydrochloride, and atropine) were given, and acetazolamide was discontinued.

Findings. The vision in the right eye is 20/30 and in the left 20/60. In the right eye there is an obvious peripheral iridectomy at the 10 o'clock position. The anterior chamber is moderately shallow, with a 3-mm. pupil. The posterior segment is entirely normal. In the left eye the chamber is moderately shallow REEL IV-3 (Reel IV-3). At the 1 o'clock position there is a peripheral iridectomy that is barely visible. The pupil is dilated to about 8 mm., and the optic nerve head is normal. The intraocular pressure in the right eye is 16 mm. Hg and in the left 30 mm. Hg as revealed by applanation tonometry.

Course. Additional cyclopentolate and phenylephrine drops were instilled, and within a few hours the intraocular tension was 25 mm. Hg as revealed by applanation tonometry in the left eye. The dosage of cyclopentolate and phenylephrine was increased to 4 times a day, and the atropine drops (2%) were continued twice daily. A regimen of acetazolamide 250 mg. 3 times a day was also begun, and in a week the intraocular pressure in the left eye was 17 mm. Hg. The dosage of acetazolamide was decreased, but the other medications were continued for the next 6 weeks, with the tensions remaining in the high teens. The anterior depth chamber measurements showed the left eye to be slightly shallower than the right.

PIGMENTARY GLAUCOMA

Krukenberg's spindle, excessive pigmentation of the trabecular meshwork, iris translucency, and open angle glaucoma characterize pigmentary glaucoma. The condition is seen predominantly in myopic patients, in males, and in the younger age groups and is usually bilateral. Although many consider it a variant of chronic open angle glaucoma, there is also evidence that it may be a type of congenital glaucoma in which there are malformations of the angle. The mechanism appears to be a degeneration of the iris and ciliary body epithelium, which results in the phenomenon of transillumination of the iris. Typically, it is the peripheral iris that shows the most marked changes. Pigment is liberated into the aqueous, giving rise to Krukenberg's spindle (or sometimes diffuse punctate deposits of pigment on the corneal endothelium) and deposition of the pigment granules on the trabecular meshwork. The latter may cause mechanical obstruction of the outflow channels, with elevation of intraocular pressure. Occasionally, the tension is elevated sufficiently to cause intermittent blurring and halos; a large diurnal variation may be present. It is not uncommon to find individuals who have the various characteristics of pigmentary glaucoma but no elevation in intraocular pressure. The response to topical corticosteroids is identical to that of primary open angle glaucoma, and water tonograms are positive in the absence of glaucoma. Patients with Krukenberg's spindles should be carefully investigated for pigmentary glaucoma. Because of the wide diurnal variations that may occur, intraocular pressures may on many occasions not be abnormal.

It is generally thought that pigmentary glaucoma, particularly in women, is more difficult to control medically than in those with ordinary chronic open angle glaucoma.

Pigmentary glaucoma

History. On routine eye examination this 43-year-old woman was found to have borderline intraocular tensions. She was asymptomatic, having never had any pain, halos, or redness of her eyes. Further examination revealed bilateral Bjerrum scotomata and nasal steps. Administration of pilocarpine drops was started in both eyes.

Findings. Vision in the right eye is 20/25 and in the left 20/30. Both eyes have almost identical findings, with prominent Krukenberg's spindles, deep anterior chambers, brown irides with some speckling of pigmentation on the anterior surface, clear media, and glaucomatous cupping of the discs. Gonioscopy shows that the iris plain is flat and that there is marked pigmentation on the trabecular meshwork overlying Schlemm's canal and lighter pigmentation above. Schwalbe's line has a scalloped appearance, with a deposit of brown pigment anterior to it. A scleral spur can be seen immediately below the heavily pigmented meshwork, and the ciliary body band is relatively lightly pigmented below the scleral spur. There are no synechia formations in the angle. On the dome of the cornea can be seen a prominent pigmentation (Krukenberg's spindle) (Reel IV-4). The intraocular pressure in the right eye is 24 mm. Hg (Schiøtz) and in the left 26 mm. Hg (Schiøtz). REEL IV-4

Course. Trials of various medications were necessitated by the patient's intolerance to strong miotics and epinephrine drops. Gradually she became more accustomed to drops, and with the addition of acetazolamide the wide swings in intraocular tension were avoided and the intraocular pressures were reduced to borderline levels. Repeated visual field examinations, however, showed some increase in the defects, and 3 years later the Bjerrum scotoma in the left eye had extended to the lower field. The irides transilluminated markedly. The vision had become only slightly reduced in the left eye and remained the same in the right. In 7 years the Krukenberg spindles had become much more pronounced, transillumination of the iris showed marked loss of pigment epithelium, and the tensions remained in the mid 20's with maximal medical therapy. Twelve years later the intraocular pressures were generally somewhat lower, the cupping was progressively deeper, but the fields remained constant.

Pigmentary glaucoma

History. Six months ago this 41-year-old man had some blurring in the right eye and was found to have glaucoma. Topical medications and acetazolamide brought his intraocular pressures to normal levels for a while.

Findings. Vision in the right eye is 20/30 and in the left 20/20. There is no injection of either eye, and the anterior chambers in both eyes are deep. Gonioscopy reveals that the angles are open, but in the right eye there is a dense deposition of pigment on the filtration meshwork overlying Schlemm's canal and there is lesser pigmentation of the remaining meshwork (Fig. 22, A). FIG. 22 A number of iris processes can be seen extending across the ciliary body band

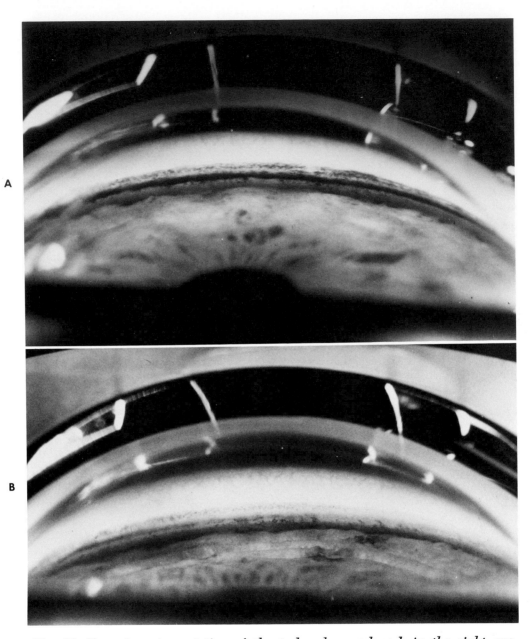

Fig. 22. *Excessive pigmentation of the trabecular meshwork in the right eye of a 41-year-old man with pigmentary glaucoma.* **A,** Gonioscopy of the right eye reveals a prominent black band representing dense pigment deposition on the portion of the trabecular meshwork overlying Schlemm's canal. Anterior to it is lightly pigmented trabecular meshwork, and just below are the scleral spur and the ciliary body band. A few iris processes are visible. **B,** Gonioscopy of the left eye shows normal pigmentation for a brown-eyed patient. The trabecular meshwork is lightly pigmented, and there are a number of iris processes extending across the ciliary body band and scleral spur onto the trabecular meshwork. The intraocular pressure is elevated only in the right eye, and a glaucomatous field change is also present.

onto the meshwork. In the left eye, pigmentation of the filtering meshwork is normal for a patient of his age with brown irides (Fig. 22, *B*). Again, there are pigmented iris processes and the angle is wide open. In both eyes the media are clear, and the fundus is normal except for the optic nerve head in the right eye, which exhibits glaucomatous cupping. Intraocular tension is 44 mm. Hg in the right eye and 21 mm. Hg in the left. Field examination shows a nasal step in the right eye.

Course. Because of the uncontrolled pressures, an Elliot trephine procedure was performed on the right eye, which over the years gradually became less functional. Six years later the intraocular pressure was found to be elevated at all times, while the pressure in the left eye remained normal without medication. Sclerotomy and iridectomy were performed on the right eye, and 4 days postoperatively there was a massive hemorrhage into the anterior chamber, which subsequently cleared, disclosing a massive vitreous hemorrhage that had completely obscured the fundus detail. Gradually this cleared, but in another 6 months there was further elevation of the intraocular pressure, and an iridencleisis with sclerectomy was performed. Eight years later the intraocular

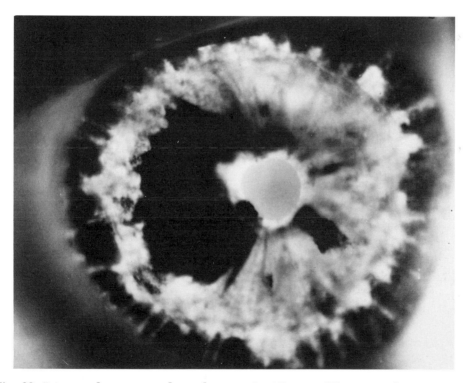

Fig. 23. *Iris translucency in the right eye of a 55-year-old man with pigmentary glaucoma.* On transillumination of the iris the red reflex of the fundus is visible in more than half of the iris. Temporally there is a large area of intact pigment epithelium, but even here the periphery of the iris partially transilluminates. Both eyes are similar, having elevated intraocular pressures, excessive pigment deposition in the trabecular meshwork, and glaucomatous cupping of the nerve head.

pressures were still controlled with the use of epinephrine (2%), but the vision had decreased to 20/60 in the right eye and 20/30 in the left.

Pigmentary glaucoma

History. About 3 weeks ago this 55-year-old man was seen because of a recurrent chalazion. He had no other ocular symptoms but was found to have glaucomatous cupping of the right disc and a tension of 52 mm. Hg (Schiøtz) in the right eye. Further investigation revealed a definite pigmentary glaucoma in the right eye and questionable glaucoma in the left. Pilocarpine (4%) in both eyes was initiated 4 times a day. In 2 weeks his intraocular pressure was still moderately elevated in the right eye; therefore, both echothiophate (⅛%) twice a day and epinephrine (1%) 3 times a day were added to his medications in the right eye.

Findings. Vision in both eyes is 20/20 with correction. In the right eye there is a moderate brown granular pigmentation on the endothelium, in a roughly vertical spindle distribution. The anterior chamber is deep and the iris normal except for a teardrop-shaped pupil. Transillumination of the iris shows a

FIG. 23 marked defect, with more than half of the pigment epithelium absent (Fig. 23). Gonioscopy reveals excessive pigmentation on the trabecular meshwork, although the pigment is not uniformly distributed. The optic nerve head is markedly cupped temporally, with no rim of normal tissue remaining, especially inferiorly. The visual field shows extensive loss, with almost the entire upper field absent and about 50% of the lower involved. In the left eye the findings are similar but less pronounced, except that the disc and the visual field are within normal limits.

Course. With maximum medical therapy the intraocular pressures remained in the 30's in the right eye but were normal in the left. Three months later a trephine filtering procedure was performed on the right eye, and except for a small postoperative hyphema there were no complications. The intraocular pressure in the right eye was somewhat elevated, and massage 4 times a day was instituted. Gradually the bleb became multiloculated, and the intraocular tension in the right eye was in the midteens despite no medication but became elevated in the left eye with maximum medication. In addition, vision was reduced due to the development of a cataract in the left eye, but the field and disc appeared to be normal. Four years later there had been no progression of the cataract. The tensions were within normal limits, and transillumination of the irides showed that they had remained the same.

PSEUDOEXFOLIATION OF THE LENS CAPSULE

Deposits of grayish white material on the anterior lens capsule, pupillary margin, iris, and trabecular meshwork characterize pseudoexfoliation of the lens capsule and may result in glaucoma (glaucoma capsulare). The characteristic material may also become deposited on the zonules, ciliary body, hyaloid face, and posterior surface of the cornea. True exfoliation of the lens capsule is seen almost exclusively in glassblower's cataract or other conditions associated with chronic exposure to infrared radiation, is rare, and is not usually associated with glaucoma. In pseudoexfoliation the common clinical finding is that of a dandrufflike material on the pupillary border and a central disc of grayish material on the anterior capsule of the lens. On dilatation of the pupil a peripheral band is also seen leaving a clear intermediate zone separating the two involved areas. Sometimes the clear intermediate zone is incomplete, having bridges of translucent material connecting the peripheral and central zones. Gonioscopy reveals that the angle is variably involved with deposition of the dandrufflike material on the trabecular meshwork and ciliary body band. The origin of the material is controversial, having at first been thought to be from the lens capsule itself. Because microscopically the lens capsule is of normal thickness, the origin was then thought to be from the pigment epithelium of the iris or ciliary body or possibly a precipitate from the aqueous. Electron microscopy has recently shown deposits within or beneath the lens capsule, indicating the possibility of a fibrillar secretion of the lens epithelium in the intermediate and peripheral portions of the anterior lens capsule.

The occurrence of pseudoexfoliation in chronic open angle glaucoma in various series has been reported to be as low as 7% and as high as 90% with considerable variation, depending on the part of the world from which the reports originate. Generally, it appears that about 20% of open angle glaucomas have pseudoexfoliation. Moreover, in patients over 50 years old the incidence of exfoliation is about the same in those with no glaucoma as in those with glaucoma. In addition, the severity of pseudoexfoliation is not correlated with the degree of glaucoma. Also, eyes with pseudoexfoliation have no more tendency toward cataract formation than those without pseudoexfoliation, and lens extraction produces no effect on the progression of the glaucoma. The mechanism of the glaucoma has now been shown to be obstruction of the outflow due to the pseudoexfoliative material, and indeed the same etiologic factor may be causing the glaucoma and the pseudoexfoliation. There seems to be good evidence that glaucoma with pseudoexfoliation of the lens capsule (glaucoma capsulare) is a distinct disease entity rather than a type of primary open angle glaucoma. Topical corticosteroid instillations indicate that the two are not genetically identical, and statistics show that pseudoexfoliation is a hereditary disease occurring in relatively high frequency in certain families.

Pseudoexfoliation

History. For at least 10 years this 84-year-old woman had poor vision in the left eye without pain or redness. Although she was advised that she could have a cataract operation, she decided against it because of her fairly good vision in the right eye.

Findings. Vision in the right eye is 20/70 and in the left light perception. The right eye appears normal except for early lens opacities composed of mainly cortical spokes. The left eye is divergent by about 20°. There is much dandrufflike material on the pupillary margin and the iris surface (Fig. 24, A). The lens is hypermature, with obvious iridodonesis. Gonioscopy reveals the angle structures to be covered with fluffy material as well as some dandrufflike deposits on the peripheral iris roll (Fig. 24, B). The intraocular pressure is 21 mm. Hg (Schiøtz) in the right eye and 18 mm. Hg (Schiøtz) in the left.

Course. The patient still declined surgery and was followed over the next

FIG. 24

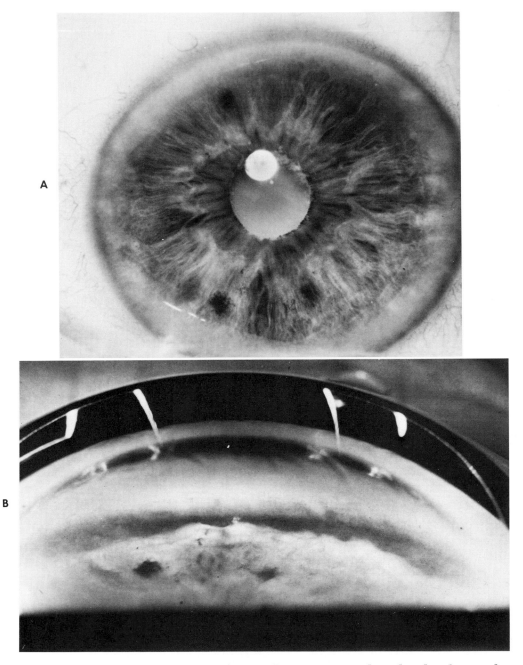

Fig. 24. *Dandrufflike material at the pupillary margin and in the chamber angle in the left eye of an 84-year-old woman with pseudoexfoliation.* **A,** On the pupillary margin are a number of fluffy white deposits, and the lens is hypermature. **B,** On the peripheral roll of the iris and covering the trabecular meshwork is much fluffy white material obscuring all the angle details. The intraocular pressure is moderately elevated, and the patient declines surgery.

2 years, during which the lens became posteriorly dislocated in the left eye, with only a moderate elevation of intraocular pressure.

Pseudoexfoliation

History. This 73-year-old woman recently noticed floaters in her left eye but had no other ocular symptoms.

Findings. Vision in the right eye is 20/30 and in the left 20/40. Both eyes are essentially the same, with normal corneas and deep anterior chambers. Around the pupillary margin are a number of fine dandrufflike deposits, and on the anterior lens capsule there are two rings of whitish material that appear to be peeling away from the surface of the lens (Fig. 25). One of these rings FIG. 25 is close to the pupillary margin, while the other is more centrally located toward the axial portion of the lens. In some places a piece of material has extended out into the anterior chamber from the lens surface. Gonioscopy reveals the angle to be wide open and to contain particles of the dandrufflike material. There is also an excessive amount of pigmentation along the trabecular meshwork. The lenses show a minimal nuclear sclerosis, and the fundus is normal. The intraocular tension is 24 mm. Hg (Schiøtz) in both eyes.

Course. Because of the borderline tensions, tonography was performed, re-

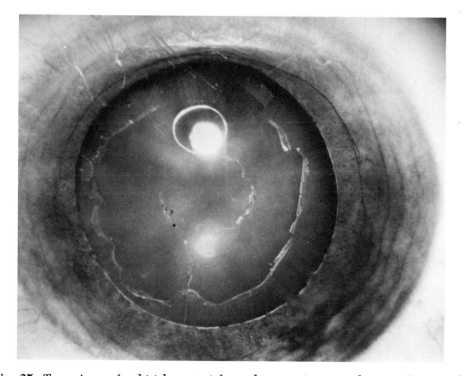

Fig. 25. *Two rings of whitish material on the anterior capsule in a 73-year-old woman with pseudoexfoliation.* With the pupil dilated, one ring of "exfoliated" material is seen close to the pupillary margin and appears to be peeling off the anterior capsule of the lens. A second ring is located near the axial portion of the lens and has the same appearance. Gonioscopy shows similar material in the anterior chamber angle and excessive pigmentation of the trabecular meshwork.

vealing the facility of outflow to be borderline as well. Six months later the intraocular tensions were still borderline. The patient was told to return in 3 months but was then lost to follow-up.

Pseudoexfoliation

History. A few months ago this 59-year-old woman was discovered to have glaucoma in the right eye and was treated with pilocarpine and acetazolamide.

Findings. Vision in the right eye is 20/80 and in the left 20/25. In the right eye the cornea is normal and the anterior chamber clear. Along the pupillary margin are a number of small grayish white dandrufflike deposits. The pupil is semidilated; there is a ring centrally of grayish deposits on the anterior capsule, with a large, somewhat rolled-up sheet of grayish material in the REEL IV-5 anterior chamber occupying the central pupillary area (Reel IV-5). This membranous material is continuous with one of a number of pieces of similar material, which are attached to the anterior capsule near the pupillary border. It is evident that previously these pieces represented a ring of deposits, a large part of which have now broken away from the anterior capsule and have floated into the anterior chamber. The central sheet represents a part of the ring that has not yet become completely free. There is moderate nuclear sclerosis, and the posterior pole appears to be normal through the lens opacities. The left eye is normal except for a minimal amount of pseudoexfoliation similar to that of the right eye.

Course. There was gradual increase in the cataract of the right eye, until a year later the vision was reduced to 20/400, at which time a cataract extraction was done without complications. Postoperatively, the vision did not improve. A macular edema appeared to be present. Fluoroangiography showed marked leakage of dye into the macular region, which is typical of cystoid macular degeneration. A year later the vision remained the same, but fluoroangiography showed less leakage of dye into the macular region.

Pseudoexfoliation

History. For about 2 years this 63-year-old woman had painless loss of vision in the right eye.

Findings. The vision in the right eye is counting fingers at 4 feet and in the left 20/30. Both eyes show essentially the same findings, except for a mature cataract in the right eye and an incipient cataract in the left. The anterior chambers are deep. Over the surface of the irides there is excessive deposition of granular pigment, and on the pupillary borders are fluffs of dandrufflike material, a few of which are also seen on the anterior lens capsule. Gonioscopy reveals that the angles are open and the irides flat. There is excessive pigmenta-
FIG. 26 tion at the root of the irides and on the angle structures (Fig. 26). The trabecular meshwork overlying Schlemm's canal is darkly pigmented, and the portion anterior to this region is heavily speckled with dark brown pigment. Anterior to Schwalbe's line there is some light deposition of brown pigment on the cornea. In a number of places in the angle are fluffs of dandrufflike material. The intraocular tension is 13 mm. Hg (Schiøtz) in the right eye and 11 mm. Hg in the left. Tonography shows a normal facility of outflow in both eyes.

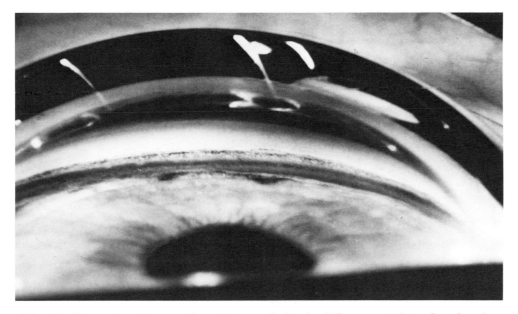

Fig. 26. *Excessive pigment deposition and dandrufflike material in the chamber angle of a 63-year-old woman with pseudoexfoliation.* The trabecular meshwork overlying Schlemm's canal is darkly pigmented, and there is heavy speckled pigmentation elsewhere, especially around Schwalbe's line. Pieces of dandrufflike material are also visible in the chamber angle. The intraocular pressure is normal in both eyes.

Course. Four months later an intracapsular cataract extraction was performed on the right eye, and the postoperative course was uneventful. Subsequently the vision was 20/40 with aphakic correction. Four months ago another refraction showed the vision to be 20/20 in the right eye, but the patient still had 20/25 vision in the left. The patient was then lost to follow-up.

Pseudoexfoliation

History. Six years ago this 84-year-old woman noticed painless loss of vision in the left eye, and 3 years ago she noticed it in the right. Recently the vision became so poor that she could not read or carry on ordinary activities.

Findings. The vision in the right eye is 20/70 and in the left 10/300. In both eyes the corneas are clear except for a marked arcus senilis. The anterior chambers are deep and the irides somewhat atrophic. Dilatation of the pupils reveals marked nuclear and cortical changes, which are more pronounced in the left eye than in the right. On the anterior capsules is a roll of dandrufflike material just inside the border of the dilated pupil. Gonioscopy shows similar material in the angles, along with excessive granular pigmentation on the trabecular meshwork and a prominent undulating line of pigmentation on the peripheral cornea (Fig. 27). The ciliary body band is easily visible in most places. The disc and macula in the right eye are seen indistinctly but appear to be normal. The intraocular tension is 24 mm. Hg (Schiøtz) in both eyes. FIG. 27

Course. Intracapsular cataract extractions were performed on both eyes, and

45

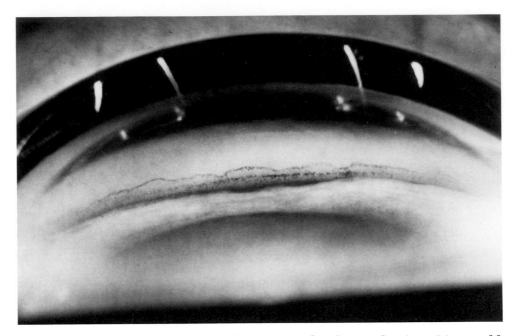

Fig. 27. *Granular pigmentation in the anterior chamber angle of an 84-year-old woman with pseudoexfoliation.* Excessive granular pigmentation is irregularly deposited on the trabecular meshwork. On the peripheral cornea is a prominent undulating line of pigment that touches Schwalbe's line in some places. The intraocular pressure was high normal, and cataracts present in both eyes necessitated cataract extractions.

the postoperative course was uneventful. With aphakic correction the patient obtained 20/25 vision in both eyes. Over the next 7 years until her death she had no ocular complaints.

Pseudoexfoliation on zonules

History. About a year ago this 68-year-old woman noticed blurring of vision in the right eye, which has progressively become worse. Also about a year ago she was found to have dandrufflike material on the pupillary margins and in the chamber angle. Her intraocular tensions were elevated in both eyes but more so in the right. Because of a mature cataract in the right eye, an intracapsular cataract extraction was done about 6 months ago, and the postoperative recovery was uneventful. She has had no drops in either eye since the cataract extraction.

Findings. Vision in the right eye is 20/20 with aphakic correction and in the left 20/20 with her ordinary correction. The right eye appears to be a normal aphakic eye with a broad-sector iridectomy superiorly. Through the gonioscope when the region of the iridectomy is viewed superiorly, white deposits can be seen on the surface of the ciliary processes and along the zonules, which REEL IV-6 extend toward the vitreous face (Reel IV-6). This appears to be identical with the material that was seen before operation along the pupillary margin and in the angle. In the left eye the dandrufflike material is still visible at the pupillary margin and in the anterior chamber angles, but the lens is clear and the fundus normal. Intraocular pressure in the right eye is 44 mm. Hg (Schiøtz) and in the left 25 mm. Hg (Schiøtz). Field examination shows the visual field of the right eye possibly to be constricted temporally and that of the left to be normal.

Course. Pilocarpine drops were initiated in the right eye, and the intraocular pressures stayed within the normal limits for the next year, at which time pressure in the left eye became elevated and was successfully treated with the same medication. Two years later the woman was found to have diabetes, and fundus examination showed waxy exudates and punctate hemorrhages. The intraocular tension gradually became elevated, and echothiophate (¼%) was required for control. A year later there was sufficient cataract progression in the left eye to warrant surgery. An unplanned extracapsular cataract extraction was performed. Postoperatively, with an aphakic correction she was able to obtain 20/30 vision. Thirteen years later (at age 83) she had 20/30 vision in the right eye and 20/20 in the left with correction, and her intraocular tensions were well controlled with echothiophate drops.

PHAKOLYTIC GLAUCOMA

Anterior chamber reaction and open angle glaucoma in the presence of a hypermature cataract characterize phakolytic glaucoma. In this condition either the capsule is broken or there is leakage of liquefied cortex through the capsule into the anterior chamber. Macrophages containing lens material block the trabecular meshwork, resulting in marked elevation in intraocular pressure. The condition is unilateral and is usually associated with a hypermature lens that is due to either trauma, senility, or a dislocated lens. There is usually marked congestion, with many cells and marked flare in the anterior chamber and sometimes iridescent crystals. The reaction may be so severe as to give the apperance of an endophthalmitis with corneal edema and severe pain, but the high tension may explain these findings. Normal or increased depth of the anterior chamber differentiates this condition from a swollen cataractous lens that has caused angle closure glaucoma. Aspiration of the anterior chamber may show the macrophages containing cortical material. Keratic precipitates and anterior and posterior synechias are rarely seen. The posterior segment is normal except for glaucomatous cupping in neglected cases.

Phakolytic glaucoma has also been referred to as phakogenic glaucoma, phakogenic ophthalmia, and phakotoxic uveitis. It must be differentiated from phakoanaphylactic uveitis, in which sensitization occurs from absorbing cortex in the same or opposite eye, producing a uveitis after a latent period. Large keratic precipitates typically seen in phakoanaphylactic uveitis are an important differential point. Treatment consists of cataract extraction even in the presence of a markedly elevated tension and an acutely inflamed eye. If a rupture of the capsule has occurred, irrigation or aspiration is imperative.

Phakolytic glaucoma

History. Twenty years ago this 85-year-old man had an intracapsular cataract extracted from the right eye, and the visual result was good. For many years he has had a cataract in the left eye but felt no need of surgery because his right

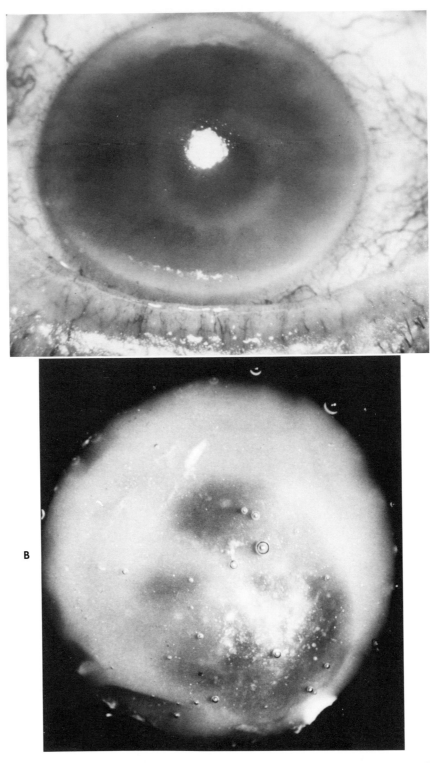

Fig. 28. *Steamy cornea and iridescent material in the anterior chamber of the left eye of an 85-year-old man with phakolytic glaucoma.* **A,** The conjunctiva is injected; the cornea is edematous; there is iridescent material in the anterior chamber; and the lens is hypermature. The intraocular pressure is 43 mm. Hg (Schiøtz). **B,** Following intensive unsuccessful medical therapy for the glaucoma, intracapsular cataract extraction shows a lens that is hypermature with a wrinkled capsule. The nucleus can be seen in the inferior portion of the lens.

eye was so good. A year ago cataract extraction was recommended, but he refused operation. Yesterday the patient noted sudden severe pain and aching in the left eye, which persisted all night.

Findings. Vision in the right eye is 20/25 and in the left light perception. The right eye is normal except for aphakia and a sector iridectomy superiorly. In the left eye there is marked conjunctival injection, and the cornea is steamy. Glycerin applied to the cornea made it possible to visualize a deep anterior chamber containing an iridescent material (Fig. 28, A). The pupil reacts to FIG. 28 light sluggishly, and the lens is hypermature. The intraocular pressure in the right eye is 17 mm. Hg and in the left 43 mm. Hg (Schiøtz).

Course. Intensive treatment with acetazolamide and topical corticosteroids was given; but the cornea became more steamy, and the eye had the appearance of endophthalmitis. An intracapsular cataract extraction was done without difficulty, and the postoperative course was uneventful. The crystalline lens after extraction showed a hypermature lens with a wrinkled capsule. The nucleus could be visualized at the bottom of the lens (Fig. 28, B). Histopathologically, there were macrophages and chronic round cell infiltration of the lens. Nine years later the vision was 20/20 in both eyes, and the intraocular pressures were 16 mm. Hg (Schiøtz).

SYNDROME OF IRIS NODULES, ECTOPIC DESCEMET'S MEMBRANE, AND UNILATERAL GLAUCOMA (COGAN-REESE SYNDROME)

Pedunculated iris nodules, glaucoma, and the histopathologic finding of a hyaline membrane characterize the Cogan-Reese syndrome. Multiple melanotic tumors of the iris in the presence of unilateral glaucoma were thought to be malignant melanomas of the iris, and enucleation was carried out in at least three reported cases. Histophathologically, the nodules were compatible with nevi and were covered by ectopic Descemet's membrane. Ectropion uveae was present in all the cases in the sector of the iris involved. Although the nodules have some similarity to those seen in neurofibromatosis, there was no evidence of systemic disease in any of the patients, and a congenital basis for the abnormalities has been proposed.

Iris nodule syndrome

History. About 2 months ago this 51-year-old woman noticed a "veil" over her left eye. An ophthalmologist told her that she had "pressure in the eye," and she was treated with drops. Later the strength of these was increased, and she was also given pills twice a day. However, there was no improvement in her symptoms.

Findings. Vision in the right eye is 20/10 and in the left 20/70, improved to 20/25 with pinhole. The right eye is normal, and the iris is light brown. In the left eye the cornea is clear except for some fine pigment granules on the endothelium, and the iris is dark brown. The pupil is irregular and displaced temporally. The entire temporal half of the iris is studded with numerous fine pedunculated dark brown masses (Reel IV-7). At the 3 o'clock position there REEL IV-7 is an extensive peripheral anterior synechia extending well onto the cornea.

The nasal half of the iris is normal in appearance. Around most of the pupil is a prominent ectropion uveae. Gonioscopy reveals excessive pigment deposits on the entire trabecular meshwork. Temporally, the meshwork is markedly obscured by the pigment, and at the 3 o'clock position an iridocorneal synechia bridges the meshwork. The posterior segment is normal, including the peripheral retina to the pars plana. Intraocular pressure in the right eye is 17 mm. Hg (Schiøtz) and in the left 48 mm. Hg (Schiøtz). The right field is normal, but the left shows a nasal constriction of the field.

Course. A ^{32}P test was negative. Because of the neoplastic appearance of the lesion, enucleation was performed, and the postoperative course was uneventful. The gross specimen of the eye showed areas of marked depigmentation of the pigment epithelium of the iris temporally. Histopathologic examination showed the temporal nodules to be compatible with nevi, and these were covered by ectopic Descemet's membrane and endothelium. There was excessive basement membrane formation on the temporal trabecular meshwork.

CHOLESTEROLOSIS BULBI

Cholesterol crystals in various parts of the eye associated with a chronic degenerative condition are referred to as cholesterolosis bulbi. The most common place for these crystals to be seen is in the vitreous, when it is usually referred to as synchysis scintillans. However, fluid vitreous may extend into the anterior chamber, producing the striking findings of glittering golden crystals floating in the anterior chamber or settling down in the form of a pseudohypopyon. Noncrystalline fatty substance tends to be lighter than aqueous and therefore floats to the upper portion of the anterior chamber, producing the effect of an upside-down hypopyon. Another source of crystalline material in the anterior chamber is from a ruptured cataractous lens of long standing. In this event both cortical material and crystals, usually cholesterol, are seen in the anterior chamber and may be difficult to distinguish from those arising from a fluid vitreous. The occurrence of cholesterol crystals in the anterior chamber is almost always in blind eyes with chronic degenerations of various types due to trauma, hemorrhage, or inflammation.

Asteroid hyalosis (asteroid hyalitis), in contrast to synchysis scintillans, is characterized by small discrete spherical yellowish white bodies (snowballs), which are usually in formed vitreous and in eyes that are otherwise healthy. Their involvement in the anterior chamber occurs only when there is prolapse of formed vitreous that contains the asteroid bodies. Vision can be reduced somewhat if the density of the bodies within the pupillary aperture is sufficiently great. Histochemical studies indicate that the bodies are made up chiefly of calcium soap.

Cholesterol in anterior chamber from old retinal detachment

History. This 57-year-old man lost his vision in the right eye because of a retinal detachment and since childhood has had poor vision in both eyes.

Findings. The right eye is blind, and the vision in the left eye is 20/80 with −8.00 correction. There is moderate injection of the bulbar conjunctiva of the right eye, with a clear cornea but a very deep anterior chamber. The

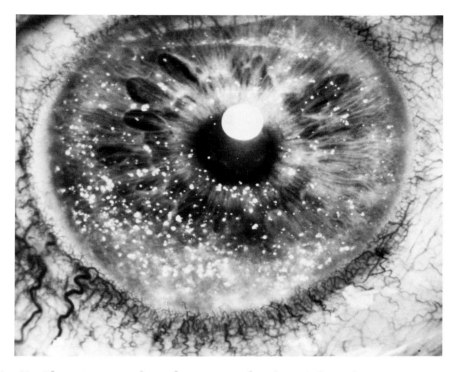

Fig. 29. *Glistening crystals in the anterior chamber of the right eye in a 57-year-old man with an old retinal detachment.* Floating free in the anterior chamber are many white crystals, some of which have settled out inferiorly. In the vitreous similar crystals can be visualized. The eye is blind from an old retinal detachment.

aqueous contains many glistening crystals, some of which have settled out inferiorly (Fig. 29). There is extensive posterior synechia formation, and the FIG. 29 lens is partially cataractous. In the vitreous can be seen crystals similar to those in the anterior chamber. In the left eye the anterior segment is normal, and the media is clear except for multiple large vitreous floaters. Fundus examination shows a large posterior staphyloma and chorioretinal macular degeneration.

Course. Two years later the crystals were still seen in the anterior chamber of the right eye. The vision in the left eye had decreased to 20/200, presumably due to increased myopic retinal degeneration.

Cholesterol crystals in anterior chamber

History. Forty years ago this 48-year-old man was struck in the left eye with a piece of cardboard, which produced a decrease of vision at that time. There was gradual further loss of vision, until 2 years ago he had no light perception. Three weeks ago he developed severe pain in the eye and was found to have many crystals in the anterior chamber.

Findings. Vision in the right eye is 20/25, and the left eye is blind. The right eye is normal. The left eye is markedly injected, and the cornea is edematous. The anterior chamber is filled with refractile golden crystals, many

FIG. 30 of which have settled in the lower half of the anterior chamber (Fig. 30). There is an iridodialysis in the upper nasal quadrant, and the pupil is miotic. The lens is cataractous, and examination of the posterior segment is impossible. Intraocular tension is 20 mm. Hg (Schiøtz) in both eyes.

Course. Enucleation of the left eye was performed, and the postoperative course was uneventful. The histopathologic diagnosis was cholesterolosis bulbi and retinal detachment with preretinal membrane.

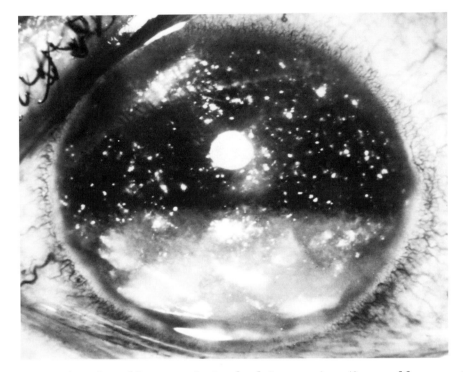

Fig. 30. *Refractile golden crystals in the left eye of a 48-year-old man with cholesterolosis bulbi.* In the upper portion of the anterior chamber golden crystals are floating freely, but in the lower portion they have layered out. As a child he was struck in the eye, and for several years he has been blind. Following enucleation, a retinal detachment was found.

Fig. 31. *Colored crystals and yellowish amorphous material in the left eye of a 69-year-old man with cholesterol in the anterior chamber.* **A,** Centrally the anterior chamber contains multicolored crystals, while superiorly there is yellowish white amorphous material. Large blood vessels course through the iris. **B,** Photomicrograph shows the anterior chamber to contain a fibrovascular tissue with crystal clefts. (H & E stain; ×400.) **C,** High-power photomicrograph reveals multiple typical cholesterol clefts. (H & E stain; ×1600.)

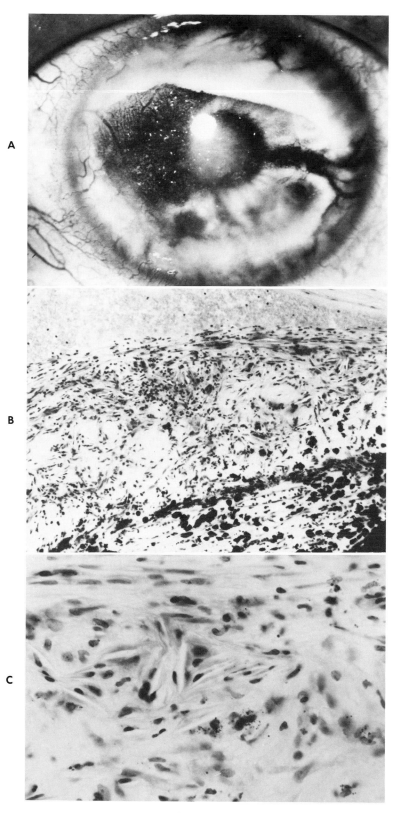

Fig. 31. For legend see opposite page.

Degenerative conditions involving the anterior chamber

Cholesterol in anterior chamber

History. Fifteen years ago this 69-year-old man developed a cataract in the left eye. According to his history, the eye had been "very poor" for at least 30 years. A year ago it became red and painful.

Findings. Vision in the right eye is 20/100 and in the left light perception. In the right eye the anterior segment is normal, the media clear, and on fundus examination a poorly defined peripapillary lesion is visible. In the left eye the cornea is clear, but the anterior chamber is extremely shallow secondary to FIG. 31 extensive peripheral anterior synechias (Fig. 31, A). Centrally there are many colored crystals floating in an otherwise clear aqueous, and peripherally there is a yellowish white amorphous material that has floated to the upper portion of the remaining anterior chamber. Large blood vessels course through the iris and the peripheral anterior synechias. The pupil is occluded, and the lens shows extensive cataractous changes.

Course. The patient was advised to have the eye enucleated, and he consented several months later. The histopathologic findings were an anterior chamber containing a fibrovascularized tissue and multiple cholesterol clefts (Fig. 31, B and C). The lens was hypermature. The retina was totally detached, with extensive gliosis and subretinal lipoidal histiocytosis.

Ruptured traumatic cataract

History. Seven years ago this 24-year-old man was injured in the right eye, which recently became irritated and watery.

Findings. The right eye is blind, and vision in the left eye is 20/15. The right eye is markedly exotropic. The cornea is clear except for a peripheral REEL V-1 stromal vascularization most marked superiorly (Reel V-1). The anterior chamber is filled with abnormal material that has separated into three distinct layers. The inferior third contains blood that appears to be undergoing organization, while the central third contains numerous shiny multicolored crystals. The upper third contains a yellow amorphous material lighter than aqueous, with the appearance of old degenerated lens cortex, possibly mixed with cholesterol. In a few places where the iris can be visualized, rubeosis iridis is present. The pupillary margins are displaced posteriorly, and through the remnant of the absorbed lens, organized vitreous can be observed. The left eye is normal.

Course. An appointment was made for the patient to return, but he was lost to follow-up.

INTERNAL VITREOUS PROLAPSE

Following intracapsular cataract extraction, dislocation or subluxation of the lens, or a complete discission of the lens, an internal prolapse of the vitreous body (vitreous hernia) may occur. The milder form is a common occurrence and generally does not lead to any complications. Unformed or semifluid vitreous usually is relatively innocuous unless the anterior chamber angle is sufficiently blocked to cause glaucoma. The most common complication is vitreous prolapse with an intact hyaloid face that is in contact with the cornea and results in endothelial damage and corneal edema. Fibrosis of the hyaloid face to the anterior surface of the cornea may occur with bullous keratopathy and permanent opacification of the cornea. Other complications of vitreous prolapse are pupillary block with secondary glaucoma, adherence of the vitreous to the corneoscleral wound, shallowing of the anterior chamber with subacute angle closure glaucoma, and the possibility of retinal detachment and macular edema secondary to vitreous adhesions resulting from inflammatory reactions in the vitreous body. Appropriate measures must be promptly taken to avoid serious, irreversible changes due to the "corneal touch."

Treatment of vitreous prolapse with corneal involvement is frequently difficult, and the exact procedure of choice is controversial. It is clear that in some cases a degree of pupillary block is involved, and maximum mydriasis should be the initial procedure in an attempt at re-formation of the shallow anterior chamber that usually exists under these circumstances. Occasionally, miosis may help hold the vitreous back, but generally it produces more pupillary block with further shallowing of the anterior chamber and is rarely successful. Hypertonic agents such as glycerol to dehydrate the vitreous have been reported to be successful and are worth a therapeutic trial. Surgical procedures include drainage of fluid vitreous through the pars plana region and air injection into the anterior chamber. In the presence of a choroidal detachment, removal of subchoroidal fluid is mandatory. Since only formed vitreous with an intact hyaloid face causes corneal edema, some have advocated incision of the anterior face. Recently the use of cocaine (5%) instilled repeatedly has caused the hyaloid face to regress remarkably in one series. This apparently is not due to the mydriatic action of the cocaine but to some other mechanism.

Vitreous in anterior chamber

History. Four years ago this 71-year-old woman had an intracapsular cataract extraction performed on her right eye, with an uneventful postoperative course and recovery of vision to 20/20. Asteroid hyalosis had been noted prior to operation. Recently she noted that her vision had become very blurred.

Findings. Vision in the right eye is 20/200 and in the left accurate light projection. The right eye is aphakic, with a complete surgical coloboma of the iris superiorly (Reel V-2). There is a prolapse of vitreous into the anterior REEL V-2 chamber, involving most of the pupillary area. This vitreous contains numerous fine, uniformly distributed particles typical of asteroid hyalosis. The fundus can not be visualized through the pupillary area due to the vitreous opacities but can easily be seen and appears entirely normal through the coloboma. The left eye is normal except for a mature cataract, which makes visualization of the posterior segment impossible. Intraocular tension is normal in both eyes.

Course. Dilating the pupil caused some of the vitreous to retract posteriorly and inferiorly and increased the patient's visual acuity to 20/50. It was further improved to 20/30 by change in her aphakic correction. Because she still complained of blurring of vision, she was advised to have the other cataract removed; however, she did not return for further treatment.

Vitreous prolapse into anterior chamber

History. About 35 years ago this 76-year-old woman had undergone bilateral cataract extractions. She did well until a month ago, when she noticed blurring of vision in her left eye.

Findings. The vision in the right eye is 20/30 and in the left counting

55

REEL V-3 fingers at 1½ feet with aphakic corrections. The right eye is aphakic and otherwise normal. In the left eye there is a large protrusion of vitreous into the anterior chamber covered by an intact hyaloid face (Reel V-3). Inferiorly there is a 1.5-mm. "hyphema" contained within the vitreous bulge. There is a small area of contact of the vitreous face with the cornea centrally, but there is no corneal edema. The aqueous contains a moderate number of cells with only a minimal flare. The vitreous body contains streaks of blood, particularly posteriorly, making visualization of the fundus impossible. Intraocular tension as shown by applanation tonometry is 17 mm. Hg in the right eye and 18 mm. Hg in the left.

Course. The patient was lost to follow-up.

Intravitreal hemorrhage in anterior chamber

History. Bilateral cataract extractions were performed on this 74-year-old woman 9 years ago. Until recently the vision in both eyes was good with her aphakic correction. However, 2 months ago she had sudden loss of vision in the left eye and was found to have a central retinal artery occlusion. A week ago she developed pain in her forehead and left temporal region, along with lacrimation. She was diabetic, and the condition was controlled by medication and diet.

Findings. The vision in the right eye is 20/25 and in the left light perception only. The right eye is aphakic but otherwise normal, and there is no pathologic condition in the fundus. In the left eye there is a moderate injection of the conjunctiva, and the cornea is diffusely hazy. The anterior chamber is deep, and the aqueous contains a moderate number of cells with some flare. Extending through the pupil into the anterior chamber and almost touching the cornea is a large globule of vitreous containing dark red blood in its dependent REEL V-4 portion (Reel V-4). There is a surgical coloboma superiorly and a peripheral iridectomy at the 2 o'clock position. The vitreous posteriorly contains much hemorrhage and makes visualization of the fundus difficult. Gonioscopy shows that about half of the angle is involved with peripheral anterior synechias, but no neovascularization is visible. Applanation tonometry shows pressures of 22 mm. Hg in the right eye and 42 mm. Hg in the left.

Course. Topical corticosteroids were instituted, which made the left eye comfortable. Six months later the blood was still trapped behind the hyaloid face, and the tension was only 31 mm. Hg (Schiøtz).

Vitreous contact with cornea

History. About a year ago this 52-year-old man had bilateral intracapsular cataract extractions. There were no complications at the time of operation, and the postoperative course was uneventful. Subsequently it was noted that the vitreous face had come forward in both eyes, and in the left eye there was a whitish membrane on the posterior surface of the cornea superiorly.

Findings. Vision in both eyes is good with aphakic correction, and the right eye is a normal aphakic eye with a slight vitreous bulge that does not touch the cornea. In the left eye superiorly there is a white area coming down on the FIG. 32 posterior surface of the cornea for about 3 mm. (Fig. 32). Slit-lamp examina-

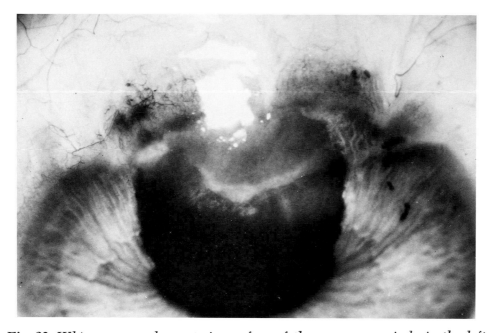

Fig. 32. *White area on the posterior surface of the cornea superiorly in the left eye of a 52-year-old man with vitreocorneal contact.* There is a white "membrane" extending on the posterior surface of the cornea superiorly, which represents the area of contact of the vitreous with the cornea, with continued good vision during the next year of observation.

tion shows vitreous coming through the coloboma superiorly and in contact with the cornea, producing the corneal opacity. The temporal pillar is also pushed forward and is touching the cornea peripherally. The remainder of the findings are normal for an aphakic eye.

Course. Over a period of the next year there was no change in the opacification of the cornea, and the patient was asymptomatic.

Vitreous contact with cornea

History. Thirteen years ago this 75-year-old man had an unplanned extracapsular cataract extraction performed in the left eye. Postoperatively there were no complications, and he obtained 20/20 vision with his aphakic correction. Three months ago he noted a foreign body sensation and some blurring of vision in the left eye, which has progressively become worse.

Findings. The vision in the right eye is 20/30 with aphakic correction and in the left 20/100. In the right eye there is no abnormality except for surgical aphakia, but in the left eye the upper third of the cornea is edematous due to vitreous extending through the surgical coloboma with adherence to its posterior surface (Fig. 33). There are many fine bullae in the epithelium of the cornea, FIG. 33 and the pupil is updrawn. Only a poor view of the fundus can be obtained. Intraocular tensions in both eyes are 18 mm. Hg (Schiøtz).

Course. A peripheral iridectomy was performed at the 4 o'clock position, and the vitreous was swept from the cornea with a cyclodialysis spatula. Air

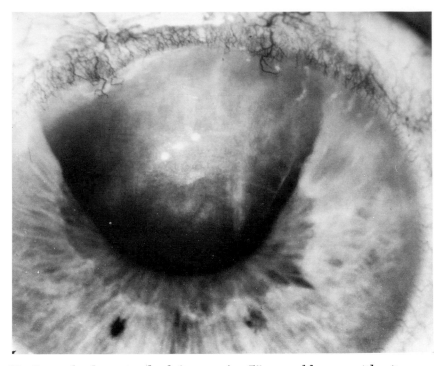

Fig. 33. *Corneal edema in the left eye of a 75-year-old man with vitreocorneal contact.* The upper third of the cornea is edematous, and the pupil is drawn up due to persistent adherence to the posterior surface of the cornea. Peripheral iridectomy and sweeping of the vitreous from the cornea eliminated the vitreous contact, but the cornea remained edematous.

was placed into the anterior chamber. Postoperatively the cornea cleared only slightly, and the bullous keratopathy persisted despite the fact that the vitreous was no longer in contact with the cornea. Because of the persistence of his symptoms, a conjunctival flap was planned, but the patient had an acute myocardial infarction and died.

Vitreous retraction with deep anterior chamber

History. Six months ago this 46-year-old woman was discovered to have chronic open angle glaucoma. Two months ago she noted loss of vision with flashes of light in the left eye.

Findings. Vision in the right eye is 20/70 and in the left perception of hand movements. In the right eye there are no abnormalities present except in the fundus, where there is an extensive equatorial lattice degeneration with one possible hole. There is no detachment. In the left eye there is moderate conjunctival injection, a clear cornea, with a markedly deepened anterior chamber REEL V-5 (Reel V-5). At the periphery there is an abrupt change in the iris plane, which sweeps forward almost at a right angle in an irregular fashion. Inferiorly there are multiple posterior synechias. The anterior chamber contains a marked flare and many cells with some pigmented keratic precipitates. The lens shows moderate nuclear sclerosis. Fundus examination shows a total detachment of the ret-

58

ina with several holes temporally. There are many thick folds and a large choroidal detachment. Intraocular pressure in the right eye is 30 mm. Hg and in the left 14 mm. Hg.

Course. Topical corticosteroids and mydriatics were administered intensively to the left eye, and there was gradual improvement in the iritis and the choroidal detachment. Two weeks later a scleral buckling procedure was performed, but reattachment was not accomplished, and a mature cataract developed in about 3 months. Careful observation was carried out on the right eye, but no surgery was required until 7 years later the patient developed a cataract, which was uneventfully extracted. The left eye was now totally blind, with marked iris atrophy, and continued to have bouts of iritis. Two years later a large choroidal detachment developed in the right eye, which required a choroidal tap. Following this, a scleral buckling procedure was done because of the retinal holes that had not yet caused any detachment. Postoperatively, the vision was reduced to 20/200 due to vitreous traction on the macular region. Over the next 5 years there was gradual continued deterioration in her central vision to counting fingers at 3 feet.

Spontaneous vitreous prolapse

History. For many years this 56-year-old man had poor vision in the left eye, and for the past 2 weeks it was painful and watery. There was an indefinite history of some sort of injury to the eye a number of years ago. Cataract extraction was performed on the right eye 6 years ago.

Findings. The vision in the right eye is 20/70 with correction, and the left eye has no light perception. The right eye shows a marked arcus senilis, with a deep anterior chamber and a surgical coloboma superiorly. The vitreous bulges through the coloboma, and the fundus is normal except for a poor foveal reflex. In the left eye there is a marked conjunctival injection and arcus senilis. The peripheral cornea is invaded with superficial vessels, and there are some fine keratic precipitates. The anterior chamber is partially filled with a bubblelike structure that almost touches the cornea and is concentric with the pupil (Reel V-6). The anterior surface of this semitransparent globular structure is cov- REEL V-6
ered by numerous minute white precipitates. Posteriorly the mass is attached to the iris around the pupil. Inferiorly there is a hypopyon, and the anterior chamber contains numerous cells and a moderate flare. The lens and posterior segment cannot be visualized, and a whitish reflex is obtained with the ophthalmoscope. Gonioscopy reveals that much of the angle is closed by peripheral anterior synechias and exudates.

Course. For several weeks the patient was treated with topical corticosteroids and mydriatics, with some improvement of the pain and redness. Three weeks later enucleation was performed, and the postoperative recovery was uneventful. Histopathologic findings were vitreous in the anterior chamber, on the surface of which were many white blood cells. There were numerous peripheral anterior synechias and Russell bodies in the iris. Posteriorly there was a generalized chorioretinal atrophy and loss of rods and cones, with an atrophic optic nerve. There was a posterior ciliary vasculitis.

Chapter 3

Traumatic conditions involving the anterior chamber

FOREIGN BODIES IN THE ANTERIOR CHAMBER

Penetration of the cornea by a foreign body that does not further penetrate into the globe is relatively common. Such a foreign body is retained in the anterior chamber, may fall to the inferior angle, and, if sufficiently small, may be undetectable except by gonioscopy. Other foreign bodies, although largely in the anterior chamber, may be caught in the cornea or be partially enmeshed in the iris stroma. Generally speaking, inert foreign bodies that are stationary in the anterior chamber cause no reaction and can be safely left in the eye. Embedded glass, plastics (methyl methacrylate), gold, silver, and platinum are well-tolerated materials; lead and zinc are less so; while iron, copper, and lime-stone cause considerable reaction. Vegetable matter such as wood usually produces a marked reaction, and organic matter in general carries a high incidence of infection. An exception is cilia, which are well tolerated and innocuous in the anterior chamber except when the follicle remains, in which case a pearl cyst can develop. In such instances one must remove the cilia and the cyst. Iron and steel foreign bodies are frequent in industrial operation, sometimes despite the use of protective goggles. High-grade steels, especially stainless steel, are relatively inert; but softer alloys break down, producing iritis and siderosis of the various tissues in the eye. Copper, if allowed to remain in the eye, produces chalcosis with degenerative effects on the ciliary epithelium, lens, and retina. Thus, even though there is only a minimal initial reaction from a copper-containing foreign body, it should be removed.

Inert foreign bodies that penetrate into the anterior chamber and fall into the inferior angle may even years later produce corneal edema in the adjacent sector by damage to the endothelium. In general, these are not fixed but can

60

move to some extent; this movement explains the occasional diurnal variation in findings. Gonioscopy of all such cases is mandatory; should the foreign body be discovered, removal is usually curative, with prompt clearing of the corneal edema unless permanent endothelial damage has occurred. In addition, the importance of diagnostic x-ray films in detecting such foreign bodies cannot be overemphasized. The absence of a detectable wound of entry does not exclude an intraocular foreign body.

Strictly speaking, the vitreous and the lens or portions of the lens in the anterior chamber are endogenous foreign bodies. Because of the occurrence of vitreous in the anterior chamber, resulting in various degenerative conditions, this is discussed in Chapter 2. Anterior dislocation of the lens is not uncommon. The entire lens may appear in the anterior chamber. This occurs in systemic diseases, such as arachnodactyly, brachydactyly, and homocystinuria, in which the zonules are weak. Congenitally dislocated lenses not associated with systemic disease are also known to dislocate anteriorly. One of the most common causes of anterior dislocation is trauma in which the zonular attachments are broken or weakened, with eventual total posterior dislocation of the lens. With the pupil moderately dilated, prolapse into the anterior chamber can occur often years after the injury. An intact lens in the anterior chamber may produce glaucoma by pupillary block or corneal edema by contact with the endothelium. With rupture of the anterior lens capsule from any cause, cortex frequently enters the anterior chamber and is well tolerated even if in contact with the endothelium. Such ruptures occur with trauma and in surgical procedures such as needling or linear extraction of a cataract. Cortex in contact with the aqueous is gradually absorbed, usually without untoward reaction. Phakolytic glaucoma (p. 47) and anaphylactic uveitis (p. 207) may occur and must be considered if glaucoma or an inflammatory reaction occurs.

Steel foreign body in chamber angle

History. Five hours ago this 30-year-old man was struck in the left eye with a steel chip. The eye was painful, but the vision was unaffected.

Findings. The vision in both eyes is 20/20. The right eye is normal. There is some injection of the left eye and a small perforating wound of the cornea near the limbus at the 3 o'clock position. The anterior chamber is formed, and no foreign body can be visualized by slit-lamp biomicroscopy. However, gonioscopic examination shows a shiny piece of steel lying in the inferior angle (Fig. 34). The lens and fundus are normal.

FIG. 34

Course. An ab externo limbal incision was made at the 6 o'clock position, and the hand magnet was used to extract the steel chip. Postoperatively there were no complications, and 2 months later the patient had 20/20 vision and was asymptomatic.

Steel foreign body in chamber angle

History. Twenty-five years ago this 45-year-old man was struck in the left eye with a fragment of steel from an ax. A traumatic cataract developed. Three operations were performed for this, but the foreign body was never recovered. Following the operations he had recurrent attacks of iritis. Five years ago he was found

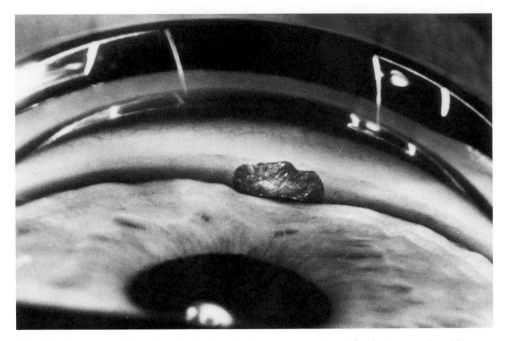

Fig. 34. *Shiny steel foreign body in the inferior angle of the left eye of a 30-year-old man.* A chip of steel has fallen to the inferior angle after perforating the cornea 5 hours ago. It was removed, and subsequently the vision was normal.

to have an intraocular pressure of 70 mm. Hg (Schiøtz) and was treated with miotics and corticosteroid drops. The eye was essentially blind.

Findings. The vision in the right eye is 20/20 and in the left eye light perception temporally. The right eye is normal and the iris is blue. In the left eye there is some conjunctival injection, and the cornea is fairly clear except for some keratic precipitates. The anterior chamber has a flare, and the iris is yellowish in color. At the 6 o'clock position the edge of a dark object can just be seen in the anterior chamber. Gonioscopy reveals a dark brown foreign body with yellow spots on its surface (Fig. 35). It lies deep in the angle and depresses the iris slightly. The angle is open, and there is excessive pigment on the trabecular meshwork. Because of lens remnants in the pupil the fundus cannot be visualized. Intraocular pressures in both eyes are 18 mm. Hg (Schiøtz).

FIG. 35

Course. Over the next 10 years the left eye developed absolute glaucoma and band keratopathy. A year later the eye became very painful due to bullous keratopathy. The eye was enucleated, and a year later the patient was comfortable, with good vision in the remaining eye.

Carborundum granule in anterior chamber

History. This 44-year-old man recalled using a grinding wheel 16 years ago when something flew off and struck him in the eye. Recently he was referred to an ophthalmologist for a question of glaucoma and was found to have a "lesion" in the inferior angle of his right eye.

Findings. The vision in both eyes is 20/25. In the right eye there is no sign of

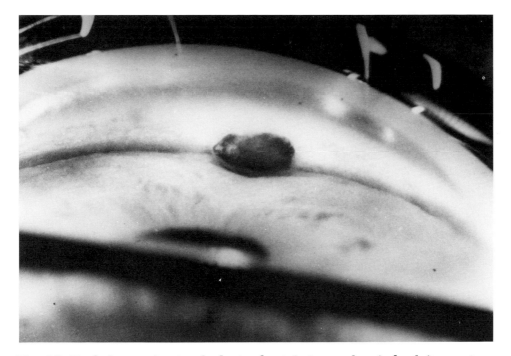

Fig. 35. *Dark brown foreign body in the inferior angle of the left eye in a 45-year-old man with a steel foreign body and siderosis iridis.* A fragment of steel from an ax perforated the cornea 25 years ago and produced a secondary cataract. Subsequently, there was iritis, and the iris became yellowish in color (siderosis iridis). He then developed absolute glaucoma and band keratopathy, and the eye was enucleated.

corneal perforation, but in the inferior angle just barely visible is the edge of what appears to be a foreign body. Gonioscopy shows the angle to be normal and wide open, but at the 6 o'clock position there is a cube-shaped structure about 1 mm. in size covered with a layer of fibrinous material (Reel V-7). There is REEL V-7 no other evidence of reaction at the point of its contact with either the cornea or iris. The remainder of the eye is normal.

Course. X-ray films showed a tiny radiopaque foreign body in the right eye. Because of the inert appearance of the foreign body, no treatment was undertaken, and the patient was lost to follow-up.

Sand granule in chamber angle

History. Twenty-five years ago a firecracker exploded near the left eye of this 32-year-old man. Twelve years ago he first noticed a red left eye, with pain, photophobia, and lacrimation. A corneal ulcer was diagnosed, and he was hospitalized and treated with antibiotics and intravenous typhoid fever therapy. However, the symptoms persisted, and 5 years later the left anterior chamber was surgically "explored" for a possible foreign body; none was found, and an iridectomy was performed. Since then there were exacerbations and remissions, with some relief with the use of Neo-Decadron drops four times a day. X-ray films for intraocular foreign bodies have always been negative.

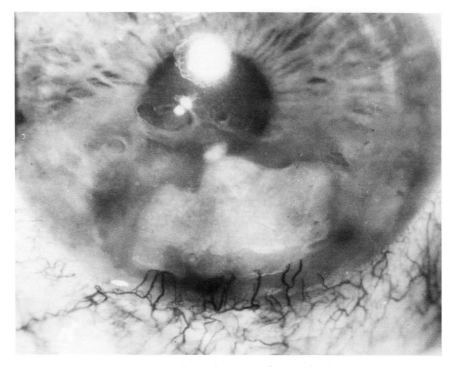

Fig. 36. *Edema and extensive bullous keratopathy of the left cornea in a 32-year-old man with a sand granule in the chamber angle.* Apparently a firecracker exploding near his eye 25 years ago caused a sand granule to penetrate the cornea. Gonioscopy (Reel VI-1) shows a semitransparent rounded mass (sand granule) just peripheral to a surgical iridectomy. Subsequently, the foreign body was removed, and a conjunctival flap was applied to the area of bullous keratopathy.

FIG. 36

REEL VI-1

Findings. The vision in the right eye is 20/15 and in the left 20/40. The right eye is normal. In the left eye there is a moderate amount of injection, and the lower cornea is edematous with extensive bullous keratopathy (Fig. 36). Peripheral vascularization from the limbus is seen inferiorly. The anterior chamber is deep and clear. There is a large peripheral iridectomy at the 6 o'clock position. Gonioscopy shows that the iridectomy is not basal, and lying in the angle just peripheral to the iridectomy is a small transparent rounded mass (Reel VI-1). The posterior segment is normal. The intraocular pressure in both eyes is 16 mm. Hg (Schiøtz).

Course. An ab externo incision was performed at the inferior limbus, and the foreign body was grasped and removed with a forceps. A conjunctival flap was placed over the inferior third of the cornea, covering the area of severe bullous keratopathy. The postoperative course was uneventful, with gradual resolution of the bullae above the edge of the conjunctival flap. As the cornea cleared, a through-and-through scar could be visualized just below the apex of the cornea, obviously the site of entrance of the foreign body. Three years later the eye was comfortable, and the vision was 20/25.

Cilium in anterior chamber

History. Four years ago this 12-year-old boy was running through the woods, when a sharp twig struck his left eye, lacerating the cornea. A cilium was noted in the anterior chamber, which had spontaneously re-formed.

Findings. Vision in both eyes is 20/25. There is a scar near the limbus at the 9 o'clock position, with some vascularization. Lying free in the anterior chamber almost against the cornea is a cilium, which extends into the angle at the 10 o'clock position (Reel VI-2). Some peripheral anterior synechias are present ad- REEL VI-2 jacent to and attached to the tip of the cilium. The pupil is distorted due to retraction toward the area of the injury. The remainder of the eye is normal.

Course. The patient was lost to follow-up.

Cilia in anterior chamber

History. One year ago this 10-year-old boy was struck in the right eye with a wire. By the time he was seen 3 days later, the anterior chamber had formed and a cilium was found lying on the iris, with its root in the inferior angle. The laceration at the 2 o'clock position near the limbus had healed. The patient was treated with systemic antibiotics and topical mydriatics and corticosteroids. Within a week there was no reaction in the eye, and the cilium was allowed to remain.

Findings. Vision in both eyes is 20/20. In the right eye an old healed wound is seen at the 2 o'clock position; the anterior chamber is clear, and in it is a cilium, the point of which reaches almost the center of the pupil, with the root disappearing in the angle (Fig. 37, A). The lens is clear and the fundus normal. FIG. 37 Gonioscopy shows that the cilium is touching the region of Schwalbe's line but that in addition there is a tip end of another cilium lying lengthwise within the angle at the 5 o'clock position (see arrow, Fig. 37, B). All angle structures are normal except for a small synechia at one end of the small cilia lying in the angle. The left eye is normal.

Course. In the next 3 years during which the patient was followed, the two cilia did not change their location or cause any reaction.

Rose thorn in chamber angle

History. Three days ago this 23-year-old man ran into a rose bush, injuring his left eye. A few hours later the anterior chamber of the left eye was found to be shallowed and the eye extremely soft, with a foreign body embedded in the sclera near the limbus. The foreign body was removed, and a conjunctival flap was placed over the wound. The anterior chamber formed, and the patient was comfortable.

Findings. The vision in the right eye is 20/15 and in the left 20/25. The right eye is normal. There is moderate conjunctival injection in the left eye, especially inferotemporally where a single catgut suture is placed through the conjunctiva and episclera. The cornea is clear and the anterior chamber of normal depth. The pupil is dilated due to mydriatic drops. Gonioscopy of the left eye reveals a brown pointed object extending through the cornea just anterior to Schwalbe's line at the 5 o'clock position (Reel VI-3). Just anterior to this REEL VI-3 foreign body, which has the appearance of the tip end of a rose thorn, is some

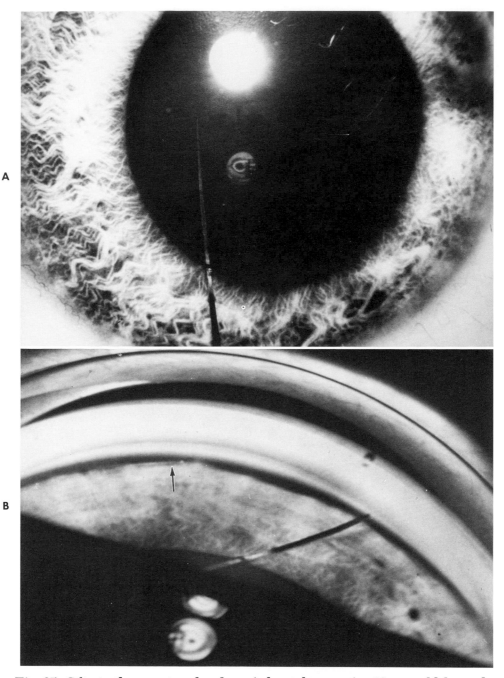

Fig. 37. *Cilia in the anterior chamber of the right eye of a 10-year-old boy who had been struck by a piece of wire.* The wire perforated the cornea and pushed two cilia in with it. **A,** One cilium lies against the iris inferiorly, and the tip end extends up into the central pupillary area. **B,** Gonioscopy shows that the end of the cilium touches the region of Schwalbe's line. In addition, the tip end of another cilium lies lengthwise in the angle (arrow).

white exudative material on the posterior surface of the cornea. The angle is open and the trabecular meshwork uninvolved. The lens and fundus are normal.

Course. In 2 months the eye was white and the patient asymptomatic. The vision was 20/15, and gonioscopy showed that a small amount of fibrous tissue had formed around the foreign body.

Cortex in anterior chamber

History. Two months ago this 52-year-old man was struck in the left eye with a wire rope. The vision was immediately decreased, but pain was slight. A gray spot appeared in the center of the eye on the day of the injury.

Findings. Vision in the right eye is 20/20 and in the left accurate light projection. The right eye is normal. The left eye is moderately injected. The cornea is clear except for several linear lacerations centrally, some of which appear to have perforated the cornea. The anterior chamber is partially filled with lens cortex, and temporally the iris is displaced forward presumably by swollen cortex located posteriorly (Fig. 38). The pupil is completely filled with cortical material, and no red fundus reflex is visible. The intraocular tension is 16 mm. Hg (Schiøtz) in the right eye and 48 mm. Hg (Schiøtz) in the left. FIG. 38

Course. Irrigation of the anterior chamber was performed through a limbal section at the 12 o'clock position. Postoperatively the pupil was free of cortical

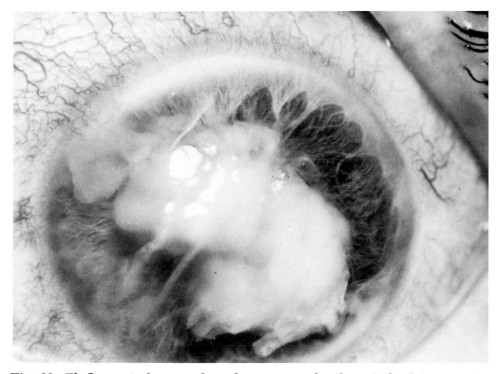

Fig. 38. *Fluffy cortical material in the anterior chamber of the left eye of a 52-year-old man who was struck in the eye by a wire rope.* The pupil and much of the anterior chamber are filled with lens cortex. Presumably the anterior capsule was ruptured when a piece of wire entered the anterior chamber.

material and was black. Some posterior synechias were present. The fundus appeared to be normal. The patient was then lost to follow-up.

Anteriorly dislocated calcareous lens

History. Seventeen years ago this 42-year-old man was struck in the right eye, resulting in intraocular hemorrhage and subluxation of the lens. Vision gradually failed. About 7 years ago he noticed a white spot in his pupil. At that time examination showed iridodonesis, posterior dislocation of a shrunken hypermature cataractous lens, and a total retinal detachment. In the past several years on a number of occasions the lens dislocated spontaneously into the anterior chamber but fell back through the pupil without causing any difficulty. Miotics were prescribed to avoid this complication, but he used the drops only intermittently. A few hours ago the lens again fell into the anterior chamber. Attempts to make it fall back through the pupil were unsuccessful.

Findings. Vision in the right eye is light perception and in the left 20/20 without correction. The right eye is only slightly injected, and the cornea is clear. There is a shrunken yellow calcareous lens lying in the inferior angle and exFIG. 39 tending up to just above the pupillary margin (Fig. 39). The iris is normal except for a prominent iridodonesis, and glimpses through the pupil reveal a detached retina. The left eye is normal. Intraocular pressure in the right eye is 18 mm. Hg (Schiøtz) and in the left 25 mm. Hg (Schiøtz).

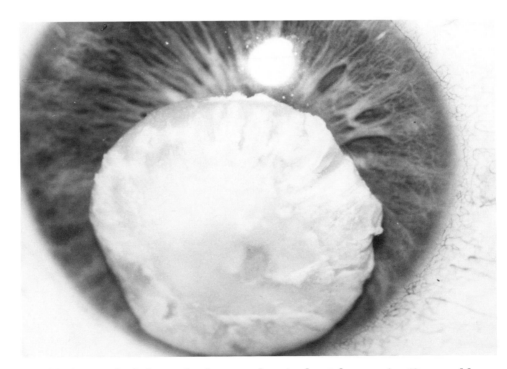

Fig. 39. Anteriorly dislocated calcareous lens in the right eye of a 42-year-old man injured 17 years ago. The entire lens, which is dislocated anteriorly and lying in the inferior angle, appears to be shrunken and calcified. Subsequently, the cataract was extracted, and the result was good.

Course. Intracapsular cataract extraction was performed without problems. The postoperative course was uneventful. Eighteen years later the patient was struck in the right eye, producing an eight-ball (black-ball) hemorrhage and causing complications for which the eye was eventually enucleated.

Soemmering's ring in anterior chamber

History. At birth this 68-year-old man had a cataract, which was presumably needled during childhood. More than 10 years ago he noticed a white spot in the pupil of the right eye. The eye was not painful.

Findings. The vision in the right eye is extremely poor, and there is minimal conjunctival injection. The anterior chamber is deep and contains in its central portion a roughly circular mass of white material with a central clear area (Fig. 40). Slit-lamp examination indicates that this is old calcified cortex surrounded by lens capsule. The pupil is only partially visible, and the posterior segment cannot be adequately examined. FIG. 40

Course. The eye remained asymptomatic, and 5 years later there was no appreciable change except for a slight decrease in the amount of cortical material contained within the capsule. The patient was then lost to follow-up.

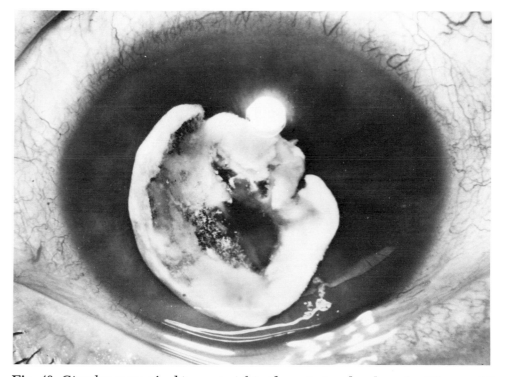

Fig. 40. *Circular mass of white material in the anterior chamber of a 68-year-old man with Soemmering's ring in the right eye.* During childhood a congenital cataract was needled, and subsequently the remaining lens dislocated into the anterior chamber. The patient is asymptomatic, and no treatment has been instituted.

Cortex in anterior chamber

History. At around age 2 this 18-year-old girl had several operations for her congenital cataracts. At age 8 she underwent needlings for pupillary membranes and has had no visual complaints until recently when the left eye again became blurred. Two months ago she again had a discission on the left eye, and the postoperative course was normal. About 2 weeks ago she was struck in the left eye, and a white piece of material became visible in the lower portion of the anterior chamber.

Findings. Vision with aphakic correction in the right eye is 20/200 and in the left counting fingers at 6 feet. In the right eye the cornea and anterior chamber are normal, and there is a round pupil with dense cortex and capsule except for a clear area centrally. Through this can be seen the fundus, which appears to be normal. In the left eye the cornea is normal, but in the inferior angle extending up toward the pupillary area is a piece of white material with an onion skin pattern typical of calcified lens cortex (Fig. 41). There is still some residual pupillary membrane centrally, which may explain the poor vision in this eye. The fundus appears to be normal. Intraocular tension in both eyes is well within normal limits.

Course. The patient was fitted with a low vision aid, obtaining a vision of 20/40 in the right eye.

FIG. 41

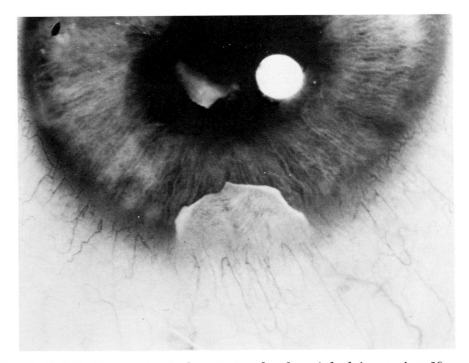

Fig. 41. *Calcified lens cortex in the anterior chamber of the left eye of an 18-year-old girl with congenital cataracts. As a young child, needlings were performed; 2 weeks ago she was struck in the left eye, at which time a piece of cortex was noted in the inferior angle.*

Portion of crystalline lens dislocated into anterior chamber

History. Twenty-four years ago this 77-year-old man had an extracapsular extraction performed on the left eye, and 4 months later he developed a retinal detachment, which was successfully reattached. Having moved away, he was not seen again until today, when he complained of recent mild irritation in his left eye.

Findings. Vision in the right eye is 20/40 and in the left 20/30 with correction. The cornea of the right eye is moderately opacified, with ghost vessels typical of old interstitial keratitis. The remainder of the eye is normal except for surgical aphakia. In the left eye there is also evidence of old interstitial keratitis. In the lower portion of the anterior chamber there is a rounded elongated structure (Reel VI-4). The central portion contains opacities typical of those seen in REEL VI-4
an immature cataract, but around this is a clear material that appears to be cortex covered by a clear capsule. Posteriorly the capsule is attached to a capsular pupillary membrane that extends behind the pupil. It is not possible to adequately see the fundus. The tension in the right eye is 14 mm. Hg (Schiøtz) and in the left 4 mm. Hg (Schiøtz).

Course. No treatment seemed necessary, and the patient was lost to further follow-up.

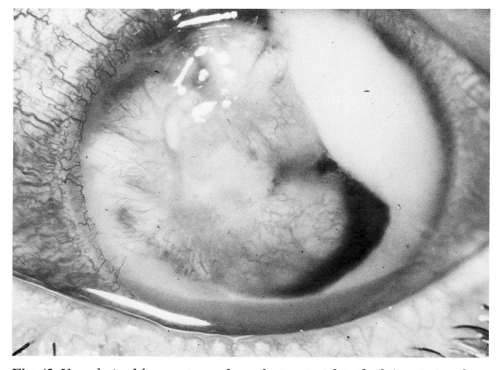

Fig. 42. *Vascularized lens cortex and purulent material in the left anterior chamber of a 30-year-old man with endophthalmitis.* The patient was struck in the eye by a nail 3 weeks ago, which resulted in a corneal perforation and rupture of the lens capsule. Despite intensive antibiotic treatment, an endophthalmitis developed, with gradual vascularization of the cortical material.

Endophthalmitis and vascularization of traumatic cataract

History. Three weeks ago this 30-year-old man was struck in the left eye by a nail he was hammering. After pulling the nail out of his eye, he could see shadows only. Ocular examination showed a perforating wound through the cornea and a cataractous lens partially in the anterior chamber. Massive antibiotics were used, but he developed a hypopyon by the next day, with an abscess of the corneal wound. There was an increase of fibrin and pus cells in the anterior chamber during the next 5 days, with swollen cortex extending into the anterior chamber. There was gradual resolution of the purulent material and the corneal abscess, but the lens cortex became vascularized.

Findings. Vision in the right eye is 20/20 and in the left light perception. The right eye is normal. The left eye shows marked conjunctival injection, and the cornea is diffusely edematous. There is a partially healed corneal perforation at the 10 o'clock position near the limbus (Fig. 42). The nasal two thirds of the anterior chamber is filled with lens cortex, the surface of which is covered by numerous fine vessels. Temporally there is a mass of purulent material. The iris and posterior segment cannot be visualized.

FIG. 42

Course. Three days later an enucleation was performed, and the histopathologic findings were perforating wound of the cornea, hypopyon, organization of lens remnants, abscess of vitreous, massive separation of the retina, and acute panophthalmitis.

HYPHEMA

An accumulation of free blood in the anterior chamber is referred to as hyphema. By far the most common cause is trauma, but spontaneous hemorrhage in the anterior chamber may be associated with intraocular neoplasms, blood dyscrasias, severe iritis, rubeosis iridis, retrolental fibrovascular membranes, and juvenile xanthogranuloma; occasionally there is no known cause. While traumatic hyphema may result from even a mild contusion, it is almost always present in severe trauma. The primary hyphema occurring at the time of the injury is frequently mild, and by gravity the red blood cells settle out inferiorly to a height of a few millimeters, while in severe hyphemas the entire anterior chamber may be filled with blood. In a secondary hemorrhage more severe bleeding is common, and complications are far more frequent. The bleeding into the anterior chamber is probably arteriolar from the root of the iris or ciliary body. Absorption of the primary hemorrhage usually occurs in 1 to 7 days, leaving no residual defect. If a secondary hemorrhage occurs, it is usually on the second to fifth posttraumatic day and can take months to absorb. Commonly, the secondary hemorrhage fills the anterior chamber and produces the so-called eight-ball or black-ball hemorrhage, this appearance being due to the dark, clotted blood in the anterior chamber. Red blood cells are ordinarily absorbed by the trabecular endothelium and the histiocytes within the meshwork of the angle as well as by the stromal cells in the iris. However, if with massive hemorrhage adequate absorption cannot take place, embarrassment of the filtration mechanism occurs, with the serious complication of secondary glaucoma. The corneal endothelium may be damaged, and hemoglobin then passes into the corneal stroma, with resultant blood staining or hematogenous pigmentation of the cornea. Occasionally, in the presence of sufficient endothelial damage, blood staining of the cornea occurs without an increase in intraocular pressure. Hematogenous pigmentation of the cornea takes many months to clear, and in most cases the vision does not completely recover. Severe hemorrhage in the anterior chamber produces a secondary uveitis with formaton of iris membranes and posterior synechias. This may result in either seclusion or occlusion of the pupil.

Treatment of traumatic hyphema is still controversial. It appears that absorption of blood from the anterior chamber is more rapid when the patient is placed on a regimen of bed rest. However, the occurrence of secondary hemorrhage in relationship to bed rest and the use of unilateral or bilateral eye pads as opposed to no padding of the eyes are still problematical. In general, no topical or systemic medication is given, but one study showed that patients treated with both pilocarpine (4%) and homatropine (1%) drops had a rapid absorption rate. The most important factor in prognosis depends on the size of the hyphema. In those involving more than three quarters of the anterior chamber volume, the incidence of increased intraocular pressure is very high (85%), and the chances of a good visual result are poor. Increased intraocular pressure is treated by the use of carbonic anhydrase inhibitors and osmotherapy; but frequently these measures are not successful, and surgical intervention is indicated. If the blood in the anterior chamber remains fluid, simple irrigation may suffice, but clotted blood requires more extensive opening of the anterior chamber and irrigation with a fibrinolytic enzyme. When the eye has recovered, gonioscopic examination will determine whether an angle recession (tear into the ciliary body) has occurred, in which case long term follow-up is obligatory. The one study reported showed that almost half of traumatic hyphema cases had "cleavage of the angle."

Traumatic hyphema

History. Four days ago this 47-year-old man was struck in the eye by a rock ejected from a power mower. He was treated with antibiotic ointment.

Findings. Vision in the right eye is 20/200 and in the left 20/20. The lids of the right eye are edematous, and there is moderate conjunctival injection. There is a 2-mm. perforating corneal laceration inferiorly, and immediately below this is a 4-mm. hyphema (Reel VI-5). The pupil is moderately dilated and fixed. The REEL VI-5 lens and vitreous are clear, and the fundus is normal. The left eye is normal.

Course. The patient was placed on a regimen of bed rest, and 3 days later most of the blood had absorbed, but there was a moderate iritis, which persisted for the next month. This was treated with mydriatics and topical corticosteroids. X-ray films were found to be negative for foreign body, and the intraocular pressure was 20 mm. Hg (Schiøtz) in both eyes. The vision was still impaired a month and a half later, and a detailed fundus examination with indirect ophthalmoscopy revealed peripheral degeneration inferiorly with evidence of old hemorrhage. This was presumably of traumatic origin. Gonioscopy revealed an angle recession nasally and inferiorly. The intraocular tension remained within normal limits for 4 months until the patient was lost to follow-up.

Old organized hyphema

History. A year ago this 53-year-old woman had a "film" over the right eye. Several months later she fell and struck the right eye, resulting in further de-

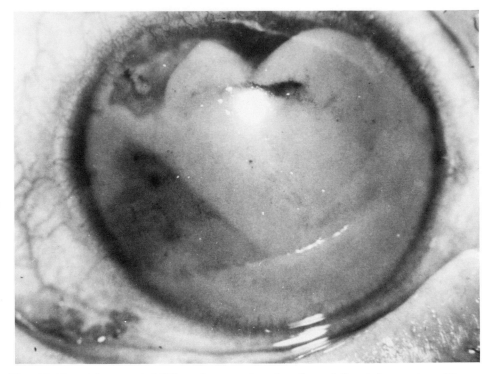

Fig. 43. *Tannish material filling the anterior chamber of the right eye in a 53-year-old woman with an old organized hyphema.* Following an injury, 4 months ago the anterior chamber was found to be filled with blood that subsequently apparently organized and produced a marked elevation in her intraocular pressure. Following enucleation, a detached retina was found histopathologically.

crease in vision. Four months ago the anterior chamber was found to be full of old blood. Recently the eye became painful, and the patient requested that it be enucleated.

Findings. The right eye is blind, and vision in the left eye is 20/20 with correction. In the right eye there is moderate conjunctival injection and some epithelial edema of the cornea, but otherwise the cornea is clear. The anterior chamber is filled with a tannish material, some of which is irregular and appears to be organized. Superiorly there is a small wedge-shaped opening through which FIG. 43 the iris can be visualized (Fig. 43). The left eye is normal. The intraocular pressure is more than 87 mm. Hg (Schiøtz) in the right eye and is 22 mm. Hg (Schiøtz) in the left.

Course. Enucleation was performed, and histopathologic diagnosis was intraocular hemorrhage of the anterior chamber and vitreous, and partially detached retina with preretinal and iris membranes. Five years later the patient had no ocular complaints.

Spontaneous hyphema

History. This 61-year-old woman stated that she awoke this morning with a "pain in my right eye." The pain lasted for several minutes, after which she noted

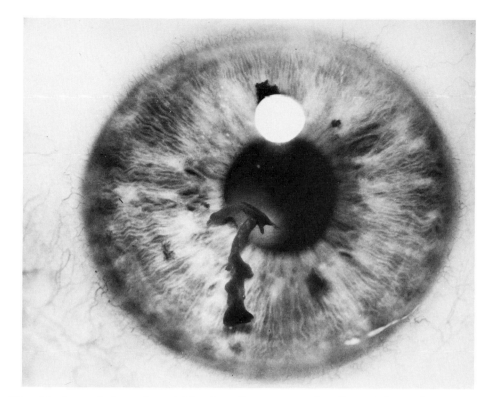

Fig. 44. *A pendulous clot of blood in the anterior chamber of the right eye of a 61-year-old woman with a spontaneous hyphema.* The patient awoke with pain and blurring of vision in her right eye. The source of the blood was not evident, but the clot was attached to the lens. No treatment was instituted, and 3 days later the clot had absorbed.

blurring of the vision in her right eye. She had no history of high blood pressure, diabetes, glaucoma, bleeding tendencies, or of being easily bruised. She had been seen 11 years previously for a red watery eye, which cleared in 1 week with no medications.

Findings. The visual acuity in both eyes is 20/30 with correction. The intraocular tension by Schiøtz tonometry is 14 mm. Hg in the right eye and 16 mm. Hg in the left. The conjunctiva of the right eye is slightly injected. Through a clear cornea a pendulous clot of blood is seen protruding inferiorly into the anterior chamber attached only to the lens near the inferior pupillary border (Fig. 44). Slit-lamp biomicroscopy reveals a few red blood cells but no flare in the anterior chamber. There are no signs of dilated iris vessels. Both pupils are equal and react briskly to light directly and consensually. There is a moderate senile nuclear sclerosis of the lens, and the posterior segment is normal.

FIG. 44

Course. With the patient receiving no therapy, the clot had resolved when she was next seen 3 days later. Over the next 3 years the patient was asymptomatic, and no systemic cause of her hyphema was discovered. The patient was subsequently lost to follow-up.

CORNEAL TRAUMA WITH ANTERIOR CHAMBER INVOLVEMENT

Probably the most common consequence of a corneal contusion is rupture or tear of Descemet's membrane. In newborn infants Descemet's membrane seems particularly susceptible, since ruptures from forceps injuries during delivery are by far the most commonly seen. The immediate picture, which may be confused with congenital glaucoma, is that of corneal edema due to infiltration of the stroma with aqueous. However, usually other evidence of forceps injury about the face indicates the source of the corneal problem. Ruptures in Descemet's membrane following forceps injuries gradually heal, with proliferation of endothelium and the formation of a new membrane across the defect. The typical finding is that of doubly refractile linear streaks, but occasionally an entire piece of Descemet's membrane may be detached from the cornea except at its two ends. In the latter situation, proliferation of endothelium and Descemet's membrane fills in the denuded portion of the posterior surface of the cornea. Thus the patient finally has a double Descemet's membrane in the traumatized region.

Proliferation of endothelium and Descemet's membrane surrounding a strand of vitreous attached to the cornea results in a so-called Descemet's membrane tube. Although this is more commonly seen in patients who have had needling operations for congenital cataracts, perforating corneal injuries can also produce the same structure. It is more commonly seen in perforating injuries sustained in childhood. It has a glassy appearance and extends from the corneal wound toward the pupillary area, with obvious proliferation of Descemet's membrane over a period of many years.

Following large corneal lacerations, one of the most serious problems is adhesion of the iris to the corneal wound, a condition known as adherent leukoma. As organization and fibrosis occurs in the healing process, the iris tissue is engulfed in the corneal wound. In many cases it is almost impossible to avoid this, and the results are loss of the pupillary opening and iris atrophy.

Formation of a corneal cyst may be associated with trauma, usually of severe degree. It is a rare occurrence. The posterior wall of a cyst may project into the anterior chamber, requiring treatment if the angle is compromised or the vision impaired.

Descemet's membrane in anterior chamber

History. At birth this 45-year-old woman was delivered by forceps, which is said to have damaged the right eye; it has been poor ever since. Two weeks ago she noted a total blacking out of her right eye and was found to have a retinal detachment.

Findings. The vision in the right eye is counting fingers at 2 feet and in the left 20/40 with a high myopic correction. Centrally the right cornea is diffusely hazy. The endothelium appears intact. There is a bridge of refractile material about 3 mm. wide attached near the limbus above and below, but reaching backward so that at midcornea it is about 2 mm. posterior to its endothelial surface REEL VI-6 (Reel VI-6). The pupil is dilated due to mydriatics, and there is a total retinal detachment with a large horseshoe tear in the superior nasal quadrant. Vision in the left eye is 20/50 with correction, and except for myopic crescents the fundus is normal in all respects.

Course. A scleral buckling procedure was performed on the right eye, but massive vitreous retraction developed postoperatively, and further surgery was considered inadvisable. Lattice degeneration of the other retina without any change was observed over a period of 2 years.

Descemet's membrane tube

History. About 15 years ago a nail struck this 58-year-old man's left eye, perforating the cornea. Subsequently his vision gradually decreased. He recently has developed severe hypertension.

Findings. The vision in the right eye is 20/20 and in the left 20/50 with correction. In the right eye there is no abnormality except that of hypertensive and arteriosclerotic retinopathy. In the left eye there is an opacity of the cornea near the limbus at the 6 o'clock position. The anterior chamber is of normal depth. The pupil is pear shaped as a result of a glassy tubular structure that curves around the inferior edge of the pupil and extends up to the corneal scar. Granular brown pigmentation is distributed on the anterior lens capsule, and there are diffuse cortical changes in the lens. Fundus examination is impossible due to the lens opacities. By gonioscopy the tube can be easily visualized inserting onto the posterior surface of the cornea (Reel VI-7). Beyond it in the angle REEL VI-7 can be seen a small pillar synechia, apparently of traumatic origin. The trabecular meshwork is covered with a moderate amount of irregular pigmentation. Intraocular tension is 18 mm. Hg (Schiøtz) in the right eye and 30 mm. Hg (Schiøtz) in the left. Central and peripheral fields are normal.

Course. The patient was treated for chronic open angle glaucoma in the left eye with pilocarpine (2%) drops 4 times a day, with good control of his intraocular pressure.

Traumatic adherent leukoma

History. Two years ago this 9-year-old boy was struck in the left eye by a stone and sustained a Y-shaped laceration extending across the entire cornea. The anterior chamber was filled with blood, and the lens could not be visualized. The cornea was successfully sutured, but a dense pupillary membrane developed, and the iris became adherent to the cornea. Large blood vessels invaded the corneal scar, and the pupillary membrane became vascularized. A month later an extensive iridectomy was done, and the adhesions to the pupillary membrane were severed. Despite topical and systemic corticosteroids and mydriatics another pupillary membrane formed, and his intraocular tension decreased to 4 mm. Hg as revealed by applanation tonometry. The eye remained soft, and the anterior chamber became progressively shallower. The remaining iris tissue became markedly atrophic.

Findings. Vision in the right eye is 20/15 and in the left light perception. The right eye is normal. In the left eye the cornea is flattened, and an extensive scar runs vertically across the central portion, with large blood vessels feeding into it from the limbal region (Fig. 45). There is an early band keratopathy extending FIG. 45 across the central portion of the cornea. The anterior chamber is shallowed, par-

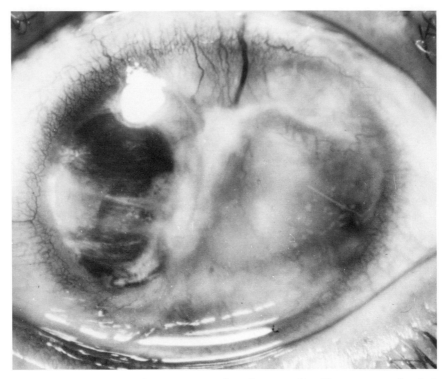

Fig. 45. *Extensive corneal scarring and iridocorneal adhesions in the left eye of a 9-year-old boy with a traumatic adherent leukoma.* The patient was struck in the eye with a stone 2 years ago, resulting in an extensive corneal laceration and disorganization of the anterior segment of the eye. Despite extensive medical and surgical treatment, a pupillary membrane formed with multiple synechias to the wound, and the eye became phthisical.

ticularly temporally, and the chamber is obliterated centrally by the adherent leukoma. Nasally an area of atrophic iris remains, but no red reflex can be obtained through this area.

Course. Over the next 5 years there was a progressive shallowing of the anterior chamber, with shrinkage and opacification of the cornea. Finally, the left eye became phthisical and blind.

Corneal cyst extending into anterior chamber

History. Four years ago this 12-year-old boy was struck in the right eye by a green apple. He developed a total hyphema with secondary glaucoma, which required irrigation of the anterior chamber. Postoperatively the eye was soft, and the angle of the anterior chamber was noted to be closed. About 6 months later he sustained another injury to the eye. This resulted in recurrent hyphema and secondary glaucoma, which were treated with bed rest and medical therapy. About a year ago a conjunctival limbal cyst was noted superiorly, which progressively became larger until 1 month ago, when multiple cysts were found, including a large cyst of the cornea.

Findings. The vision in the right eye is 20/400 and in the left 20/20. In the right eye there is a large multiloculated cyst of the conjunctiva superiorly, with the appearance of a direct extension into an intracorneal cyst involving the upper nasal quadrant of the cornea (Reel VII-1). The cyst is situated about mid- REEL VII-1 way in the corneal stroma, leaving anterior and posterior walls of about equal thickness. In the inferior portion of the cyst is a collection of grayish amorphous sediment. The remainder of the cornea and anterior chamber is clear, but the lateral and inferior portions of the iris show marked atrophy, being blue in contrast with the normal brown of the remaining iris. The lens contains anterior and posterior subcapsular opacities and some cortical changes. Fundus examination is normal. The left eye is normal in all respects. Intraocular tension is 23 mm. Hg (Schiøtz) in the right eye and 20 mm. Hg (Schiøtz) in the left.

Course. Aspiration of the corneal cyst and a partial excision of the conjunctival cyst were carried out. During the procedure it became clear that the two cysts communicated. Postoperatively the corneal cyst did not recur, and the intraocular tension remained normal with the use of topical epinephrine drops. When the patient was last seen 5 years postoperatively, his vision had remained the same and cyst had not recurred.

Chapter 4

Medical and surgical iatrogenic conditions involving the anterior chamber

EPITHELIALIZATION OF THE ANTERIOR CHAMBER (EPITHELIAL DOWNGROWTH)

The presence of a white membrane on the posterior surface of the cornea in a hypotonic eye with a fistula characterizes epithelialization of the anterior chamber (epithelial downgrowth). Its occurrence is most common after a cataract extraction, but it may follow other operative procedures or trauma. Corneal epithelial proliferation through a wound tract or an area of faulty closure results in the extension of epithelium into the anterior chamber. Corneal epithelium regenerates rapidly and intensively and can creep through a wound into the anterior chamber where it grows as a sheet of white tissue. It usually first appears on the posterior surface of the cornea but later on the iris, the vitreous face, and the iridocorneal angle as well. In the early stages the eye is usually soft, with a wound leak; but later when the draining fistula is closed by epithelium or synechias, a severe intractable glaucoma develops. Symptoms of epithelial downgrowth can occur any time from a few weeks to many years. The thin, veillike membrane on the upper portion of the cornea spreading downward has a thickened advancing edge frequently with beadlike prominences along it. As the condition advances, the iris, vitreous, and iridocorneal angle become involved. The vision becomes reduced, not only due to the membrane over the pupillary area, but to the corneal edema that is always present over the area of epithelialization.

Sometimes the first sign of epithelialization is the presence of an irritated eye with a low-grade iritis, a very frequent finding. Later the membrane becomes vascularized; and as it advances, corneal edema and intractable glaucoma develop from involvement of the filtering meshwork. Occasionally the eye remains hypotonic if the fistula persists, and eventually the eye becomes phthisical.

The most important aspect of treatment is prophylaxis, since technical errors at the time of surgery account for the vast majority of cases. Recent advances in surgical materials, instrumentation, and technique will certainly decrease the incidence. In one series 16% of all eyes enucleated following cataract extraction showed epithelialization of the anterior chamber; often the condition had not been diagnosed before enucleation. An increased awareness of the various diagnostic features of the condition should lead to an earlier diagnosis and a better prognosis. A number of techniques, including curetting or performing a penetrating keratoplasty of the involved cornea, employing cryotherapy photocoagulation, cauterizing the involved areas, and excising the iris, have been used to eliminate the epithelium in the anterior chamber. Recently, a technique combining cryoprobe freezing of the involved posterior corneal surface, extensive excision of the affected iris, removal of the vitreous face, and excision of the fistula has resulted in success in more than one fourth of the cases.

Epithelialization of anterior chamber

History. Four months ago this 59-year-old man underwent an intracapsular cataract extraction with three Kirby sutures of 6-0 silk, with no conjunctival flap. Nine days after the operation two of the sutures had already fallen out, and the third was removed 2 days later, but the anterior chamber remained formed. The eye continued to be irritable, and cornea striae persisted. At 3 weeks, when the patient had vision of 20/40 with a pinhole, there was a small area of whitish membrane on the endothelial surface at the 2 o'clock position. Corticosteroid and atropine drops were given, but irritability and redness persisted. Three months after the operation there was obvious epithelial downgrowth on the vitreous face as well as on the cornea.

Findings. The right eye is apparently normal, but the left has marked conjunctival injection. The cornea is clear except for a whitish membrane, which extends halfway down on the endothelium and has a thickened, irregular border from the 10 o'clock to the 3 o'clock position (Reel VII-2). Superiorly there is deep peripheral vascularization of the cornea. The anterior chamber contains moderate cells and flare, and on the vitreous face is a dense, white membrane except for a 2-mm. area temporally. A white band of tissue extends from the vitreous face up to and through the limbal region at the 1 o'clock position to lie on the surface of the conjunctiva. REEL VII-2

Course. A tab of white tissue at the limbus was excised. A persistent fistulous tract acted as a safety valve against an increased intraocular pressure. The eye continued to be irritable, and a month later the anterior chamber was found to be full of heavy white exudate. Enucleation was performed, and the histopathologic findings were a purulent endophthalmitis and epithelialization of the anterior chamber.

Epithelialization of anterior chamber

History. Three years ago this 68-year-old man had an intracapsular cataract extraction performed on the left eye. Five months later a gray area was noted on the cornea. This subsequently developed into a clearly defined picture of epithelialization of the anterior chamber. A radical operation to remove the epithelium was anticipated, but further examination showed a large hole and detachment of the retina. This was surgically reattached; but shortly thereafter another hole developed, and this led to total detachment and loss of light perception. Enucleation was performed 2 months later. A month ago because of failing vision, an intracapsular cataract extraction was performed on the right eye. The postoperative course was uneventful, but about 3 weeks later the patient developed an iritis. A week ago he complained of blurred vision, and epithelialization of the anterior chamber was noted.

Findings. The vision in the right eye is 20/100, and the left eye is anophthalmic. The right eye is moderately injected. However, the cornea is clear except for an area extending from the 10:30 to the 1 o'clock position that has a hazy membranous appearance and a thickened beaded anterior edge (Fig. 46). A positive Sidell test shows a leak at the limbus at the 12 o'clock position. Superficial vessels invade the cornea in this region. There are minimal cells

FIG. 46

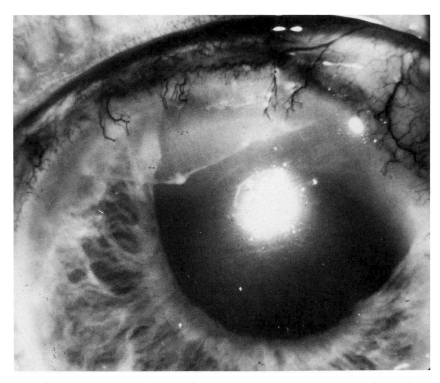

Fig. 46. *A hazy membrane superiorly on the posterior surface of the right cornea in a 68-year-old man with epithelialization of the anterior chamber.* An area of whitish material extends downward from the superior limbus and has a thickened beaded anterior edge. One month ago the patient had a cataract extraction, and a week ago the vision became blurred. Subsequently, the epithelium was excised from the cornea and an iridectomy performed. Five years later there was no recurrence.

and a trace of flare in the anterior chamber. The vitreous face is intact at the level of the pupil. The fundus shows some peripapillary choroidal atrophy and myopic changes.

Course. Over the period of the next week it appeared that there was some increase in the epithelialization of the cornea, so an excision of the epithelial tissue of the anterior chamber and iridectomy were performed. The postoperative course was uneventful, and 2 months later vision of 20/40 was obtained with an aphakic correction. Over a period of the next few years there was some development of edema of the upper portion of the cornea and resultant loss of vision. In addition, it appeared that the retina had developed further myopic degeneration; finally, 5 years later the vision was reduced to 20/400, but there were no signs of recurrence of the epithelialization.

Epithelialization of anterior chamber

History. Three years ago this 52-year-old woman had an uneventful intracapsular cataract extraction in the left eye. Three chromic catgut sutures were used for closure of the wound. When the patient was discharged, her vision was 20/20 with correction. The postoperative course was uneventful until the first outpatient visit, when a shallow anterior chamber and a choroidal detachment were observed. However, the anterior chamber re-formed without treatment. Because the vision was good in the right eye she did not use an aphakic correction, and her first untoward symptoms were a foreign body sensation associated with photophobia and tearing beginning about 3 months ago.

Findings. Vision in the right eye is 20/20 and in the left counting fingers at 4 feet. In the left eye there is moderate conjunctival injection, and the cornea is diffusely edematous superiorly. There is epithelial bedewing and one area of epithelial loss at the 12 o'clock position near the limbus (Fig. 47, A). FIG. 47 Extending almost halfway down on the posterior surface of the cornea is a membrane that has a thickened lower border. This membrane can be seen extending down onto the vitreous face as well. The complete coloboma superiorly is distorted, and laterally a grayish membrane can be seen extending onto it. Gonioscopy shows that the iris pillars are pulled laterally, and the membrane can be seen sweeping over the superior angle structures onto the vitreous face and iris. About 4 hours of the clock inferiorly are uninvolved. No leak of the wound area can be demonstrated. Only a hazy view of the fundus can be obtained. The right eye is normal, with a clear media and normal fundus. Intraocular pressure as revealed by applanation tonometry is 19 mm. Hg in the right eye and 28 mm. Hg in the left.

Course. An anterior chamber tap revealed typical epithelial cells (Fig. 47, B). A radical operative procedure was carried out in which the retrocorneal membrane was curetted, the iridectomy was enlarged, and the angles were curetted. Immediately postoperatively the eye did well, but in 2 months there was evidence of further epithelialization and fibrovascular membrane formation. A year later there was no remaining anterior chamber, and the eye was painful and blind. Enucleation was performed. Histopathologic examination showed the anterior chamber to be lined by epithelial cells that had in some places caused a dense adherence of the cornea to the iris (Fig. 47, C).

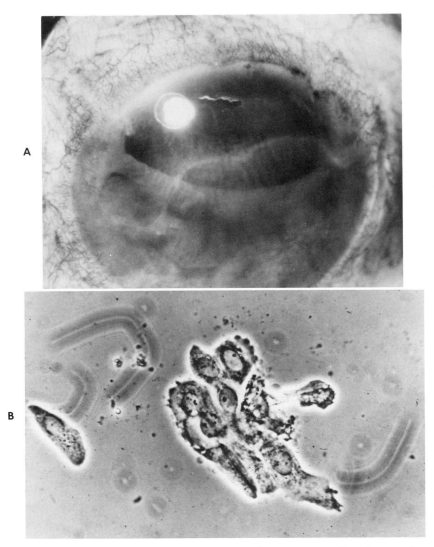

Fig. 47. *Extensive membrane formation in the anterior chamber and corneal edema in the right eye of a 52-year-old woman with epithelialization of the anterior chamber.* **A,** Whitish membranes extend halfway down on the posterior surface of the cornea and onto the vitreous face and iris. At the 12 o'clock position there is epithelial loss near the limbus, and the superior cornea is diffusely edematous. Three years ago the patient had an uneventful intracapsular cataract extraction, and 3 months ago she developed photophobia and tearing. **B,** Typical epithelial cells are seen in the aqueous removed by anterior chamber tap. (No stain, ×1600.) Despite a radical operative procedure to remove the epithelium from the anterior chamber, there was recurrence, and an enucleation was performed. **C,** Histopathologic examination shows the anterior chamber to be lined with epithelial cells, with a dense adherence of cornea to iris. (H & E stain; ×400.)

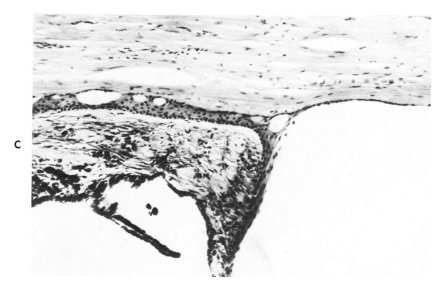

c

Fig. 47, cont'd. For legend see opposite page.

DESCEMET'S MEMBRANE IN ANTERIOR CHAMBER

During a surgical procedure Descemet's membrane can be caught in the process of instrumentation, causing a tear or detachment of the membrane from the posterior surface of the cornea. This may result in a piece of the membrane hanging from the cornea or occasionally in one that is totally free and lying in the anterior chamber. One common mechanism causing it occurs when the tip of the scissors used to enlarge the wound inadvertently catches Descemet's membrane. Stripping of Descemet's membrane from the cornea also very commonly occurs in cyclodialysis procedure where the spatula used to dislodge the scleral spur is inserted between Descemet's membrane and the stroma. Although the immediate result may be edema of the cornea, generally the endothelium proliferates over the denuded area, apparently laying down new Descemet's membrane. Months later it may be impossible to tell where the defect occurred.

Occasionally during penetrating keratoplasty a portion of the host Descemet's membrane in the area of the trephination is advertently allowed to remain in the eye. If there is a total retention of the intact host Descemet's membrane, a complete double Descemet's membrane results, usually producing an edematous graft and necessitating a regraft. If there is only a partial retention of the host Descemet's membrane, the graft may remain clear and the result good.

So-called Descemet's membrane tubes occur as a result of proliferation of endothelium and Descemet's membrane around a strand of vitreous attached to the cornea, usually in patients who previously have had needling operations for congenital cataracts. Sometimes they occur following a perforating corneal injury. The condition is discussed in more detail in Chapter 3.

Medical and surgical iatrogenic conditions

Descemet's membrane in anterior chamber

History. About 4 years ago this 77-year-old woman underwent a cyclodialysis procedure in the left eye for glaucoma. Since then the tension has been within normal limits without the use of medications. There is a history of a possible operative procedure such as cyclodiathermy on the right eye about 10 years ago.

Findings. Vision in the right eye is light perception and in the left 20/100. The right eye shows a small nonreactive pupil, and gonioscopy reveals partially closed angles with trabecular synechias. The fundus cannot be visualized due to the small pupil that will not dilate. In the left eye the anterior chamber REEL VII-3 contains a curled-up piece of Descemet's membrane lying inferiorly (Reel VII-3). In addition, there is a piece of stripped off Descemet's membrane that is still attached to the cornea at the 4 o'clock position near the cyclodialysis cleft. The pupil is small and unreactive and will not dilate due to posterior syncehia formation at the pupillary margin. However, through the small pupil it is apparent that the patient has an immature cataract. The tension in the right eye is 16 mm. Hg (Schiøtz) and 18 mm. Hg (Schiøtz) in the left.

Course. Because of gradual diminution of vision in the left eye, an intracapsular cataract extraction was performed, and there were no complications. At the time of the patient's discharge, the procedure appeared to have a good result; the patient was then lost to follow-up.

Descemet's membrane in anterior chamber

History. Eighteen years ago this 48-year-old woman was found to have a markedly elevated intraocular pressure in the right eye, with extensive field changes and marked glaucomatous cupping. The diagnosis was chronic juvenile glaucoma in the right eye, and cyclodialysis was performed in an attempt to control the pressure. Two trephine procedures were also carried out, which brought the tension into the 30's; but the patient's vision remained very poor. Recently the tension in her left eye also became elevated.

Findings. Vision in the right eye is light perception and in the left 20/20 with correction. In the right eye the anterior chamber is fairly deep, and there are FIG. 48 two peripheral iridectomies superiorly (Fig. 48). Lying in the anterior chamber just below the iridectomy at the 10 o'clock position is a piece of glassy membrane that is rolled up, with the upper end lying against the iris. There are no indications in the cornea as to the site of origin of this piece of Descemet's membrane. The pupil is miotic, and a moderately advanced cataract makes the fundus examination impossible. Gonioscopy shows a number of peripheral anterior synechias in the region of the iridectomies and multiple synechias from the 6 o'clock to the 9 o'clock position, presumably the area of cyclodialysis. In the left eye the anterior chamber is of average depth, the iris normal, and the media clear. Fundus examination reveals a normal disc. Visual field examination is normal. The intraocular tension in the right eye is 39 mm. Hg and in the left 20 mm. Hg (Schiøtz).

Course. With medical treatment the intraocular pressure in the left eye was controlled, and when the patient was last seen at age 65 her vision in this eye was still 20/20 and the intraocular pressure in the left eye 20 mm. Hg (Schiøtz).

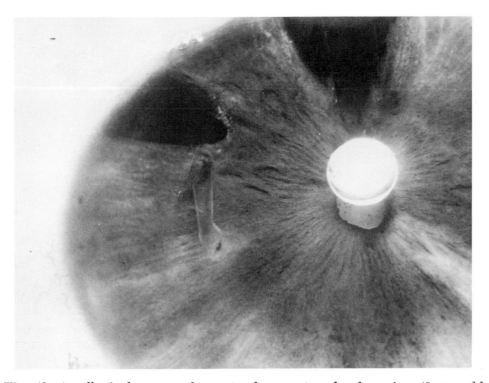

Fig. 48. *A roll of glassy membrane in the anterior chamber of a 48-year-old woman with Descemet's membrane in the anterior chamber.* Lying on the iris just below a peripheral iridectomy is a piece of Descemet's membrane entirely free from the cornea. The patient underwent a cyclodialysis and two trephine procedures for her glaucoma. Subsequently, the piece of Descemet's membrane was noted.

Retained host Descemet's membrane following keratoplasty

History. Since she was a teen-ager this 31-year-old woman was known to have lattice dystrophy. Her vision became markedly reduced in both eyes, and 18 months ago a penetrating keratoplasty was performed on her left eye. Eight months ago a penetrating keratoplasty was performed on the right eye, although this eye was amblyopic due to an esotropia in childhood. Her father and paternal uncle were known to have lattice dystrophy.

Findings. Vision in the right eye is 20/100 and in the left 20/30 without correction. In the right eye there is a 6.5-mm. penetrating graft that is compact and clear. Around the graft can be visualized irregular refractile lines in the corneal stroma, typical of lattice dystrophy. The remainder of the examination is negative. In the left eye there is a 7-mm. penetrating full-thickness graft, with a slight superficial haziness of the graft centrally. At the edge of the graft, particularly between the 7 and 10 o'clock positions there is some diffuse edema. Behind the nasal half of the graft is a wrinkled glassy membrane that attaches to the nasal edge of the graft but is otherwise floating free from it (Reel VII-4).   REEL VII-4
Again, around the graft can be seen refractile irregular lines in the corneal

stroma, typical of lattice dystrophy. The anterior chamber is deep, the pupil dilated due to mydriatics, and the media and posterior fundus are normal.

Course. During the next 6 months vision in the right eye remained at 20/100, and vision in the left became reduced to 20/60, although there was no change in the transparency of the graft.

Descemet's membrane tube

History. In childhood this 42-year-old man underwent needlings in both eyes for congenital cataracts. For about a month vision was poor in the right eye. The left eye was blind.

Findings. Vision in the right eye is 5/300 and in the left no light perception. In the right eye the cornea is clear except for two scars near the limbus at the 2 and 9 o'clock positions. Attached to these scars are tubular-appearing structures that extend approximately two thirds of the way across the anterior chamber to-

REEL VII-5 ward the vitreous face (Reel VII-5). Extending from the vitreous face is a strand of vitreous, which in each case is attached to the ends of the tubes, and the vitreous can then be seen extending into the tube. Remnants of the pre-existing congenital cataract are present in the temporal portion of the pupillary opening. Fundus examination shows a detached retina above and temporally. The left eye is phthisical.

Course. The patient had a scleral buckling procedure performed, but a month later the retina again detached and a second scleral buckle was done. Four months later the retina was still attached, and the vision was counting fingers at 4 feet. The patient was then lost to follow-up.

POSTOPERATIVE ANTERIOR CHAMBER FOREIGN BODIES

Blood, following surgery or from other causes, is probably the most common foreign body in the anterior chamber. Postoperative hyphema is common and relatively innocuous, particularly in cataract surgery. In glaucoma filtering procedures it may be more serious if sufficiently large to produce an inflammatory reaction within the filtering bleb. Massive postoperative hyphemas have essentially the same complications as those occurring with trauma; these are discussed in Chapter 3. However, there is a further complication due to the limited ability of the surgical wound to withstand the force exerted on it by a high intraocular pressure; therefore, lowering of the intraocular pressure cannot be delayed too long.

The ophthalmic surgeon may be responsible for leaving a foreign body in the anterior chamber, inadvertently or by design. Some foreign bodies, such as cotton fibers and pieces of cilia are minute and innocuous, while others may cause complications. Rubber particles inadvertently irrigated into the anterior chamber from a rubber irrigating bulb have been known to produce an iritis, and silicone fluid intended to be in the vitreous cavity can produce corneal edema if in the anterior chamber. As a rule, ointments with a petrolatum base are inert but may remain for many years in the anterior chamber. Water soluble ointments are absorbed rapidly with no reaction, except when in very large amounts, in which case a "violent iritis" may result. Talc powder and even starch particles from surgical gloves or disposable drapes give rise to a granulomatous reaction.

Undoubtedly the most controversial postoperative foreign body in the anterior chamber is the intraocular lens used following cataract extraction. Those surgeons employing the procedure are enthusiastic, while others feel that modification of such a satisfactory operation as cataract extraction is not indicated. Although Ridley first attempted to use his artificial lens (pseudophakos) more than 30 years ago, not until recently has the procedure been used rather extensively, with the development of the iris fixation type of artificial lens. The currently employed lenses have a smaller bulk and superior resistance to physical or chemical degradation within the anterior chamber, which also contributes to a greater rate of success. The procedure is used with both the intracapsular and extracapsular extractions, and both have their advantages and disadvantages. The lenses are generally placed in the eye immediately following the cataract extraction, in the same operative procedure or, less frequently, after an interval. The haptic portion of the lens is supported chiefly by the iris, although the hyaloid face in the intracapsular technic and the posterior capsule of the lens in the extracapsular technic also offer some support. The optical portion of the lens is generally made of polymethylmethacrylate, and the haptic portion consists of loops made of various materials. Apparently, when the lens is used with the extracapsular procedure, there is less likelihood of dislocation of the lens, but the occurrence of a secondary cataract requires a needling procedure in a number of cases. One group reports excellent results in extracapsular extractions for congenital cataracts. When the lens is used with the intracapsular procedure, most of the patients are placed on a regimen of miotics to avoid dislocation of the lens should the pupil dilate. When dislocation does occur, it is apparently a minor complication, and in most instances the lens can be replaced with a minimum of difficulty by manual manipulation or needling. More serious complications may require removal of the lens; this was necessary in 6% of the patients in one series. The most common complication is recurrent iritis, which may be associated with glaucoma and hypopyon. In the majority of cases this condition can be controlled with topical corticosteroids. With the advent of the iris fixation lens, such as the Binkhorst iris clip lens and the iris plane lens (Copeland), persistent postoperative corneal edema is almost nonexistent. Apparently, cystic macular edema is no more common than in the ordinary cataract extraction, and there is reason to believe that retinal detachments are less common than those following ordinary cataract extraction. The advantages of pseudophakia are an image size that closely approximates the phakic eye, with a minimal refractive error following surgery. The field is of normal size. Some lenses have been in situ for up to 10 years, and a large number up to 5 years, and late complications are surprisingly rare. One group who use the intracapsular procedure restrict the use of the implant to patients over 70 years of age and limit the use of the implant in the second eye if a 4- to 5-year successful interval has elapsed since the lens was implanted in the first eye. Several groups have made unusually careful long-term follow-up studies, which indicates that the use of the pseudophakos is relatively safe and has distinct advantages.

Postoperative hyphema

History. A few months ago this 35-year-old woman noted blurring of vision, which caused her to go to an ophthalmologist. Although her vision was only slightly reduced, she had markedly elevated intraocular tension and extensive field loss in both eyes. Medical therapy was unsuccessful in reducing her tensions appreciably, so 1 month ago an iridencleisis and anterior sclerectomy were performed on the right eye. A week later the same procedures were carried out on the left eye. In another week the tension had already reached its previous levels, so a transfixion of the nonfiltering bleb in the right eye was performed. There was a postoperative hyphema with more than half the anterior chamber filled with blood. Because the tension remained elevated in the left eye and because of the shallow anterior chamber, a posterior sclerotomy and re-formation of the anterior chamber with air were performed.

Findings. Both eyes show elevated, thickened blebs superiorly and surgical colobomas. The right eye contains a hyphema that extends almost to the lower FIG. 49 edge of the pupil (Fig 49). In the left eye the chamber is shallow, and there is a small air bubble present. Tension is 21 mm. Hg (Schiøtz) in the right eye and 46 mm. Hg (Schiøtz) in the left eye.

Course. A week later a cyclodialysis was performed in the left eye because of persistently elevated intraocular tension. Subsequently, the tensions in both eyes remained well controlled with medical therapy. A mature cataract de-

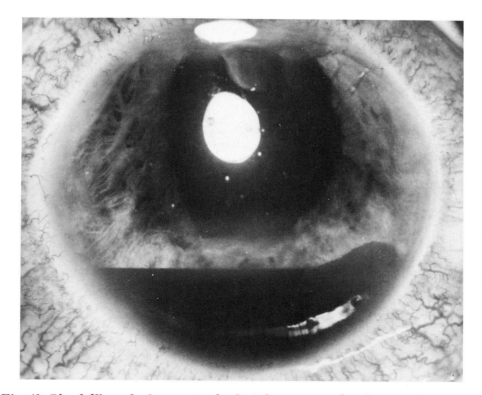

Fig. 49. *Blood filling the lower one third of the anterior chamber in a 35-year-old woman with a postoperative hyphema.* Superiorly there is a thickened bleb, and there is a surgical coloboma of the iris. A month ago the patient underwent an iridencleisis and anterior sclerectomy, and 2 weeks later she had a transfixion of a nonfiltering bleb. This was followed by bleeding into the anterior chamber, which subsequently cleared; but further surgery was required for the glaucoma.

veloped in the right eye 4 years later, and a planned extracapsular cataract extraction was performed. Postoperatively, a pupillary membrane developed, and the tension was frequently elevated into the 30's and 40's. Because the vision was only hand movements, no further therapy was attempted on this eye. Ten years later a cataract extraction was performed on the left eye. Following extraction, the best corrected vision at that time was 20/200, with an intraocular pressure of 12 mm. Hg (Schiøtz).

Rubber particles in anterior chamber

History. About a month ago this 67-year-old man had an unplanned extracapsular cataract extraction performed on the left eye. Two days postoperatively he had severe pain, and within another day total hyphema developed, with a markedly elevated intraocular tension. A small portion of the wound was opened, and gentle irrigation was performed to remove some of the blood from the anterior chamber. There was gradual absorption of the residual blood; when the patient was discharged a week later, the anterior chamber was almost clear with no signs of recurrent bleeding. There was continued clearing of the anterior chamber so that by a month later there were no signs of bleeding. However, there was some foreign bodies noted in the anterior chamber of the surface of the iris.

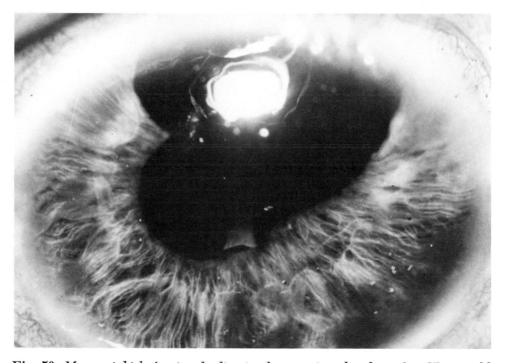

Fig. 50. *Many pinkish foreign bodies in the anterior chamber of a 67-year-old man with rubber particles in the anterior chamber.* Following a cataract extraction a total hyphema developed, which required irrigation of the anterior chamber. As the residual blood absorbed, rubber particles (presumably from the rubber irrigating bulb) were visible on the iris. They caused no reaction.

Findings. Vision in the right eye is 20/50 and in the left 20/20 with aphakic correction. In the right eye the anterior segment is normal, but the lens shows lenticular opacities, both spokes and water clefts. The posterior segment is normal. In the left eye the anterior cornea is normal and the anterior chamber clear. There is a large surgical coloboma, and lying on the iris and extending into the anterior chamber are twenty or more pinkish foreign bodies that seem to be causing no reaction (Fig. 50). There are few foreign bodies on the intact vitreous face just above the pupillary opening. The vitreous is clear and the fundus normal. The intraocular tension in both eyes is normal.

FIG. 50

Course. The patient was lost to follow-up.

Silicone bubble in anterior chamber

History. This 63-year-old man had cataract extractions performed in both eyes 3 years ago. Six months later a retinal detachment developed in the right eye, and two scleral buckling procedures were performed unsuccessfully. The eye became blind. Three months ago the left eye, which had had 20/25 vision, developed a retinal detachment, and this was successfully operated by a scleral buckling procedure. A week ago a redetachment occurred due to a massive vitreous re-

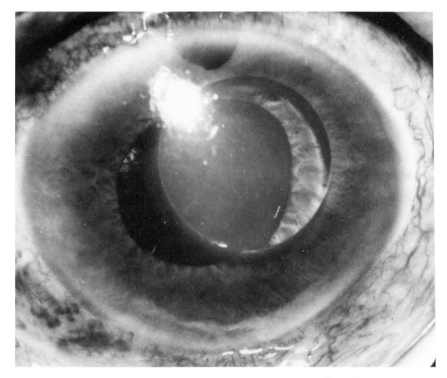

Fig. 51. *A large globule of silicone fluid in the anterior chamber of a 63-year-old man who had a silicone injection into the vitreous cavity.* Three months ago the patient had a retinal detachment repaired, but 1 week ago a redetachment occurred with massive vitreous retraction. Silicone fluid was injected into the vitreous cavity. Now a globule has appeared in the anterior chamber. Corneal edema is avoided by the patient's sleeping on his stomach.

traction, and a revision of the scleral buckle was done with injection of silicone in the vitreous cavity. Today silicone fluid was noted in the anterior chamber.

Findings. In the right eye there is a total retinal detachment. The left eye is markedly injected due to the recent operative procedure. The cornea is clear and the anterior chamber of normal depth. There is a peripheral iridectomy superiorly, and in the central portion of the anterior chamber involving most of the pupillary area is a large globule of silicone fluid (Fig. 51). Behind it is formed vitreous at the level of the pupil. Fundus examination shows the retina to be reattached. FIG. 51

Course. Although the retina remained reattached, the vision stayed at about counting fingers at 8 to 10 feet. No attempt was made to remove the silicone fluid from the anterior chamber, and it caused no apparent difficulty. Subsequently, the silicone implant used for the scleral buckle became exposed, and finally it was removed. A year later the retina was still attached, and vision remained the same. Two years later the retina was attached superiorly but detached inferiorly due to massive vitreous retraction. The vision was counting fingers at a few feet. The patient avoided corneal edema by sleeping on his stomach, which kept the silicone fluid from being in constant contact with the endothelium.

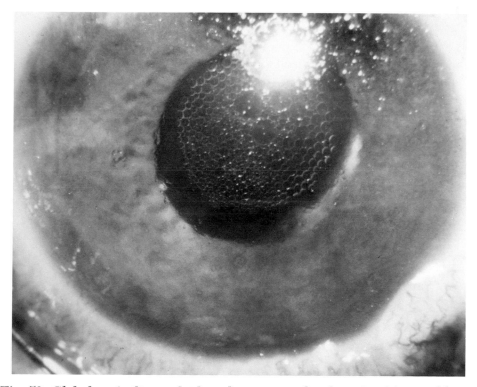

Fig. 52. *Globules of silicone fluid in the anterior chamber of a 24-year-old man with intravitreal silicone injection for recurrent retinal detachment.* A month ago the patient had a retinal detachment, which resulted in massive vitreous retraction following two operative procedures. Some of the silicone fluid injected in the vitreous cavity broke up into globules and appeared in the anterior chamber.

Silicone fluid in anterior chamber

History. This 24-year-old man had operations for bilateral congenital cataracts at age 7. Three years ago he developed a retinal detachment in the right eye, for which he had two operations. A month ago he developed a retinal detachment in the left eye, and he has had two operations, which resulted in a massive vitreous retraction. The subretinal fluid was released and intravitreal silicone fluid injection performed.

Findings. Vision in the right eye is questionable light perception and in the left hand movements at 2 to 3 feet. The entire retina in the right eye is detached and displaced superiorly. In the left eye the anterior chamber contains many small globules of silicone fluid, which collect at the apex of the cornea FIG. 52 when the patient is prone (Fig. 52). A large globule of silicone fluid fills the vitreous cavity. There is total retinal detachment, numerous vitreous attachments, and one hole somewhat posterior to the equator.

Course. A week later it was obvious that the preretinal vitreous band had been broken, and a retinal tear could be seen just behind the old buckle. Another scleral buckling was performed, resulting in reattachment of the posterior pole. The patient returned to the referring doctor and was lost to follow-up.

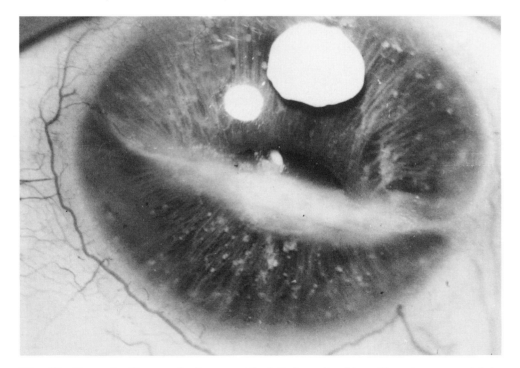

Fig. 53. *Central adherent leukoma and globules of white glistening material in the anterior chamber of a 46-year-old man who 9 years ago had an extensive laceration of his cornea.* Ointment was placed in the eye, and spontaneous healing occurred, with ointment remaining in the anterior chamber. The large globule superiorly moved freely but caused no reaction.

Ointment in anterior chamber

History. Nine years ago this 46-year-old man was struck in the left eye, breaking his glasses and severely lacerating his cornea. At the hospital he refused admission but did allow atropine drops and mercury bichloride (1:3,000) ointment with a petrolatum base to be placed in his eye and a dressing to be applied. When he was seen again 2 days later, it was found that the laceration had spontaneously healed and that globular masses of white material were trapped in the anterior chamber. Three weeks later some of these globules had coalesced into one large globule superiorly. Six months later there was no appreciable change in the appearance of the ointment in the anterior chamber, and the eye showed no reaction. With an aphakic correction and pinhole the vision was 20/40. He was then lost to follow-up until today.

Findings. Vision in the right eye is 20/30 and in the left hand movements only. The right eye is normal. The cornea of the left eye has an adherent leukoma that starts at the 10 o'clock position and extends to the 3:30 position (Fig. 53). About half of the pupillary opening is obstructed by the scar. The  FIG. 53 anterior chamber is shallow, and superiorly there is a large globule of white glistening material. Elsewhere there are numerous small globules of similar-

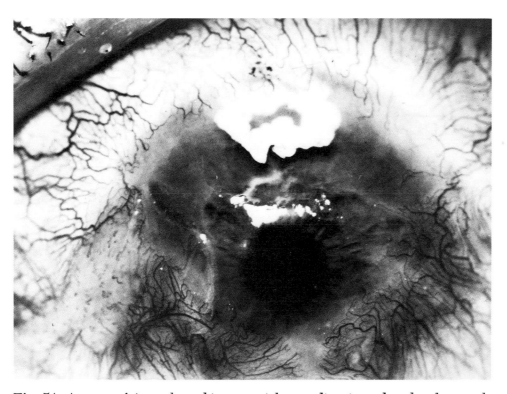

Fig. 54. *A mass of irregular white material extending into the chamber angle superiorly in a 66-year-old man with ointment in the anterior chamber.* During an excision of the recurrent carcinoma in situ, perforation of the limbal region occurred superiorly. Antibiotic ointment was used at the end of the operation and subsequently was found in the anterior chamber. Gradually, it broke up into several pieces and partially disappeared.

appearing material caught in the anterior iris stroma. The remaining pupillary area is aphakic, and there is one white globule against the vitreous face. With movement of the head the large globule at the 12 o'clock position moves freely from side to side.

Course. In a week the patient was again seen, and it was decided that no surgical treatment was indicated.

Ointment in anterior chamber (postoperatively)

History. Two years ago this 66-year-old man had a foreign body removed from his left eye, at which time a growth was noted on the eyeball. Two months later this tumor was excised and was found to be a carcinoma in situ. Within the next year the tumor recurred three more times, and each time an attempt was made at total excision. A week ago the third recurrence was excised, and during the procedure the anterior chamber was inadvertently entered at the 12 o'clock position. Routinely, antibiotic ointment was placed in the eye at the termination of the operation. The anterior chamber re-formed spontaneously, but a white mass of irregular material was noted in the superior portion of the anterior chamber.

Findings. The vision in both eyes is about 20/50, although determination of the exact vision is difficult due to a language barrier. The right eye is normal, but the left is moderately injected, with the peripheral cornea superficially vascularized. In the superior angle is a mass of irregular white material, which disappears under the limbus (Fig. 54). The anterior chamber is of normal depth. The posterior segment is normal.

FIG. 54

Course. During the next month the foreign material in the anterior chamber broke up into several pieces, and some disappeared. Because surgical intervention was thought to be contraindicated due to thinning of the cornea, x-radiation (60 kv.) was given despite the risk of producing a radiation cataract. At first there was a marked iritis with posterior synechia formation, but 3 months later the eye was white and there seemed to be a complete resolution of the residual tumor tissue. The patient was then lost to follow-up.

Anterior chamber implant in albino

History. Two years ago this 13-year-old albino girl had an anterior chamber implants placed in both eyes. There was slight improvement in the visual acuity, and she had no difficulty until 3 weeks ago, when she was accidentally struck in the right eye and was found to have a hyphema. During the next 3 weeks she continued to bleed, and intraocular tension remained in the 30's and 40's despite medical treatment with acetazolamide and Premarin. Yesterday the anterior chamber was entirely free of blood, but last night there was again fresh bleeding.

Findings. The vision in the right eye is hand movements and in the left is 20/200. In the right eye there is a 2-mm. hyphema, and the upper portion of a light blue plastic implant can be visualized. The remainder of the eye is difficult to see due to the blood in the anterior chamber. The tension is 30 mm. Hg (Schiøtz). In the anterior chamber of the left eye is a light blue-colored plastic implant, which extends across the anterior chamber into the angles at the 3 and 9 o'clock positions (Fig. 55). Centrally there is a round opening corre-

FIG. 55

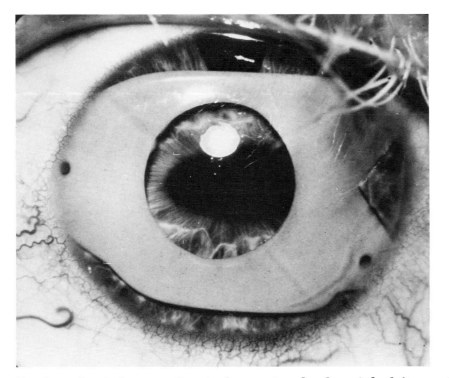

Fig. 55. *Blue-colored plastic implant in the anterior chamber of the left eye of a 13-year-old albino girl.* Two years ago this patient had anterior chamber implants placed in both eyes. Following trauma to the right eye, she developed recurrent bleeding, and the implant was removed. Only slight improvement of vision resulted from the use of the implants.

sponding to a normal pupil, but the pupil is elongated. Superiorly there is also a peripheral iridectomy.

Course. The implant was removed from the right eye, and postoperatively the anterior chamber remained deep and clear with no further bleeding. The patient was then lost to follow-up.

Intraocular lens (pseudophakos)

History. Four months ago this 80-year-old man had an extraction of a mature cataract in his left eye, with insertion of a Federov iris-clip lens. The postoperative course was uneventful.

Findings. Vision in the right eye is 20/40 and in the left 20/20 with a −1.00 sphere. Except for arcus senilis, the cornea is clear and the anterior chamber deep. There are two peripheral iridectomies superiorly. On the surface of the iris is a convex plastic lens; around the periphery of this lens are three rodlike projections, on the posterior surface of which there are six points that extend through the pupillary opening (Fig. 56). These points cause the pupil to have a FIG. 56 hexagonal shape.

Course. The patient was followed for 2 years and there was no change in his vision.

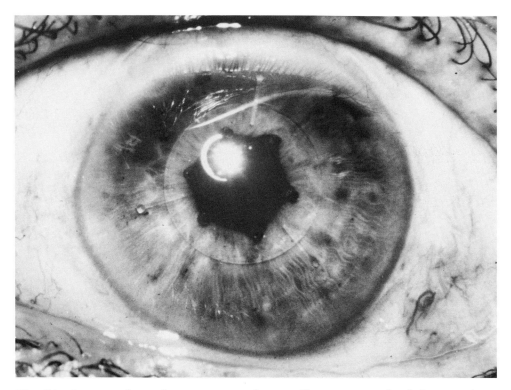

Fig. 56. *Convex plastic lens covering the pupillary area in the left eye of an 80-year-old man with an intraocular lens (pseudophakos). Four months ago the patient had a mature cataract extracted and a Federov iris-chip lens inserted. The vision with correction is 20/20, and the pupil is hexagonal in shape due to the six points of the lens.*

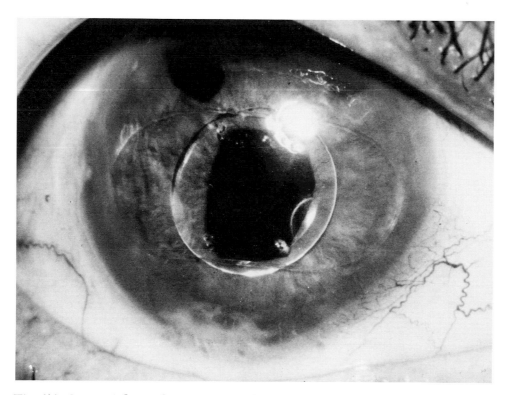

Fig. 57. *Convex plastic lens covering the pupillary area in the right eye of a 74-year-old woman with an intraocular lens (pseudophakos).* Following a cataract extraction 3 years ago the patient had a Binkhorst iris-clip lens inserted. Two loops of fine plastic wire extend almost to the angles at the 3 o'clock and 9 o'clock positions. The resulting vision was 20/40.

Intraocular lens (pseudophakos)

History. Three years ago this 74-year-old woman had a cataract extraction performed on a mature cataract in the right eye. A Binkhorst iris-clip lens was inserted, and the postoperative course was uneventful.

Findings. Vision in the right eye is 20/40 and in the left 20/50. In the right eye the cornea is clear except for an opacity caused by a peripheral anterior synechia at the 6 o'clock position. The anterior chamber is of normal depth, and there are two large peripheral iridectomies superiorly. Over the pupillary area and lying on the anterior surface of the iris is a convex plastic lens from which extend a pair of clips composed of fine plastic wire reaching almost to the angle at the 3 and 9 o'clock positions (Fig. 57). Four small plastic projections FIG. 57 from the back side of the lens extend through the pupil and cause the pupil to have a square shape.

Course. The patient was followed for a period of 5 years; good vision was maintained, and there were no complications.

Bibliography for part one

Alkemade, P. P. H.: Dysgenesis mesodermalis of the iris and the cornea, Assen, Netherlands, 1969, Royal Van Gorcum Ltd.

Ashton, N., Shakib, M., Collyer, R., and Blach, R.: Electron microscopic study of pseudo-exfoliation of the lens capsule, Invest. Ophthal. 4:141-161, Apr. 1965.

Becker, B., and Shaffer, R. N.: Diagnosis and therapy of the glaucomas, St. Louis, 1965, The C. V. Mosby Co.

Binkhorst, C. D.: Power of the prepupillary pseudophakos, Brit. J. Ophthal. 56:332-337, Apr. 1972.

Binkhorst, C. D., Kats, A., and Leonard, P. A. M.: Extracapsular pseudophobia, Amer. J. Ophthal. 73:625-635, May 1972.

Chandler, P. A., and Grant, W. M.: Lectures on glaucoma, Philadelphia, 1965, Lea & Febiger.

Chandler P. A., Simmons, R. J., and Grant, W. M.: Malignant glaucoma, medical and surgical treatment, Amer. J. Ophthal. 66:495-502, Sept. 1968.

Cogan, D. G., and Reese, A. B.: A syndrome of iris nodules, ectopic Descemet's membrane and unilateral glaucoma, Docum. Ophthal. 26:424-433, 1969.

deVeer, J. A.: Pathologic findings in cases of retained nonmetallic foreign bodies, Amer. J. Ophthal. 31:615, 1948.

Donaldson, D. D., and Smith T. R.: Descemet's membrane tubes, Trans. Amer. Ophthal. Soc. 64:89-109, 1967.

Duke-Elder, S.: System of ophthalmology. Vol. 8, Diseases of the outer eye; conjunctiva, cornea and sclera, St. Louis, 1965, The C. V. Mosby Co.

Duke-Elder, S., and McFaul, P. A., editors: System of ophthalmology. Vol. 14, Injuries. Part 1, Mechanical injuries, St. Louis, 1972, The C. V. Mosby Co.

Duke-Elder, S.: Textbook of ophthalmology. Vol. 6, Injuries, London, 1954, Henry Kimpton.

Gass, J. D.: Surgical excision of persistent hyperplastic primary vitreous, Arch. Ophthal. 83:163-168, Feb. 1970.

Giles, C. L., and Bromley, W. C.: Traumatic hyphema, a retrospective analysis from the University of Michigan teaching hospitals, J. Pediat. Ophthal. 9:90-94, May 1972.

Gorin, G., and Posner, A.: Slit-lamp gonioscopy, Baltimore, Md., 1961, The Williams & Wilkins Co.

Horven, I.: Exfoliation syndrome, Arch. Ophthal. 76:505-511, Oct. 1966.

Jaffe, N. S.: Current status of intraocular lenses, Eye Ear Nose Throat Monthly 51:290-296, Aug. 1972.

Jerndal, T.: Dominant goniodysgenesis with late congenital glaucoma, a re-examination of Berg's pedigree, Amer. J. Ophthal. 74:28-32, July 1972.

Joseph, N., Ivry, M., and Oliver, M.: Persistent hyperplastic primary vitreous at the optic nerve head, Amer. J. Ophthal. 73:580-583, Apr. 1972.

Laibson, P. R.: Inferior bullous keratopathy and unsuspected anterior chamber foreign body, Arch. Ophthal. **74**:191-197, Aug. 1965.

Levene, R. Z.: Glaucoma, Arch. Ophthal. **85**:227-251, Feb. 1971.

Levene, R. Z.: A new concept of malignant glaucoma, Arch. Ophthal. **87**:497-506, May 1972.

Lichter, P. R.: Iris processes in 340 eyes, Amer. J. Ophthal. **68**:872-878, Nov. 1969.

Lichter, P. R., and Shaffer, R. N.: Iris processes and glaucoma, Amer. J. Ophthal. **70**:905-911, Dec. 1970.

Mann, I.: Developmental abnormalities of the eye, Philadelphia, 1957, J. B. Lippincott Co.

Maumenee, A. E., Paton, D., Morse, P. H., and Butner, R.: Review of 40 histologically proven cases of epithelial downgrowth following cataract extraction and suggested surgical management, Amer. J. Ophthal. **69**:598-603, Apr. 1970.

McDonald P. R., and Ashadian, M. J.: Retained glass foreign bodies in the anterior chamber, Amer. J. Ophthal. **48**:747-750, Dec. 1959.

Pearce, J. L.: Long-term results of the Binkhorst iris clip lens in senile cataract, Brit. J. Ophthal. **56**:319-331, Apr. 1972.

Perkins, E. S.: Glaucoma in the younger age groups, Arch. Ophthal. **64**:882-891, Dec. 1960.

Pohjanpelta, P., and Hurskainen, L.: Studies on relatives of patients with glaucoma simplex and patients with pseudoexfoliation of the lens capsule, Acta Ophthal. **50**:255-261, 1972.

Rakusin, W.: Traumatic hyphema, Amer. J. Ophthal. **74**:284-292, Aug. 1972.

Rieser, J. C., and Schwartz, B.: Miotic-induced malignant glaucoma, Arch. Ophthal. **87**:707-712, June 1972.

Riise, D.: Congenital leucoma of the cornea (Peters's anomaly), Acta Ophthal. **42**:1063-1069, 1964.

Scheie, H. G., and Fleischhauer, H. W.: Idiopathic atrophy of the epithelial layers of the iris and ciliary body, Arch. Ophthal. **59**:216-227, Feb. 1958.

Scheie, H. G., and Yanoff, M.: Peters' anomaly and total posterior coloboma of retinal pigment epithelium and choroid, Arch. Ophthal. **87**:525-530, May 1972.

Sugar, H. S.: Pigmentary glaucoma, Amer. J. Ophthal. **62**:499-506, Sept. 1966.

Sugar, H. S., and Airala, M. A.: Introduction of some ophthalmic atropine ointments into the anterior chamber, Ann. Ophthal. **4**:367-374, May 1972.

Thorkilgaard, O., and Moestrup, B.: Contusion-angle deformity, its incidence and appearance, Acta Ophthal. **45**:51-56, 1967.

Weiss, D. I., and Shaffer, R. N.: Ciliary block (malignant) glaucoma, Trans. Amer. Acad. Ophthal. Otolaryng. **76**:450-461, Mar.-Apr. 1972.

Wolter, J. R.: The histopathology of Descemet's membrane tubes, J. Pediat. Ophthal. **9**(1):39-42, 1972.

Wolter, J. R., and Makley, T. A.: Cogan-Reese syndrome, J. Pediat. Ophthal. **9**(2):102-105, 1972.

Part two

IRIS

The function of the iris is that of a diaphragm within the image-forming portion of the eye. The diaphragm has a variable opening, the pupil, which is a circular aperture located slightly nasally and below the center of the optical axis of the eye. The aperture's size, or pupillary opening, varies with the amount of light impinging on the retina. Contraction of the pupil occurs not only with an increase in light but also in the act of accommodation for near focus. The smaller pupil increases the depth of focus of the eye and also reduces aberrations in the refracting system. Anatomically, the iris is situated between the two refracting components of the eye—the cornea and the lens. The anterior chamber is separated from the posterior chamber by the iris; the pupillary portion touches the anterior surface of the lens; and the base is attached to the anterior end of the ciliary body. The peripheral iris roll represents the beginning of the angle recess (p. 1).

The iris is one of three portions of the uveal tract; and although divided regionally, it is developmentally and structurally indivisible from the ciliary body and choroid. Probably the most important function of the uveal tract is to provide nourishment for the globe through its blood supply from the posterior arteries and to a lesser extent from the anterior ciliary arteries.

The surface of the iris is made up of numerous iris fibrils, which vary considerably in appearance within a given iris and also from patient to patient. The presence of contraction furrows, crypts, and various degrees of pigmentation results in prominence of the trabeculated appearance. Often the radial-coursing blood vessels are visible extending to the base of the iris. In the darkly pigmented iris the appearance is smooth and velvety, the only apparent surface structures being the contraction furrows and the collarette. The latter represents a minor vascular circle of the iris and separates the pupillary zone from the ciliary zone. The collarette is characterized by a ring of slightly elevated, irregularly scalloped tissue about 1.5 mm. from the pupillary border. The ciliary zone is composed of two layers of stroma, the anterior and the posterior leaves; in the pupillary zone the anterior layer atrophies shortly after birth. Pupillary remnants, which are commonly seen, almost invariably arise from the collarette. Contraction furrows and iris crypts are often prominent in the more peripheral portion of the ciliary zone of the iris. Crypts also occur in the pupillary zone, where they are larger and deeper than the peripheral type.

The anterior border of the layer of the iris consists of a condensation of stromal cells and is not a continuous layer. The dilator and sphincter muscles are situated deep to the stroma and are ectodermal in origin, in contrast to the stroma, which is mesodermal. Thus the muscles are derived from the epithelial layer of the iris, the sphincter having been produced by complete transformation of epithelial cells into muscle fibers and the dilator representing an incomplete transformation. The deepest layer of the iris is the pigment epithelium, which is continuous posteriorly with the superficial layer of the ciliary epithelium. The thinnest portion of the iris is at the last iris roll, or root of the iris just central to the angle recess. This roll may interfere with visualization of a portion of the angle recess and occasionally with even the scleral spur and some of the trabecular meshwork. Histologically, the stroma is of particular interest in that it contains a rich vascular supply, nerves, melanocytes, clump cells, and an abundance of acid mucopolysaccharide. The arrangement of the iris stromal tissue allows for rapid expansion and contraction. The blood vessels are thick walled and thus have a remarkably low permeability in the noninflamed eye. However, in the presence of inflammation (iritis) the vessel walls do become permeable, and the blood-aqueous barrier is lowered.

In the absence of inflammation, trauma produces remarkably little tissue reaction, and thus there is no fibroblastic proliferation or scar tissue formation; an iridectomy or tear of the iris will remain practically the same over a period of many years. However, in the presence of inflammation and toxins, the stimulus for fibroblastic proliferation is present. In hemorrhage involving the iris, the absorption of blood is usually complete, and there are no residual signs. Because of the extreme vascularity of the iris, it is not surprising that systemic diseases (including toxic and allergic reactions) produce a marked reaction in the iris (as well as in the rest of the uveal tract), with the well-known signs and symptoms of iritis. The inflammatory reaction may result in anterior and posterior synechias, pupillary membranes with a secluded pupil, distortion and atrophy of the iris, and secondary glaucoma due to involvement of the trabecular meshwork.

Chapter 5

Congenital conditions of the iris

CONGENITAL ANISOCORIA, POLYCORIA, CORECTOPIA, AND DYSCORIA

Abnormalities of the pupil in size, shape, and position are referred to by various terms and frequently cause few symptoms or none.

An inequality of the size of the pupils, referred to as anisocoria, is a relatively frequent finding. Often the difference in size is only 0.5 mm., but sometimes it may be as much as 2 mm. The condition may be transmitted as an irregular autosomal dominant trait; it is not usually associated with other congenital anomalies, and the patient is usually asymptomatic.

The appearance of more than one pupil is defined as polycoria. True polycoria, in which two or more pupils occur surrounded by sphincter muscle, is a rare condition; but pseudopolycoria, in which there is only one pupil with a true sphincter and there are other holes with the appearance of a pupil, is fairly common. In pseudopolycoria the apparent reaction of such holes to light and medication is probably secondary to movements of the single sphincter of the iris. This condition may be transmitted as an autosomal dominant characteristic. It may also be seen congenitally in Rieger's and rubella syndromes. In adults the most common cause of pseudopolycoria, other than trauma, is probably essential iris atrophy.

A deviation of the pupillary aperture away from the center is referred to as corectopia. The normal pupil is situated slightly down and in from the center of the iris, but in corectopia (ectopia pupillae) displacement may be in any direction and is almost invariably bilateral. Commonly it is symmetrical, being equal and opposite in the two eyes. Frequently the pupil is also oval or irregular, but occasionally it retains its round appearance with a normal sphincter. If the displacement of the pupil is very great, there is usually decrease in vision, and the eyes are usually myopic. Ectopia lentis is commonly associated with the defect, and in some cases it occurs as a dominant mendelian characteristic.

Congenital conditions of the iris

Congenital abnormality of the shape of the pupils is referred to as dyscoria. The condition is usually bilateral; the pupils are often slitlike; and the appearance of the pupils may vary considerably with contraction and dilatation associated with light and dark. The sphincter of the iris may be abnormal or absent along some portions of the pupillary opening; this may explain the abnormal shape. Atypical colobomas and congenital aphakia have been reported to be associated with the condition. The vision is usually not markedly affected when dyscoria alone exists.

Anisocoria

History. This 54-year-old woman was seen for treatment of recurrent chalazia and was incidentally found to have a pupillary abnormality. Examination of her relatives revealed the remarkable finding of enlarged oval pupils in only the left eye of the following family members: the patient's father, two of her five siblings, all four of her children, and eight grandchildren.

Findings. The vision in both eyes is 20/20 without correction. The right eye is

FIG. 58   normal, including a round pupil, which reacts to light and accommodation (Fig. 58, *A*). In the left eye the pupil is larger than normal and oval (Fig. 58, *B*). It reacts minimally to light, both direct and consensual, but more completely to accommodation. The iris is normal and is the same color as the fellow eye. The remainder of the eye is normal.

Corectopia

History. Since childhood this 72-year-old man had poor vision in the right eye. For a number of years he was also known to have abnormal pupils.

Findings. The vision in the right eye is counting fingers at 4 feet and in the

FIG. 59   left 20/30. The pupil of the right eye is pear shaped and displaced nasally (Fig. 59, *A*). The iris is normal, but there is pigment on the anterior capsule and nuclear sclerosis of the lens. The left eye also has an elliptical pear-shaped pupil, which is slightly displaced superotemporally (Fig. 59, *B*). At the upper edge of the pupil is a posterior synechia, and the lens shows moderate nuclear sclerosis. Gonioscopy reveals no abnormality in either eye. The intraocular pressure is 20 mm. Hg (Schiøtz) in both eyes.

Course. The patient did not return for follow-up.

Dyscoria

History. For many years and probably since birth this 62-year-old man had abnormal pupils. Four years ago he was discovered to have chronic open angle glaucoma in both eyes and has been treated medically with a moderate degree of success. Recently echothiophate (¼%) drops, epinephrine (1%) drops, and acetazolamide have been required for the control of the tension in both eyes.

Findings. Vision in the right eye is 20/30 and in the left 20/25 with correc-

FIG. 60   tion. The pupil of the right eye is centrally located but irregular in shape (Fig. 60, *A*). The iris tissue in the region of the sphincter is irregular in thickness and in some places is covered by a granular brown pigmentation. The remainder of the iris is normal, and gonioscopy reveals normal wide open angles. Examination of the media shows a moderate nuclear sclerosis, and the disc is saucerized.

Text continued on p. 111.

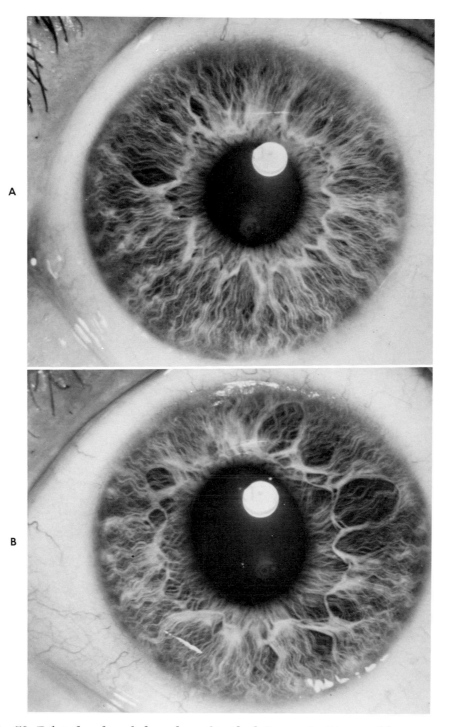

Fig. 58. *Dilated and oval-shaped pupil in the left eye of a 54-year-old woman with anisocoria.* **A,** The right eye has a normal round pupil. **B,** The left pupil reacts minimally to light, is larger, and is oval in shape. The abnormality is familial.

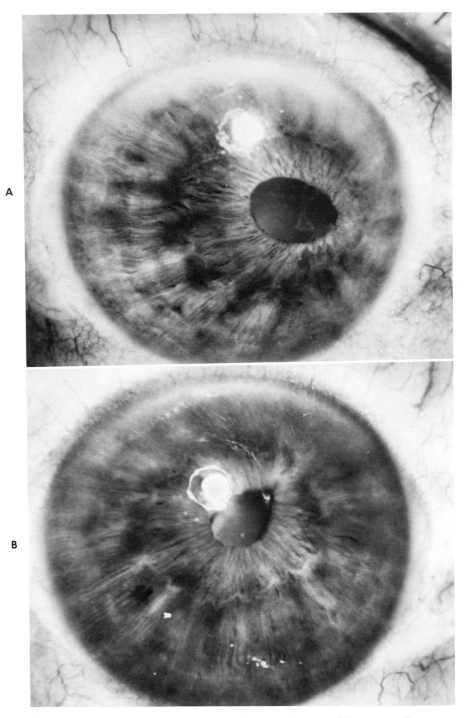

Fig. 59. *Pear-shaped and displaced pupil in a 72-year-old man with corectopia.* **A,** The right pupil is ovoid and displaced nasally. **B,** The left pupil is also pear shaped and only slightly displaced.

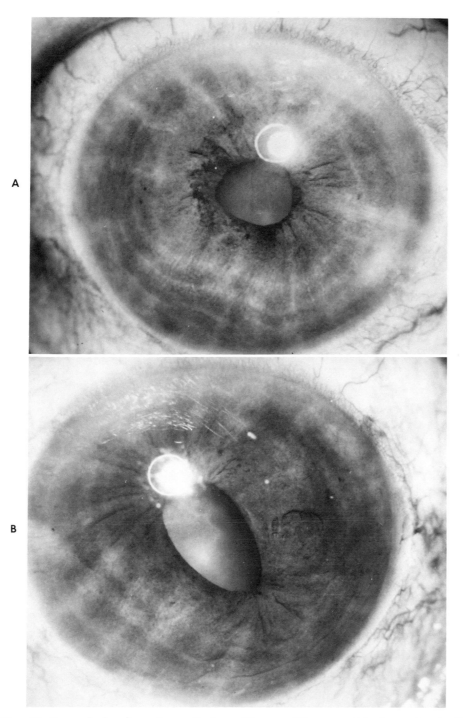

Fig. 60. *Irregularly shaped pupils in a 62-year-old man with dyscoria.* **A,** The right pupil is centrally located but irregular in shape and has varying thickness of the sphincter muscle. **B,** The left pupil is vertically elongated, with some portions appearing to have no iris sphincter. The pupillary abnormalities were probably present since birth; only recently did the patient develop chronic open angle glaucoma.

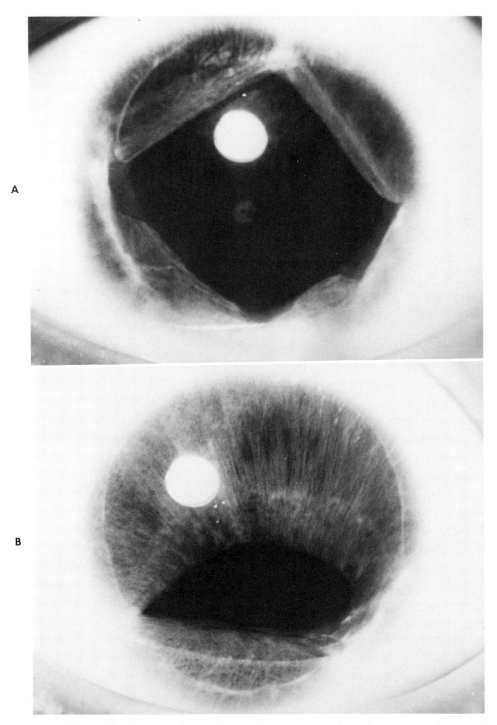

Fig. 61. *Markedly abnormal pupils in a 6-year-old girl with congenital dyscoria.* **A,** The right pupil is diamond shaped, and the iris is hypoplastic, with a prominent ectropion uveae. **B,** The left pupil is irregularly elliptical and displaced inferiorly. The prominent posterior embryotoxon (Axenfeld's anomaly) extends around most of the circumference of the cornea. The patient had a nystagmus and decreased vision, with the same ocular findings as in her identical twin.

110

In the left eye the pupil is oval shaped and the iris grossly irregular (Fig. 60, B). The pupil is vertically elongated, and the region along the sides of the pupil is markedly thinned, giving the impression that there is no sphincter. However, peripheral to the pupillary margin there is an area in which the iris is elevated and irregular as if excessively heavy sphincter muscle tissue existed in this region. Gonioscopy reveals the angles to be wide open but to show some excessive pigmentation. The lens contains moderate nuclear sclerosis, and the disc is minimally saucerized. The intraocular tension by applanation tonometry is 28 mm. Hg in the right eye and 18 mm. Hg in the left. The fields are normal in both eyes.

Course. For 6 years the intraocular pressures were well controlled in the left eye but were frequently elevated in the right. There was some increase in the cupping of the right disc, but in spite of this the fields remained normal.

Dyscoria

History. One of identical twins, this 6-year-old girl was noted to have abnormal pupils at birth. Subsequently she was also noted to have a nystagmus and decreased vision. The twin had almost identical ocular abnormalities.

Findings. The vision in the right eye is 20/60 and in the left 20/100. There is a pendular nystagmus. In the right eye the cornea is only about 8 mm. in diameter, and the limbal region is poorly defined. The anterior chamber is very shallow, and the pupil is diamond shaped (Fig. 61, A). The iris is hypoplastic, FIG. 61 and there is a prominent ectropion uveae at three of the points of the diamond. Iridocorneal adhesions are present particularly at the 4 and 9 o'clock positions, and there is a posterior embryotoxon (Axenfeld's anomaly) from the 9 o'clock to the 12 o'clock position. The lens has a fine diffuse punctate opacification of the nucleus, and the posterior pole is normal. In the left eye the cornea is 9 mm. in diameter, and there is a prominent posterior embryotoxon (Axenfeld's anomaly) extending almost the entire circumference of the cornea (Fig. 61, B). The anterior chamber is shallow and the iris irregularly elliptical and inferiorly displaced. A minimal amount of ectropion uveae is visible. The lens contains fine punctate opacities in the nucleus, and the posterior pole is normal. By gonioscopy the angles are open and normal in a number of areas, and typical iridocorneal adhesions are seen attaching to the thickened Schwalbe's line.

Course. Four months later there had been no change in the patient's ocular status, and she was then lost to follow-up.

PERSISTENT PUPILLARY MEMBRANE

Strands or layers of iris tissue remaining in the pupillary area after birth characterize a persistent pupillary membrane. This is a common finding and represents a failure of atrophy of the arcades and their associated mesodermal tissue. The remnants consist of the remains of obliterated blood vessels and mesoderm. They are quite common in newborn infants (95%) but are much less common in adults due to absorption. They are likely to be permanent, however, if present after the first year of life.

Clinically, they are seen in various forms. When contact with the iris is maintained, they are seen as strands attaching to the superficial layer of the iris at the collarette. In addition, they may be attached to the anterior capsule of the lens, forming a white plaque at the site. At other times they may attach to the posterior surface of the cornea. The rest of the eye is usually normal. Treatment is usually unnecessary.

Persistent pupillary membrane

History. This 3½-year-old boy was seen because of a peculiar-appearing pupil of the right eye.

Findings. The vision appears to be good in both eyes. In the right eye the anterior segment is normal except for the iris. From the collarette arise a number of dense strands of tissue, which extend out somewhat into the anterior
FIG. 62   chamber and across the pupillary opening interconnecting with each other (Fig. 62). As far as can be determined, the lens is normal. In the left eye a few persistent pupillary remnants also are present; the eye otherwise appears normal.

Course. The patient was lost to follow-up.

Congenital pupillary membrane

History. Fifteen years ago this 69-year-old man was found to have pupillary membranes in both eyes; he had normal vision in the right eye and slightly

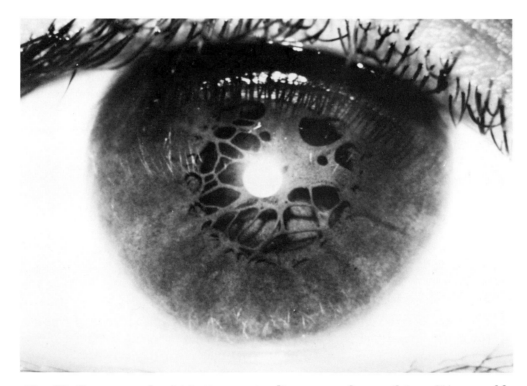

Fig. 62. *Dense strands of iris tissue extending across the pupil in a 3½-year-old boy with persistent pupillary membrane.* Arising from the collarette is a dense meshwork of interconnecting pupillary iris strands, which appears to cause no interference with vision.

reduced vision in the left. After he had been treated with 2% epinephrine (Adrenalin) injected subconjunctivally, the pupillary membranes were partially detached from the pupillary margin, and there was slight improvement of the vision in the right eye. Recently his eyes felt "scratchy."

Findings. Vision in the right eye is 20/40 and in the left 20/100 with correction. In the right eye there is a papillomatous lesion of the upper lid. The only other abnormality is that of the pupil, which has a filmy membrane attached to the pupillary margin except from the 8 o'clock to the 12 o'clock position (Fig. 63, A). A number of pigment granules are distributed on the FIG. 63 surface of the membrane and the lens. The pupil is small and reacts poorly to light. Behind the membrane some diffuse lens opacities can be discerned, and the fundus cannot be visualized. In the left eye the findings are similar to those of the right, except the anterior chamber is shallower and the pupillary membrane denser (Fig. 63, B). It is detached from the pupillary margin only from the 9 o'clock to the 11 o'clock position. The lens shows some diffuse opacification, and the fundus cannot be seen. Intraocular pressure is 15 mm. Hg (Schiøtz) in the right eye and 25 mm. Hg in the left.

Course. The patient was next seen 9 years later, when he complained that his vision was very poor. His intraocular pressures were found to be 20 mm. Hg (Schiøtz) in the right eye and 42 mm. Hg in the left. Vision was reduced to 20/200 in the right eye and hand movements in the left. Gonioscopy revealed that the anterior chamber was very shallow in the left eye and that the angle contained many fine peripheral anterior synechias. The angle in the right eye was not narrow and contained excessive uveal meshwork. A therapeutic trial of pilocarpine (2%) drops five times a day in the left eye brought the intraocular pressure down to 26 mm. Hg (Schiøtz) in a week. However, when the patient was seen 2 months later, the intraocular pressure was again elevated, and he was advised to have a full iridectomy and possible cataract extraction in the left eye. The patient declined surgery, and the strength of the pilocarpine was increased in the left eye, resulting in reduction of intraocular pressure to 27 mm. Hg (Schiøtz). He was then lost to follow-up.

Congenital pupillary membrane and cataract

History. At birth this 1-month-old female infant was found to have a small right eye with a white mass in the pupil.

Findings. In the right eye the cornea is clear, with a diameter of about 9 mm. The anterior chamber is shallow due to a forward bulging of the iris and lens. The iris has prominent radial vessels throughout, and many of these extend into the pupil and onto the surface of the lens (Reel VII-6). In the lens REEL VII-6 there is a dense anterior subcapsular opacity near the pupillary margin at the 7 o'clock position; this extends through to the posterior portion of the lens, where there is a vascularized retrolenticular membrane. The iris stroma is hypoplastic and is absent in some places at its periphery. The left eye appears to be normal.

Course. As the child grew, a pendular nystagmus developed in both eyes. This was present in all directions of gaze. Fourteen years later the vision in the right eye was no light perception and in the left 20/100 with correction. There was a pendular nystagmus in both eyes, which was made worse with attempted

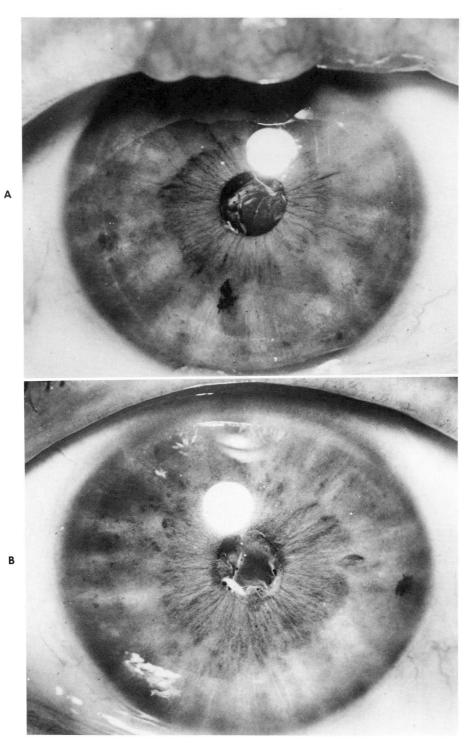

Fig. 63. *Filmy tissues in the pupils of a 69-year-old man with congenital pupillary membranes.* **A,** In the small pupil there is an irregular membrane that is partially attached to the pupillary border. **B,** A denser membrane is firmly attached to the pupillary border and has pigment granules on its surface.

fixation. The cornea of the right eye was clear except for some peripheral opacification and vascularization. The anterior chamber was shallow due to a prominent forward bowing of the iris especially in its midregion, which is typical of iris bombé (Reel VII-7). The pupillary region was completely adherent REEL VII-7 to a dense white cataract. The entire iris appeared atrophic and at the periphery contained no pigment. The angle of the anterior chamber appeared open. The eye was definitely microphthalmic. The left eye was normal except for a pale disc.

Congenital pupillary membrane and microphthalmia

History. Since birth this 11-year-old boy had poor vision and abnormal-appearing eyes.

Findings. Vision in the right eye is hand movements and in the left counting fingers at 2 feet. There is a gross pendular nystagmus. The right cornea is 4.5 mm. in diameter, and its superficial layers are diffusely vascularized. The iris is covered by a yellowish fibrous membrane. There are both peripheral and central anterior synechias. Pupillary membrane remnants are present, and the lens is cataractous. In the left eye the cornea is 8.5 mm. in diameter. In the interpalpebral region there is some early band keratopathy, and superiorly there is superficial vascularization at the periphery of the cornea. The iris is yellowish and appears atrophic, and the pupil is semidilated. Fine strands of stromal tissue extend across into the pupillary area, and one passes vertically across the entire pupil (Reel VIII-1). A few small white opacities are in the lens nucleus, REEL VIII-1 but the lens is otherwise clear. Because of the pendular nystagmus, examination of the retina is difficult, but it appears that there is some type of retinal dysplasia.

Course. Over the next 3 years the vision remained the same. However, the patient developed total blacking out of vision on standing up, which lasted for a few minutes, with return to normal vision thereafter. No change in his ocular status was found, and it was decided that his blackouts were due to episodes of transient hypotension.

Congenital pupillary membrane

History. At birth this 16-year-old boy was noted to have opacities of both pupils. It was obvious that he had profound mental retardation. The parents, including their ocular status, were normal; one older sibling was also normal.

Findings. In both eyes the corneas are about 9 mm. in diameter, and the pupillary margins are irregular. In the right eye there are fine tenuous bands of iris tissue extending from the pupillary margin across the pupil, and there is one large opacity on the anterior capsule of the lens attached to the pupillary margin superiorly. In the left eye there are many fine tenuous strands of iris tissue extending from the collarette into the central area of the pupil and attaching to the anterior capsule of the lens, which is irregularly opacified (Fig. 64). Deep in the lens there is an irregular indistinct opacity. Evaluation of the FIG. 64 posterior segment is impossible.

Course. There was no change in the ocular status of the patient; but as he became older, the profound mental retardation became more apparent. More-

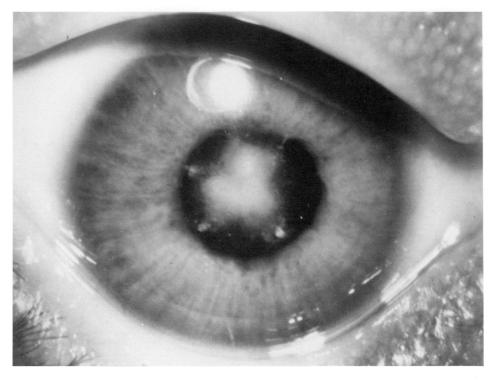

Fig. 64. *Fine strands of iris tissue attached to an anterior capsular cataract in the left eye of a 16-year-old boy with a congenital pupillary membrane.* The strands of pupillary membrane arise from the collarette and become incorporated in the anterior capsular opacity centrally. The left pupil also has fine tenuous bands of persistent pupillary membrane, but there is no cataract.

over, a younger sibling was born with persistent pupillary membrane material attaching to the anterior capsule of the lens and with lenticular opacities very similar to those of the patient. There was every indication that he too was profoundly mentally retarded.

Congenital pupillary membrane

History. This 5-year-old girl was born with a white reflex in the pupil of the left eye. The mother reported that the white spot seemed to be getting larger and that the child tended to bump into things on the right.

Findings. Vision in the right eye is 20/40 and in the left 15/200. Both eyes are normal except for the pupillary abnormality in the left eye. This consists of a continuous sheath of iris stromal tissue arising from the temporal half of the collarette and extending to the center of the lens, where it is attached to a dense white opacity of the anterior lens capsule. With mydriatics the nasal half of the pupil dilates normally, while the temporal half remains small due to the iris attachments to the lens capsule (Fig. 65).

FIG. 65

Course. Mydriatic drops were used to produce a larger pupillary opening, and the right eye was continuously patched for 6 weeks, resulting in some improvement in vision of the left eye. Cycloplegic refraction showed a moderate

116

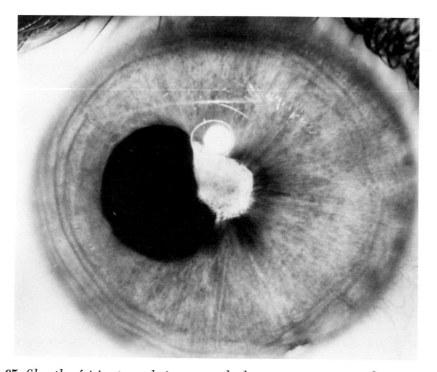

Fig. 65. *Sheath of iris stromal tissue attached to an anterior capsular cataract in a 5-year-old girl with a congenital pupillary membrane.* The pupillary membrane arises from the collarette and extends to a central dense white capsular cataract. The defect causes a marked decrease in the visual acuity.

hyperopia and astigmatism in the left eye, and glasses were prescribed. The patient was then lost to follow-up.

Congenital pupillary membrane

History. Since birth this 9-year-old boy had a "growth" over the pupil of the right eye. No change in the size of the lesion has been noted since that time.

Findings. Vision in the right eye is 20/25 and in the left 20/20. Both eyes are normal except for a pupillary membrane in the right eye, which arises from the collarette and attaches to the anterior capsule lens at its apex (Fig. 66). There FIG. 66 are a total of six strands of iris stroma, which vary in size and attach at a common point, producing a small white anterior capsule lens opacity. The remainder of the iris is normal.

Course. The patient was lost to follow-up.

Persistent pupillary membrane

History. Upon awakening this morning this 75-year-old woman found that she was "blind" in the left eye. Over a period of the next 2 hours there was some improvement in the vision, but it was still very hazy.

Findings. Vision in the right eye is 20/60 and in the left 20/100. The right eye

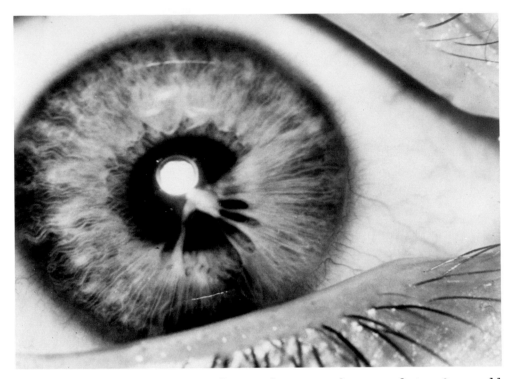

Fig. 66. *Strands of iris tissue attaching to the anterior lens capsule in a 9-year-old boy with a congenital pupillary membrane.* About six strands of persistent pupillary membrane tissue arise from the collarette and attach at a central common point on the anterior lens capsule.

is normal except for some posterior cortical opacities and drusen of the macula. In the left eye there is a mass of hemorrhage involving about two thirds of the pupil and extending nasally over the iris (Fig. 67). A small hyphema is present. Arising from the collarette superiorly is a strand of iris tissue containing a single blood vessel and disappearing into the upper temporal portion of the clot. The remainder of the iris is normal. There are some posterior cortical opacities, and a poor view of the fundus is obtained.

FIG. 67

Course. In 2 days the clot decreased to about one fourth of its original size, and in 3 more days only a small speck of clot remained attached to an elliptical-shaped piece of pigmented tissue in the center of the pupil (Reel VIII-2). This pigmented mass, typical of iris pigment epithelium, was attached to the anterior lens capsule and to a persistent pupillary strand located superiorly and contained a blood vessel. Four days later no blood remained, and with refraction 20/50 vision was obtained in each eye. Four years later there had been no recurrence of the hemorrhage, but there was a decrease of vision in both eyes due to lens opacities and early macular degeneration.

REEL VIII-2

CONGENITAL IRIS COLOBOMA

Localized incomplete or complete absence of the iris at birth is referred to as a congenital iris coloboma. These defects are usually divided into two types,

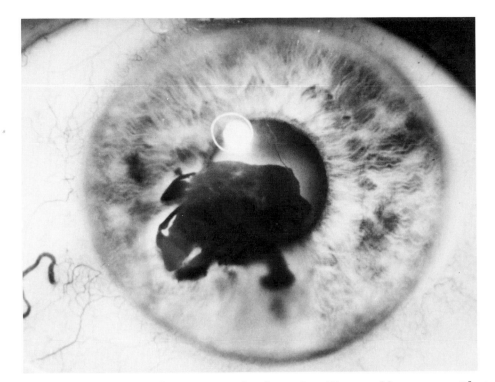

Fig. 67. *Blood clot in the anterior chamber of a 75-year-old woman with a persistent pupillary membrane.* Covering most of the pupillary area is clotted blood, and extending from the collarette superiorly to the edge of the clot is a single strand of iris containing a blood vessel. Five days later (see Reel VIII-2) almost complete absorption of the clot had occurred, and a piece of pigmented tissue in the center of the pupil was visible. Attached to this was the persistent pupillary strand of tissue containing the blood vessel. The patient had no further difficulty.

typical and atypical. Typical colobomas extend downward or down and in from the pupil, while atypical ones extend in any other direction. The typical colobomas usually involve the ciliary body, which is often continuous with a coloboma of the choroid. They are secondary to the defect in closure of the optic cup that produced the choroidal and retinal coloboma. The atypical colobomas, on the other hand, usually involve only the iris. They may involve the ciliary body but only rarely reach the choroid.

In both types the defect in the iris is triangular, with the base of the triangle toward the pupillary margin. When a ciliary body defect is associated with the iris coloboma, the two are usually separated by a bridge of normal iris tissue. It is also common to find tags of persistent pupillary membrane attached to the stroma of the iris at the edge of the gap, and in many cases abnormal pigmented tissue occupies the apex of the gap at the corneoscleral junction. The rest of the iris is normal, and the sphincter is usually present and active except at the notch. Often there are associated defects of the lens, such as coloboma of the lens, gaps in the suspensory ligament, and capsular or lamellar opacities.

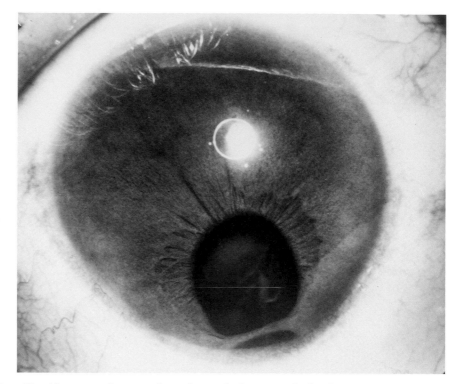

Fig. 68. *Absence of iris inferiorly and downward displacement of pupil in a 50-year-old woman with bilateral congenital iris colobomas.* There is total lack of iris tissue inferiorly except for a small strand of iris bridging the coloboma.

The defect may be hereditary. Vision is usually good, although in some patients myopia or astigmatism of high degree is present. Two possible causes of the defect exist: either there is a localized failure of a portion of the ectodermal margin of the optic cup, or there is undue persistence of fetal mesoderm producing a secondary inhibition of growth of the ectoderm in contact with it.

Congenital iris coloboma

History. Since birth this 50-year-old woman had abnormal pupils, but until 1 year ago her vision was good enough to enable her to drive an automobile and read newspapers. Recently there was gradual painless decrease in vision.

Findings. The vision in each eye is 20/400. The anterior segments are normal except for the pupils, which are displaced downward and nasally, and the iris, which is colobomatous inferiorly. In the right eye a strand of iris tissue bridges across the coloboma (Fig. 68). Both lenses show marked nuclear sclerosis and posterior subcapsular opacities. Fundus examination reveals a choroidal coloboma in the inferior nasal quadrant of both eyes. Gonioscopy shows flat iris planes and total lack of iris in the region of the coloboma. Intraocular pressure is 18 mm. Hg (Schiøtz) in both eyes.

FIG. 68

Course. Intracapsular cataract extraction was performed on the right eye, and the postoperative course was uneventful. Two months later the patient obtained 20/50 vision in the right eye with an aphakic correction.

120

Congenital coloboma of the iris, lens, and choroid

History. This 23-year-old woman had been born 2 months prematurely with congenital cataracts. At age 3 a cataract extraction was done on the right eye, which developed phthisis bulbi and was enucleated. She also had a cleft palate, which was repaired during infancy. With a high myopic and astigmatic correction the vision in the left eye has remained between 20/40 and 20/70.

Findings. The right eye is anophthalmic, and vision in the left is 20/50. In the left eye there is a prominent inferior iris coloboma (Reel VIII-3). In the coloboma REEL VIII-3 can be seen a notch in the inferior edge of the lens, with at least 3 mm. of the lens absent at the 6 o'clock position. Zonules can be seen bridging the defect, and there is a dense white opacity involving the nucleus of the lens. Another opacity is just under the anterior capsule in the axial region. Fundus examination reveals a large coloboma extending from the ora down almost to the optic nerve head. Within the coloboma are two deep posterior staphylomas. Gonioscopy shows the angle to be wide open, but there is an excessive number of pigmented iris processes in the angle. The intraocular pressure is 21 mm. Hg (applanation tonometry), and the facility of outflow is borderline normal.

Course. Over the next 2 years the evidence from repeated tonography and intraocular tensions indicated that the patient probably did not have glaucoma.

Congenital anterior synechia and lens coloboma

History. Since birth this 14-year-old girl has had a brown right eye and a blue left eye. The vision in the right eye has always been poorer than in the left.

Findings. Vision in the right eye is 20/40 with correction and in the left 20/20. In the right eye a large peripheral anterior synechia extends onto the cornea about 2 mm. Adjacent to the synechia is a dark brown area of thinned iris stroma contrasting with the remaining light yellow-brown iris. By gonioscopy the stroma of the iris is firmly attached to the cornea, producing a broad truncated synechia at the 6 o'clock position (Reel VIII-4). Elsewhere the angle REEL VIII-4 is wide open, and there are a number of iris processes extending across the ciliary body to occasionally reach Schwalbe's line. Also clearly visible is a notch in the inferior portion of the crystalline lens, which extends above the lower edge of the pupillary margin. The fundus appears to be normal. The left eye is normal, and the iris is blue.

Course. Cycloplegic refraction showed the right eye to have a high mixed astigmatic error, but with this correction there was little improvement in the vision. Subsequently, glasses were given to the patient, but she did not wear them. Five years later she was slightly myopic in the left eye, and the refractive error of the right had remained unchanged.

CONGENITAL HYPOPLASIA

Thinning of the iris stroma when present at birth represents congenital iris hypoplasia. The extent of the hypoplasia may be extreme, or it may be limited to a small portion of the iris. Furthermore, the depth of the hypoplasia may vary in that only the anterior leaf or, on the other hand, the entire thickness of the mesodermal stroma may be affected. In marked hypoplasia the ectodermal pigment and the sphincter are easily visible. This produces a whitish gray ring several millimeters wide surrounding the pupil and causes the peripheral iris to be dark brown or almost black in color. Localized defects may appear as "iris pits" or as sector-shaped defects that may contain free-floating stromal fibers. Larger areas of free-floating fibers may be seen as a senile change in the condition known as iridoschisis (p. 225). Excessive hypoplasia of the anterior leaf or underdevelopment of the entire mesodermal portion of the iris may be an isolated defect, but either condition is frequently associated with congenital or systemic diseases. The peripheral stroma of the iris is commonly hypoplastic in mongolism and is often seen along with Brushfield's spots (p. 136). More extreme hypoplasia of the iris stroma is seen in association with the rubella syndrome consequent to maternal rubella during the first trimester of pregnancy. In such cases the hypoplasia may be so marked as to involve pigment epithelium. It may result in a pseudopolycoria. In some instances of the rubella syndrome, the iris progressively and slowly becomes more atrophic throughout life.

Hypoplasia or total absence of the iris sphincter is a rare condition and, as expected, produces a defect in pupillary constriction. A surprising fact is that these pupils are not generally semidilated.

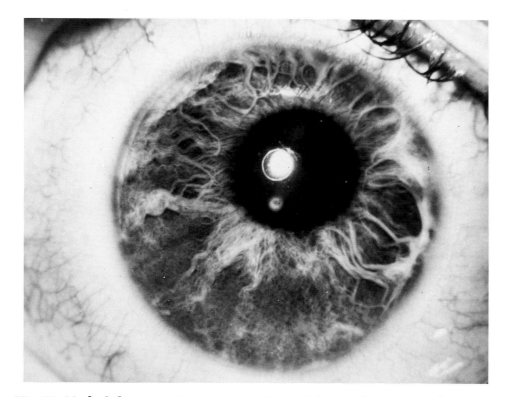

Fig. 69. *Marked thinning of iris stroma and a peripheral white ring in the cornea of an 18-year-old boy with congenital iris hypoplasia and posterior embryotoxon. The pupil was ovoid and displaced upward, with markedly hypoplastic iris stroma inferiorly. On the posterior surface of the cornea at the periphery is a thickened Schwalbe's line most apparent from the 9 o'clock to the 12 o'clock position.*

Congenital iris hypoplasia and posterior embryotoxon

History. This 18-year-old boy had a piece of steel strike the left eye and, as an incidental finding, it was discovered that he had unusual pupils and irides.

Findings. Vision in the right eye is 20/60 and in the left 20/15. The right eye is slightly injected, the cornea clear, and the anterior chamber of moderate depth. The pupil is ovoid and displaced upward and nasally (Fig. 69). There is FIG. 69 marked thinning of the iris stroma, particularly inferiorly and temporally, and a prominent white ring can be seen near the periphery of the cornea both nasally and temporally. By gonioscopy the angle is abnormal with peripheral anterior synechias, most of which bridge the trabecular meshwork and attach to the anteriorly displaced prominent Schwalbe's line. There is a small anterior polar cataract; the fundus is normal except for a myopic crescent. In the left eye there is a foreign body at the 9 o'clock position at the limbus, but the eye is otherwise normal in all respects. Intraocular pressure is 19 mm. Hg (Schiøtz) in both eyes.

Course. The steel foreign body was removed, and the recovery was uneventful.

Congenital hypoplasia of iris sphincter

History. Some time ago this 35-year-old man noted that his right pupil was larger than his left. Five of his children were examined, and two of them were found to have an identical lack of tissue in the sphincter region.

Findings. The vision in both eyes is 20/20. The eyes are normal in all respects except for the irides. The pupil of the right eye is 4 mm., and that of the left is 3 mm. At the pupillary margin there is a prominent edge of pigment epithelium of the iris extending slightly onto the anterior surface of the iris (ectropion uveae). In the right eye iris tissue in the region of the sphincter extending out to the collarette is markedly thinned so that pigment epithelium is visible through the small amount of remaining stroma (Reel VIII-5). This REEL VIII-5 imparts an appearance of concavity to the sphincter region. The sphincter region in the left eye has an identical appearance, except that the pupil is appreciably smaller. The right pupil does not react to light; the left does, but to a lesser extent than normal. Both react somewhat to accommodation. Methacholine (Mecholyl) (2½%) has no effect on either pupil, but there is normal dilatation with atropine and miosis with pilocarpine (4%). Transillumination indicates a loss of pigment epithelium in the midzone of the iris, and gonioscopy reveals an open angle containing a prominent uveal meshwork. The fields are full in both eyes. There is no refractive error.

Iris atrophy due to maternal rubella

History. During the third month of pregnancy the mother of this 36-year-old man had rubella. At 9 years of age he was found to have iris atrophy bilaterally and poor vision in the left eye. When he was 12 years of age, it became clear that there was some mental retardation. About this time refraction showed a marked anisometropia, which explained the amblyopia in his left eye. Hearing tests showed a "chronic adhesive deafness." Although the vision remained the same over a period of 20 years, comparison of photographs showed that the iris atrophy had increased in that where areas of stromal iris atrophy had previously revealed an intact pigment epithelium, dehiscences of the pigment epithelium had occurred, exposing the anterior capsule of the lens.

Findings. Vision in the right eye is 20/30 and in the left 20/100. In the right eye there is a marked arcus senilis and a deep anterior chamber. The iris is markedly atrophic throughout; but from the 6 o'clock to the 10 o'clock position no stroma remains, and pigment epithelium is exposed (Fig. 70). At the 8 o'clock position the pigment epithelium is completely atrophied, leaving a wide slitlike dehiscence, which exposes the anterior lens capsule. The sphincter is represented by a prominent white ring bordering the pupil, which is irregular and slightly ovoid. The media are clear, and the fundus is normal. In the left eye there is moderate conjunctival injection and a prominent arcus senilis, with an excessively dense infiltration of lipid substance between the 4 and 6 o'clock positions (Reel VIII-6). The anterior chamber is deep and the iris stroma markedly atrophic. Between the 3 and 4 o'clock positions there is a wide slit of total absence of iris pigment epithelium, revealing the anterior capsule of the lens. The sphincter of the iris is prominent and the pupil irregular and ovoid.

FIG. 70

REEL VIII-6

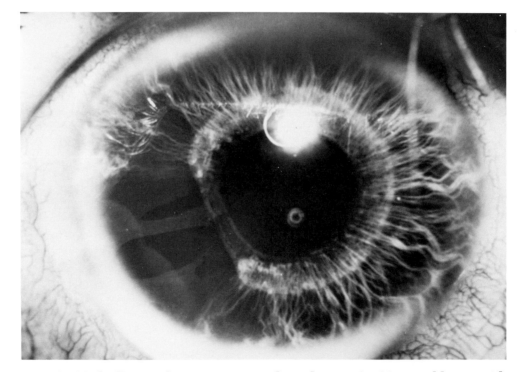

Fig. 70. *Markedly atrophic iris stroma in the right eye of a 36-year-old man with iris atrophy due to maternal rubella.* In some places only iris pigment epithelium remains, and at the 8 o'clock position there are several slitlike openings in which there is total iris atrophy. In the left eye there is a similar appearance, but in addition there is an area of excessive lipid infiltration of the cornea (see Reel VIII-6).

The media are clear, and the fundus is normal. Intraocular tension is 18 mm. Hg (Schiøtz) in both eyes.

Course. The patient was lost to follow-up.

CONGENITAL ECTROPION UVEAE

Eversion of the pigment epithelium of the iris characterizes ectropion uveae, caused by shrinkage of a fibrovascular membrane on the anterior surface of the iris. In true ectropion uveae the sphincter muscle, stroma, and pigment epithelium are all everted. The exposure of the pigment epithelium gives a brown color to the anterior surface of the pupillary portion of the iris. The same appearance may be obtained by proliferation of the pigment epithelium onto the anterior surface of the iris without eversion of the pupil. Congenital defects of the iris commonly cause ectropion uveae; one of these defects is the presence of a nevus of the iris close to the sphincter. Some congenital systemic diseases, such as neurofibromatosis, commonly cause ectropion uveae; in late rubeosis, particularly diabetic rubeosis, a marked ectropion uveae commonly occurs.

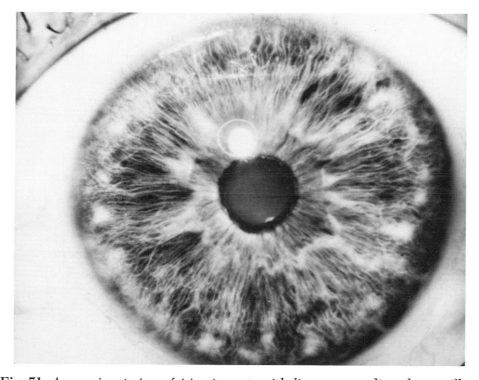

Fig. 71. *A prominent ring of iris pigment epithelium surrounding the pupillary margin in the right eye of a 58-year-old man with congenital ectropion uveae.* The irregular dark pigment epithelium extends to the level of the inner border of the sphincter pupillae muscle. There is central corneal edema and several areas of thinning of the iris stroma, suggesting an early essential iris atrophy of Chandler's type.

Congenital conditions of the iris

Congenital ectropion uveae

History. This 58-year-old man experienced blurring of the vision in his right eye over the past month for which he consulted his ophthalmologist. At that time examination showed central corneal edema, normal intraocular tension, questionable iris atrophy, and questionable endothelial dystrophy in the right eye. The patient was treated with hypertonic saline ointment at bedtime. He denied having eye pain, halos, or a red eye.

Findings. The vision in the right eye is 20/20 and in the left eye 20/15. The intraocular pressures by Schiøtz tonometry are 17 mm. Hg in both eyes. On general ocular examination the pupils are equal and react briskly to light and accommodation. Along both pupillary margins is a prominent ring of iris pigment epithelium extending to the level of the inner border of the sphincter muscle of the pupil. The right iris is light blue, with questionable early atrophy in the midperipheral zone at the 1, 3, and 9 o'clock positions (Fig. 71). Ringing the entire extreme periphery are numerous 1- to 2-mm. white clumps of anterior iris stroma tissue (Kruckmann-Wolfflin bodies). Slit-lamp examination of the right eye reveals a mild degree of fine guttate change in the corneal endothelium and central epithelial edema. The left cornea is normal. There is early nuclear sclerosis of the lenses, but the posterior segments are normal. By gonioscopy the angles are normal except for a slight increase in the pigmentation of the angle meshwork in the right eye.

FIG. 71

Course. When the patient was seen 2 years later, he had discontinued his ocular medication. In spite of definite corneal edema, with several bullae primarily in the center of the cornea, the patient's vision in the right eye was 20/40 with glasses, corrected to 20/30 with pinhole, and in the left 20/20 with glasses. The intraocular pressures were 17 mm. Hg (Schiøtz), and there had been no progression in the ocular abnormalities found on his previous visits. It was felt that the patient had an early essential iris atrophy of Chandler's type. The patient was subsequently lost to follow-up.

Congenital ectropion uveae

History. This 4-year-old boy had a vague history of a red painful right eye on several occasions. It was also noted that the right pupil was different from the left.

Findings. Vision in the right eye is 20/200 and in the left 20/30. In the right eye the cornea is clear and the anterior chamber of normal depth. However, the iris is grossly abnormal in that extending in from the pupillary margin to cover all the sphincter region is a dark brown pigmented material, with a scalloped border (Reel VIII-7). There is no clearcut collarette, and the peripheral iris is hypoplastic. Fundus examination reveals deep cupping, with some normal rim remaining. Gonioscopy shows thinning of the iris at the root and an anterior insertion of the iris in some areas. There is no closure of the angle or peripheral anterior synechia formation. The left eye is normal. Intraocular pressure in the right eye is 34 mm. Hg (Schiøtz) and in the left 20 mm. Hg (Schiøtz).

REEL VIII-7

Course. Intensive medical therapy was unsuccessful in maintaining a normal intraocular pressure, so two goniotomy procedures were carried out, after which the intraocular pressure remained within normal limits for 2 years. With subsequent elevation of pressure in the right eye at 26 mm. Hg (Schiøtz) medical therapy was again instituted; but despite this the pressure became even more elevated, and two more goniotomy procedures were necessary in the next 6 months to keep the intraocular pressure controlled. A year later medical therapy with epinephrine (2%), echothiophate (¼%), and acetazolamide was required to keep the intraocular pressure in the high teens. Visual fields showed a nasal step in the right eye, and the vision remained the same as when the patient was first seen.

CYSTS OF THE IRIS

Spontaneously occurring cystic structures in the iris and ciliary body are generally considered congenital even though they may not become manifest until adult life. Free-floating pigment cysts of the anterior chamber are derived from iris pigment epithelium.

The least common of the iris cysts are the intrastromal (ectodermal) type, which occur on the anterior surface of the iris and are lined by stratified or irregular layers of cylindrical and cuboidal cells. They are similar to inclusion cysts of the iris in that they have a thin anterior wall and a posterior wall made up of compressed iris stroma. They may become so large as to fill the anterior chamber and produce glaucoma by virtue of involvement of the trabecular meshwork. Total excision is the most satisfactory treatment, with photocoagulation or cryotherapy as an alternative.

Cysts of neuroectodermal origin occur on the posterior surface of the iris and in the ciliary body epithelium. Iris pigment epithelium is made up of two epithelial layers between which spaces that represent persistent remnants of the lumen of the primary optic vesicle may commonly be observed. This is particularly true at the pupillary margin, which is the last region to close and which contains the marginal sinus of von Szily. The latter explains the frequent occurrence of congenital cysts at the pupillary margin, which are easily visible and often serial. These have an appearance of dark brown rounded multiple masses frequently encircling the pupillary opening and occasionally almost occluding it. If the cysts become too extensive, there is a self-compensatory mechanism whereby the light entering the eye is reduced, causing the pupil to dilate. Iris pigment epithelium cysts arising peripheral to the spincter produce a bulge of the iris that is smoothly rounded, but there is no noticeable change in the iris stroma. Cysts near the root of the iris may cause occlusion of the angle and must be differentiated from cysts and tumors of the ciliary body. The diagnosis depends on observation of the posterior chamber, with a maximally dilated pupil, through the gonioscope. Transillumination may help differentiate these tumors from solid masses.

Free-floating cysts in the anterior chamber undoubtedly arise from iris pigment epithelium. They are asymptomatic and float freely in the anterior chamber. They produce no reaction and, when small, usually lie in the inferior angle. With the patient's head inverted, they gradually float to the superior angle, and blurring of vision occurs as they cross the pupillary area. Although many cysts appear to stay the same size over long periods of time, others have been noted to enlarge gradually, finally encroaching on the pupillary area. Histopathologically, the cyst wall consists of a single layer of typical posterior iris pigment epithelium.

Cysts of the ciliary body are also congenital; they are frequently bilateral. Commonly they project forward, pushing the root of the iris against the trabecular meshwork. When sufficiently numerous they produce a subacute angle closure glaucoma by pushing the iris against the angle structures. They are discussed in more detail in Chapter 12 (p. 328).

Treatment of cysts of the iris pigment epithelium is usually unnecessary. However, such cysts in exceptional cases can cause glaucoma due to pupillary block. Puncture of the cyst with a needle knife is usually successful in relieving the glaucoma. After puncture, recurrences do not ordinarily occur. Cysts of the peripheral iris and ciliary body involving the angle structures may require a large basal iridectomy to avoid angle closure glaucoma. If free-floating cysts of the anterior chamber involve the pupillary area, they can be removed.

Flocculi are also congenital structures, but generally not cystic. Their appearance is that of black nodules growing in grapelike clusters at the pupillary margin, arising from the pigment epithelium of the iris. Usually stationary throughout life, they occasionally become detached to float free in the aqueous.

Congenital intrastromal iris cyst

History. For 2 years this 19-year-old girl was aware of a black spot in her right eye. For the past 3 weeks she had pain over her right eye and blurring of vision when reading.

Findings. Vision in the right eye is 20/50 and in the left 20/20. In the right eye at the 7 o'clock position is a cystic-appearing lesion that begins just inside FIG. 72 the pupil and extends into the angle (Fig. 72, A). From this lesion there is an outpouring of thick mucoid material with granules of pigment dispersed throughout it. This material fills the lower half of the anterior chamber. Gonioscopy reveals a small rounded red mass in the angle at the end of the cystic lesion. Elsewhere the angle is open, and the trabeculum is darkly pigmented. The fundus is normal except for pulsations of the retinal arteries on the disc. The left eye is normal. The intraocular tension is 69 mm. Hg (Schiøtz) in the right eye and 17 mm. Hg (Schiøtz) in the left.

Course. Pilocarpine (4%) drops were instituted every 3 hours in the right eye. The intraocular pressure gradually fell to the 30's and remained there

---

Fig. 72. *Gradually progressive cystic lesion in the right eye of a 19-year-old girl with a congenital intrastromal iris cyst.* **A,** At the 7 o'clock position a cyst within the iris stroma is producing a thick mucoid material that is partially filling the anterior chamber. The intraocular pressure is markedly elevated. Subsequently, an Elliot trephine procedure was performed after medical treatment for glaucoma had failed. A year later (see Reel IX-1) the cyst had enlarged, and drops were required to control her tension. **B,** In another 6 months the cystic structure had tripled in size and extended almost to the pupillary margin. A heavily pigmented mass had developed at the periphery of the iris. Following iridocyclectomy, she had no further difficulty.

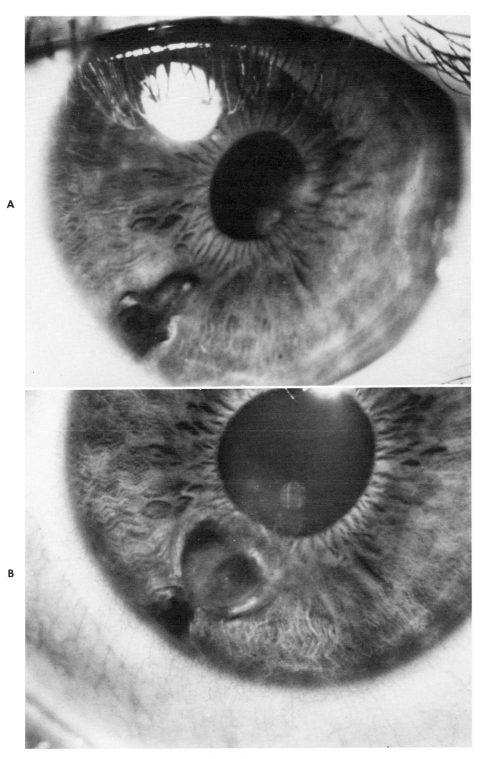

Fig. 72. For legend see opposite page.

for several days. When the patient was seen 3 weeks later, the intraocular pressure has risen to 55 mm. Hg (Schiøtz), with no appreciable change in the appearance of the iris lesion. An Elliot trephine procedure was performed superiorly, and the postoperative course was uneventful. For about a year the intraocular pressure remained in the normal range but then became elevated, and again pilocarpine was required to control the pressure. At the same time there was a gradual increase in the size of the gelatinous mass and the REEL IX-1 cystic structure in the iris (Reel IX-1). Six months later the intraocular pressure had risen to 40 mm. Hg (Schiøtz), and the cystic structure had about tripled in size and extended almost to the pupillary margin (Fig. 72, B). In addition, a heavily pigmented mass had developed at the periphery of the iris. An iridocyclectomy was performed, and all the involved iris and the adjacent ciliary body were removed. Only part of the gelatinous material filling the lower portion of the anterior chamber was removed, and postoperatively this caused no difficulty. The histopathologic diagnosis was congenital epithelial cyst of the ciliary processes and iris. When the patient was last seen 10 years later, the vision was 20/20 in both eyes and the intraocular pressure 18 mm. (Schiøtz). Fields were also normal.

Congenital intrastromal iris cyst

History. On routine examination the iris of this 55-year-old woman was found to have a cystic-appearing lesion. Eight months ago an attempt was made to destroy the cyst with cryotherapy applications. Four months later there was a recurrence of the cyst.

Findings. Vision in both eyes is 20/20. The right eye is normal. In the left eye at the periphery of the iris in the 6 o'clock position is a cystic-appearing structure, which by slit-lamp biomicroscopy can be seen to have a thin anterior REEL IX-2 wall and a densely pigmented posterior wall (Reel IX-2). The cyst is ovoid in shape and about 3 mm. in diameter. With a maximally dilated pupil the posterior surface of the iris is seen to be depressed backward toward the ciliary processes, but the ciliary body is entirely normal. The lens is clear and the fundus normal.

Course. The cyst was excised through a limbal incision, and there were no complications. Histopathologic diagnosis was iris cyst. Four months later the patient was asymptomatic, and there were no signs of recurrence of the cyst.

Congenital intrastromal iris cyst

History. This 39-year-old man went to his opthalmologist because of tired eyes. He was unaware of any abnormality of the left iris.

Findings. Vision in both eyes is 20/30. The right eye is normal, but at the 2 o'clock position the left iris has a pigmented lesion involving the pupillary FIG. 73 margin (Fig. 73). There is a prominent ectropion uveae, and the iris lesion is somewhat elevated and covered with fine pigment granules. The total size of the lesion is about 2 mm. in diameter. The remainder of the eye is normal. Intraocular pressure in both eyes is 25 mm. Hg (Schiøtz).

Course. A ^{32}P test indicated no significant difference in uptake between the corresponding areas in each eye. Basal iridectomy was performed, and the histo-

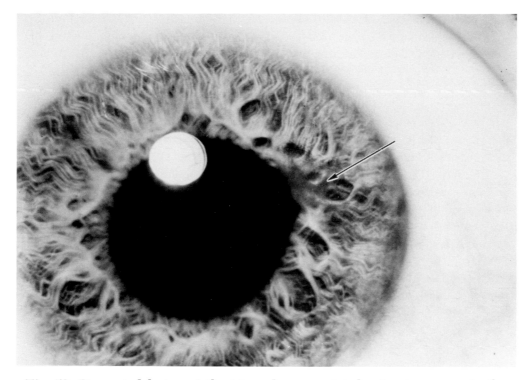

Fig. 73. *Pigmented lesion of the iris and an associated ectropion uveae in the left iris of a 39-year-old man with a congenital intrastromal iris cyst.* The somewhat elevated iris lesion is covered with fine pigment granules (arrow) and is adjacent to an area of ectropion uveae. A stromal cyst with a fibrous capsule was found in the iridectomy specimen.

pathologic diagnosis was a cyst of the iris stroma with a fibrous capsule. Postoperatively the patient did well, and 3 years later the vision and tensions in both eyes were normal.

Congenital stromal iris cyst

History. About a year ago this 64-year-old man was found to have a cyst in his left eye. This gradually covered the pupil and caused considerable decrease in vision.

Findings. Vision in the right eye is 20/20 and in the left hand movements. The right eye is normal. In the left eye there is mild conjunctival injection. The cornea is clear. The upper two thirds of the anterior chamber contains a large cyst that covers the entire pupillary area and has an almost transparent anterior wall (Reel IX-3). The cyst appears to arise out of the superior angle REEL IX-3 and is composed of one large lobule and a smaller one nasally. Tension by applanation tonometry is 15 mm. Hg in the right eye and 32 mm. Hg in the left.

Course. The cyst was aspirated and the cyst wall incised. In about 3 months the cyst recurred to its original size. An excision now was performed in which all the involved iris and the cyst were removed. Immediately postoperatively there were no complications; but gradually some lens opacities developed, and 2 years later the vision was 20/70. Because of slight elevation of intraocular pressure, epinephrine (1%) drops were used, resulting in adequate control of pressure. Histopathologic findings were idiopathic epithelial cyst of the iris stroma.

Iris pigment epithelium cyst

History. Recently this 67-year-old woman noted blurring of vision in her left eye. Examination by her ophthalmologist revealed a cyst at the pupillary margin in the left eye; and when the pupil was dilated, similar cysts were found in the right eye.

Findings. The vision in the right eye is 20/20 and in the left 20/30. The anterior segements of both eyes are normal except for the finding of pigmented cysts at at the pupillary margin. In the patient's right eye the cysts are not visible until the pupil is dilated, at which time an elongated black rounded structure can be seen extending from the 5 o'clock to the 8 o'clock position along the pupillary margin (Fig. 74). The iris is elevated in the region of the cyst, which transilluminates easily. The lens shows moderate cortical changes and some early posterior subcapsular opacification. The fundus is normal. In the left eye two small cysts are visible at the pupillary margin

FIG. 74

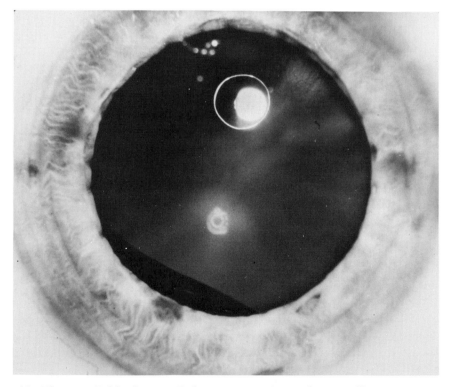

Fig. 74. *Elongated black rounded structure along the pupillary margin in a 67-year-old woman with a cyst of the iris pigment epithelium.* From the 5 o'clock to the 8 o'clock position, with the pupil dilated, a black cystic structure, which transilluminates easily, is visible. Similar cysts are present in the other eye. Over the next 2 years the cysts remained stationary.

between the 2 o'clock and 5 o'clock position in the undilated pupil. When the pupil is dilated, these can be seen to extend into the pupillary area about 3 mm. and also transilluminate easily. The lens shows more advanced changes, with considerable posterior subcapsular opacities. The iris is pushed anteriorly in the region of the cyst. By gonioscopy it can be seen that the cysts in both eyes close the angle completely, while in areas not involved with the cyst the angle is wide open. With dilated pupils the applanation tension is 18 mm. Hg in both eyes.

Course. During the next 2 years the cataract in the left eye progressed almost to maturity and caused marked loss of vision. One of the cysts had become adherent to the anterior lens capsule. The cyst in the right eye remained stationary, as had the cataract. A year later an uneventful intracapsular cataract extraction was performed on the left eye, at which time one of the cysts was grasped with a capsular forceps and a portion of it removed. Postoperatively the vision in the left eye with a cataract correction was 20/20. A number of adhesions of the pupillary border to the hyaloid face developed, but these seemed to be unassociated with the cysts.

Congenital iris cyst

History. One and a half years ago this 44-year-old woman was seen by her ophthalmologist because of severe left-sided headaches associated with temporary loss of vision. The exact cause of the headaches was not determined, but an iris cyst in the left eye seemed to be unrelated.

Findings. Vision in the right eye is 20/20 and in the left 20/15. In the left eye there is a single dark brown elongated cyst of the pupillary margin extending from the 7 o'clock to the 10 o'clock position. The remainder of the eye is normal. In the right eye there are four cysts of the pupillary margin, which are similar to the one seen in the left eye except that there is one in each quadrant (Fig 75, *A*). Again, the remainder of the eye is normal. FIG. 75 The intraocular pressures are 21 mm. Hg (Schiøtz) in the left eye and 14 mm. Hg (Schiøtz) in the right.

Course. The pupil of the right eye was dilated, and a continuous cyst extending around the entire pupillary margin was found. Gonioscopy showed it to be compressed between the anterior capsule of the lens and the sphincter of the iris (Fig. 75, *B*). Pilocarpine (4%) drops were given several times in the right eye to constrict the pupil, and the patient was sent home. The next day she developed aching in the right eye; finally a week later she was seen by her ophthalmologist, who found an intraocular pressure of 42 mm. Hg (Schiøtz). Pilocarpine (2%) drops were given at frequent intervals, and the intraocular pressure was reduced to 12 mm. Hg (Schiøtz) and maintained at that level with the patient receiving pilocarpine three times a day. The intraocular pressure in the left eye was not elevated.

Iris flocculus

History. Six years ago this 55-year-old man had an attack of acute iritis in the right eye for which no cause was ever found. Except for a posterior synechia superiorly, there were no sequelae of the attack, and the patient was

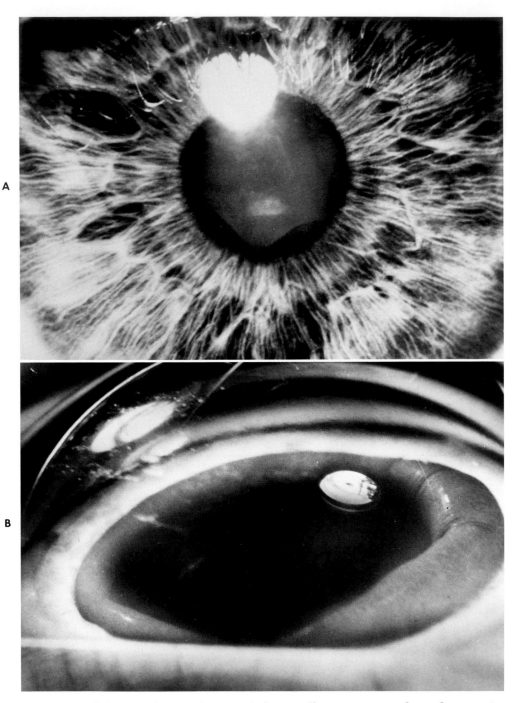

Fig. 75. *Dark brown elongated cysts of the pupillary margin in the right eye of a 44-year-old woman with congenital iris cysts.* **A,** In the right eye, four cysts in the iris pigment epithelium extend inward from the pupillary border and occlude a small portion of the pupillary aperture. **B,** With the pupil dilated, there is a continuous cyst around the entire pupillary margin. It is compressed between the anterior lens capsule and the sphincter of the iris and subsequently caused an acute attack of glaucoma.

asymptomatic since the attack. Today he was seen for a foreign body sensation in his right eye.

Findings. Vision in both eyes is 20/20. In the right eye there is mild conjunctival injection, but no foreign bodies of the conjunctiva or cornea can be found. Arising from the pupillary margin at about the 7 o'clock position is a solid-appearing pigmented structure hanging down over the anterior surface of the iris more than halfway to the limbus (Fig. 76). The structure is the color and texture of iris pigment epithelium and has an irregular nodular shape like a string of grapes. Superiorly there is a posterior synechia. The media are clear, and the fundus is normal. The left eye is normal.   FIG. 76

Course. The patient was treated with antibiotic ointment and was subsequently lost to follow-up.

Free-floating cyst

History. For many years this 30-year-old man had noted an object floating in his left eye. He was entirely asymptomatic.

Findings. The vision in both eyes is 20/20. The right eye is normal, but in the left there is an oval-shaped dark brown cystic-appearing structure lying in the inferior angle (Reel IX-4). This structure changes position slowly   REEL IX-4
with change in position of the patient's head so that with his head upside down,

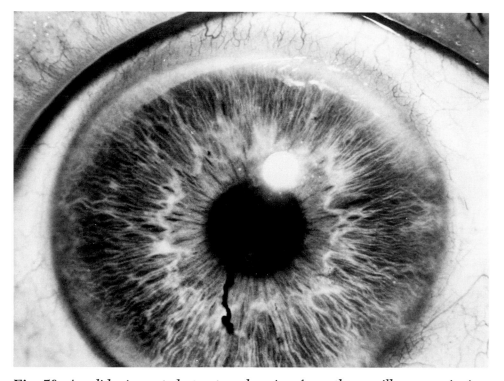

Fig. 76. *A solid pigmented structure hanging from the pupillary margin in a 55-year-old man with an iris flocculus.* The structure has an irregular nodular shape like a string of grapes and has the color and texture of iris pigment epithelium.

the object slowly floats to the superior angle. The iris is normal, and with the pupil dilated no cyst of the iris or ciliary body can be seen. The remainder of the eye is normal.

Course. Over several years the cyst did not change in size or appearance. There was no irritation or inflammatory response caused by the cyst at any time.

Free-floating iris cyst

History. About 15 years ago this 29-year-old woman had an attack of acute uveitis in the right eye, and she had a recurrence of this several weeks ago. As an incidental finding, a cyst in the anterior chamber was noted.

Findings. Vision in the right eye is 20/25 and in the left 20/20. In the right eye there is moderate conjunctival injection, and on the posterior surface of the cornea inferiorly are a number of nonpigmented keratic precipitates. Lying in the inferior angle is a smoothly rounded, somewhat oval cystic struc-

FIG. 77 ture (Fig. 77, A). Its surface is covered with an irregular brownish pigment. The iris is normal and the pupil dilated due to mydriatics. On the surface of the anterior capsule of the lens are a number of pigment granules; the posterior segment is normal. By gonioscopy the cystic structure can be seen lying in the angle, and except for some increased pigmentation of the trabecular meshwork no abnormalities of the angle are present (Fig. 77, B). The cyst moves freely within the anterior chamber, changing position with movement of the patient's head. The left eye is normal.

Course. The patient's iritis subsided; and when she was lost to follow-up months later, there was no change in the appearance of the cyst or in its mobility within the anterior chamber.

MONGOLISM

Mongoloid facies, mental retardation, cataracts, and iris abnormalities are common findings in mongolism. This congenital defect is due to a chromosomal abnormality in which there is a trisomy of the 21 chromosome pair, resulting in a total of 47 chromosomes. Apparently the extra chromosome is due to a nondisjunction of a pair of chromosomes of the ovum. That old ova may be more prone to nondisjunction explains the fact that the average age of women bearing mongoloid infants tends to be about 10 years above the random average childbearing age. Patients with mongolism typically have mental retardation, small skulls, and abnormalities of the eyelids. In contrast to persons of the Mongolian race, patients with mongolism characteristically have a short, wide palpebral fissure that is positioned obliquely in an upward and outward direction. Large bilateral epicanthal folds are present, along with a flat face and small nose with a depressed bridge. The ears are malformed, the tongue is thick, and the hands are small and have a transverse straight line formed across the palm. Hypogenitalism is frequent, and congenital heart defects occur.

Between the ages of 1 and 10 years, approximately 75% of all patients with mongolism develop a cataract characterized by small whitish flecks or rounded opacities in the adolescent nucleus (punctate cataract). Opacity of the anterior Y suture is also often present.

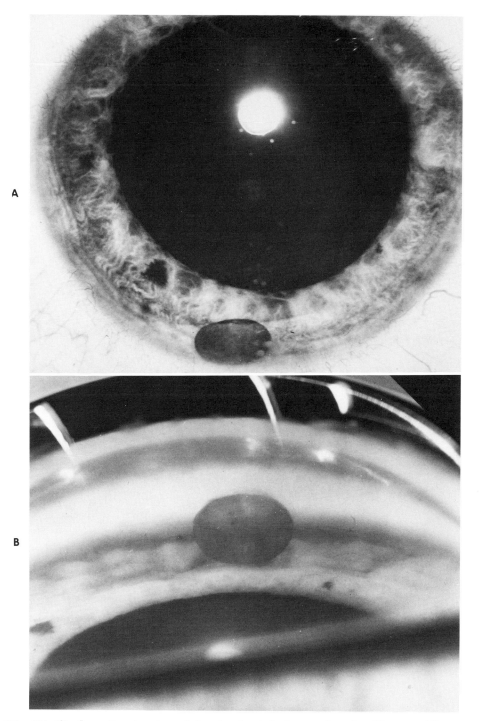

Fig. 77. *Oval cystic structure lying in the inferior angle of a 29-year-old woman with a free-floating iris cyst.* **A,** The cyst is only partially visible and is light brown due to its surface being covered with an irregular brownish pigment. **B,** By gonioscopy the cyst can be seen lying in the inferior angle. It moves freely with change of position of the patient's head.

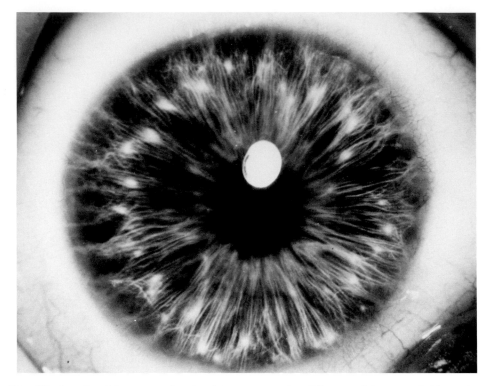

Fig. 78. *Small white spots in the iris stroma of a 25-year-old mongoloid patient with Brushfield's spots.* About 20 well-delineated spots are in the midzone of the blue iris, which exhibits a moderate degree of hypoplasia.

Approximately 85% of all patients with mongolism have white spots (Brushfield's spots) that form a ring on the anterior surface of the iris. These represent condensations of iris stroma and are frequently associated with a hypoplasia of the peripheral iris. They are more distinct, more numerous, and closer to the pupillary margin than are the similar-appearing opacities sometimes seen in normal persons (Kruckmann-Wölfflin bodies).

Brushfield's spots in mongolism

History. This 25-year-old mongoloid patient has no ocular complaints.

Findings. The patient's I.Q. is 17. Both eyes are blue and are normal except for the iris, which exhibits about 20 small, well-delineated white spots in the anterior stroma. These are in the midzone of the iris and have an appearance of

FIG. 78 dense stromal tissue. (Fig. 78). The peripheral iris is dark blue and exhibits a moderate degree of iris hypoplasia. The lens contains a number of fine punctate cortical opacities.

Course. The patient was lost to follow-up.

Brushfield's spots in mongolism

History. This 5-year-old mongoloid patient has no ocular complaints.

Findings. The patient's I.Q. is 42. The eyes appear to be normal except for

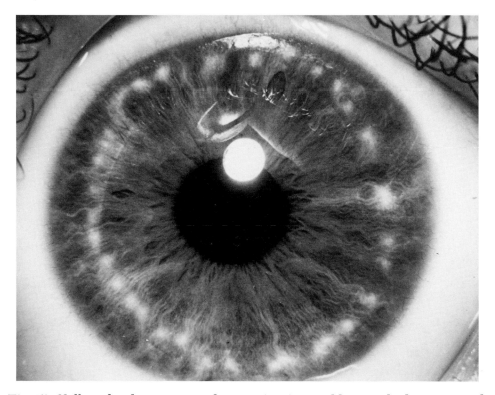

Fig. 79. *Yellowish white spots in the iris of a 5-year-old mongoloid patient with Brushfield's spots.* About 35 spots are distributed in a ring formation in the anterior stroma of a brown iris.

the irides, which are brown and exhibit about 35 yellowish white spots that appear to be condensations of the anterior iris stroma (Fig. 79). These spots FIG. 79 are distributed in a ring formation at the outer portion of the middle third of the iris. The lens is clear.

Course. The patient was lost to follow-up.

ALBINISM

Decrease or absence of melanin in the skin, hair, and eyes, associated with pendular nystagmus, characterizes oculocutaneous albinism. Inheritance is an autosomal recessive trait, and the basic defect is a partial or total reduction of melanin deposition within melanosomes. The defect is in the enzymatic conversion of the amino acid tyrosine to melanin. Ocular albinism is a condition in which the congenital hypomelanosis is limited to the eye; the metabolic defect is unknown. Inheritance is generally a sex-linked recessive trait.

In both types of albinism the outstanding ocular finding is a marked pendular nystagmus, presumably due to a congenitally defective macula. The visual acuity is very poor. Myopia and astigmatism are common. A diagnostic finding is iris translucency by scleral transillumination, due to thinned or absent iris pigment epithelium. It is interesting that a parent of an albino may also show some degree of hypopigmentation of the skin and partial translucency of the iris without any other ocular defect. Histopathologically, the eyes appear normal except for absence of uveal melanocytes and a marked hypopigmentation of the retinal pigment epithelium.

Treatment of the albino is universally unrewarding. Glasses incorporating temporal shields for use out of doors make the patient more comfortable but do not improve the vision. Opaque scleral contact lenses with only a central clear aperture have not improved the vision or decreased the nystagmus.

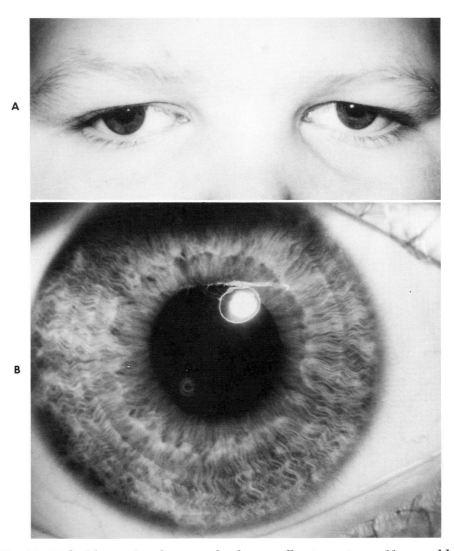

Fig. 80. *Light blue irides that completely transilluminate in an 11-year-old boy with oculocutaneous albinism.* **A,** The patient's complexion is very light, and he has light brown hair. **B,** The irides are normal in appearance and are very light blue. **C,** Transillumination reveals complete transmission of the red reflex except for the sphincter. **D,** Transillumination of the mother's irides shows transmission of the red reflex except for the sphincter and an iris nevus. The patient had markedly decreased vision, with a pendular nystagmus.

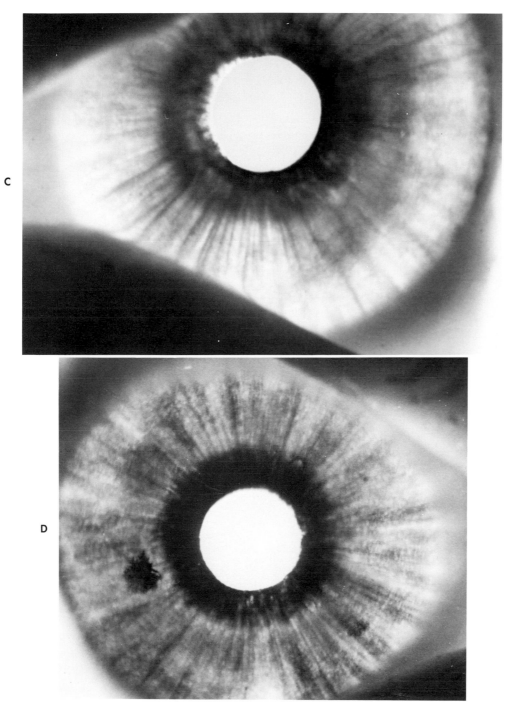

Fig. 80, cont'd. For legend see opposite page.

Oculocutaneous albinism

History. Shortly after birth this 11-year-old boy was noted to have nystagmus and poor vision. Recently the patient had diplopia and was found to have an exotropia. Examination of the boy's mother showed that she had good vision and no nystagmus, but on transillumination of her irides the red reflex was seen in all except the sphincter region (Fig. 80, *D*). Her skin was normally pigmented, and she had dark brown hair.

Findings. The vision in both eyes is about 20/300. The patient's complexion FIG. 80 is very light, and he has light brown hair (Fig. 80, *A*). The extraocular movements are full, and there is an exotropia. There is a pendular nystagmus in all directions of gaze. The iris is light blue and has a normal appearance (Fig. 80,

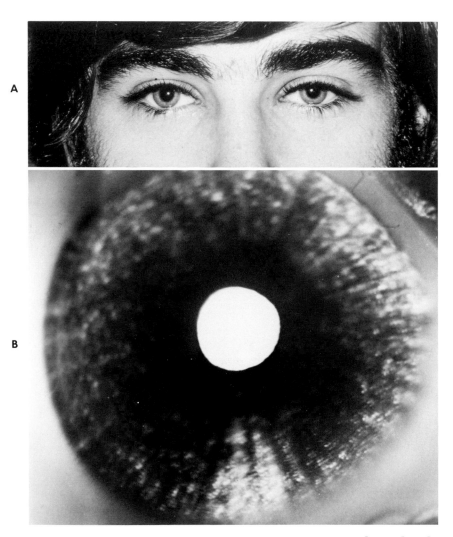

Fig. 81. *Light blue irides and partial transillumination of the red reflex in a 20-year-old man with ocular albinism.* **A,** The skin is moderately pigmented and the hair dark brown. **B,** There is a moderate degree of absence of pigment epithelium shown by scleral transillumination. The patient has a constant pendular nystagmus, decreased vision, and a pale fundus.

B). On transillumination of the irides there is complete transmission of the red reflex except in the sphincter region (Fig. 80, *C*). The fundi are normal.

Ocular albinism

History. Since infancy this 20 year old man had a searching type of nystagmus. At age 2 he was examined under general anesthesia and found to have a markedly tessellated fundus typical of albinism. The vision in both eyes remained poor. No one else in the family had a similar ocular defect.

Findings. The patient's hair is dark brown and the skin moderately pigmented (Fig. 81, *A*). The vision in both eyes is 20/200. There is a constant FIG. 81 pendular nystagmus in all directions of gaze, which is converted to a jerk nystagmus on extreme lateral conjugate gaze. The anterior segments are normal except for the irides, which are light blue and show a moderate degree of absence of pigment epithelium by scleral transillumination (Fig. 81, *B*). The peripheral iris transilluminates almost completely, while the sphincter region is opaque. The fundi are light, and the choroidal circulation is easily visible. In the macular region there appears to be no pigment epithelium, and there is no foveal reflex.

Course. Refraction indicated that the patient needed a small myopic astigmatic correction, which improved his vision to 20/100 in each eye.

RIEGER'S SYNDROME

Hypoplasia of the iris, abnormalities of the iridocorneal angle, bilaterality of ocular defects, and usually dental defects comprise the findings now generally referred to as Rieger's syndrome (dysgenesis mesodermalis of the iris). The iris defects may be limited to hypoplasia of the stroma, with a normal pupil; but more commonly (in at least 75% of the cases) there is marked hypoplasia, and atrophy of the iris and angle anomalies occur almost universally. The iris changes may result in a corectopia, polycoria, or dyscoria. Occasionally the iris abnormalities are so marked that only a few residual remnants of iris tissue remain. Posterior embryotoxon (Axenfeld's anomaly) is a common associated finding. The angle anomalies are highly variable, ranging from minimal changes, as seen in primary congenital glaucoma, to extensive fibrous adhesions and abnormal tissue obscuring the normal angle structures. The cornea may have an ill-defined limbal region.

The most common dental anomaly is associated with hypoplasia of the maxilla and gives the impression of prognathism. Because of this hypoplasia, the maxillary incisors and second bicuspids are the teeth that are most frequently absent. In addition, microdontia, enamel hypoplasia, and peg or conical teeth may be present. Although it is not universally accepted that dental anomalies are a part of the syndrome, in most affected families they are a prominent feature. The condition is inherited as an autosomal dominant trait. The primary pathogenesis is an early disturbance of mesodermal differentiation, which subsequently causes incomplete or disturbed cleavage.

Treatment of ocular abnormalities is primarily concerned with glaucoma, which develops in well over half of the patients with Rieger's syndrome. Generally, the onset of glaucoma occurs within the first 2 decades, but occasionally it is congenital. Medical therapy may be sufficient; but various types of glaucoma operations, including filtering procedures and goniotomies, may be necessary to control the tension. Recent reports indicate that goniotomy is seldom of value and that external trabeculectomy may be the treatment of choice. Generally, glaucoma in Rieger's syndrome is easier to control than congenital glaucoma. Rarely, there is some progression of the iris defects after birth; in this instance, Rieger's syndrome may be confused with bilateral essential iris atrophy (p. 214).

Rieger's syndrome

History. This 32-year-old man had no complaints except for slight blurring of vision in the left eye.

Findings. Vision in the right eye is 20/15 and in the left 20/40. In both eyes the corneas are clear and the anterior chambers deep. Both irides are flat, and the stroma is markedly hypoplastic, making the sphincter muscle readily visible. The pupils are irregular and somewhat ovoid. The posterior segments are normal. Gonioscopy shows a marked persistence of uveal meshwork and an anterior REEL IX-5 insertion of the iris in some places (Reel IX-5). Elsewhere the angle is unusually deep and contains tortuous blood vessels. Tension as revealed by applanation tonometry is 28 mm. Hg in the right eye and 30 mm. Hg in the left. The profile of the face shows a small premaxilla, giving the appearance of prognathism. The patient has congenital absence of the permanent maxillary anterior and second bicuspid teeth.

Course. Pilocarpine (2%) drops were initiated, and the intraocular pressure was promptly reduced to 14 mm. Hg as revealed by applanation tonometry. Other members of the family were examined, and all three of the patient's sons were found to have abnormal irides and a hypoplastic premaxilla with associated dental abnormalities. The patient's 7½-year old son had temporally displaced FIG. 82 pupils and an elliptical opening extending nasally (Fig. 82, A). He also had glaucoma in one eye. The 10-year-old son had extremely hypoplastic irides, with a temporally displaced pupil and a total loss of iris inferiorly. In addition, there were extensive peripheral anterior synechias adjacent to the iris defects (Fig. 82, B). The intraocular pressure in both eyes was elevated but with pilocarpine drops was reduced to normal range. The third son, 9 years of age, had such hypoplastic irides that only about 10% of the iris remained in his right eye and 25% in his left. He did not have glaucoma. Two daughters and the mother were normal, but a paternal uncle and grandmother had similar ocular and dental abnormalities.

CONGENITAL ANIRIDIA

A congenital and usually hereditary partial absence of the iris characterizes congenital aniridia. It is a relatively rare condition in which the iris is extremely rudimentary. The term aniridia is correct only in the clinical sense, for a short stump of the iris is always hidden behind the corneoscleral margin. In true aniridia the cornea is of normal size and curvature, the lens is normal, and the rim of iris and concentric zonule are visible all around. In a very few patients the visual acuity is normal; but in the majority it is poor, and there is nystagmus and absence of the foveal reflex.

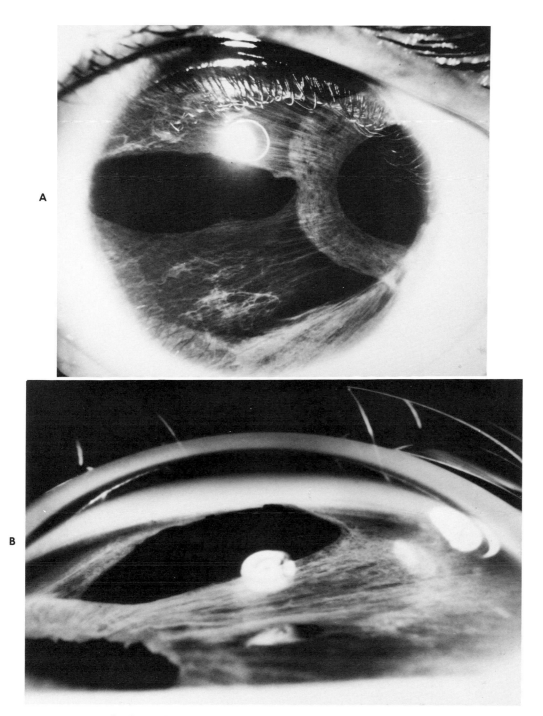

Fig. 82. *Marked iris hypoplasia, displacement of pupils, and anterior chamber angle anomalies in a family with Rieger's syndrome.* The premaxilla of all the involved members of the family is hypoplastic. The father (see Reel IX-5) has hypoplastic irides, with persistence of the uveal meshwork seen gonioscopically. Glaucoma is present in both eyes. **A,** The 7½-year-old son has temporally displaced pupils and a total absence of iris stroma nasally. Glaucoma is present in one eye. **B,** The 10-year-old son has displaced pupils and irides that are extremely hypoplastic. Gonioscopy reveals extensive peripheral anterior synechias. He has glaucoma in both eyes. The mother and two daughters are normal, but other relatives of the father have similar ocular and dental abnormalities.

In the region of the corneoscleral junction there is a short stump of iris often adhering to the posterior surface of the cornea. This adherence may interfere with the function of Schlemm's canal and explains the extreme likelihood that patients with congenital aniridia will develop glaucoma in middle life and sometimes earlier. The clump of iris present consists of ectodermal and mesodermal elements. The condition is usually bilateral but often of different degrees in the two eyes, and it has an irregular dominant hereditary pattern. A small but very significant number of patients with Wilms' tumor have aniridia.

Partial aniridia

History. This 9-year-old girl was seen because of headaches. Her parents had been aware of a defect of the iris of her left eye. Three of the six children in her family had iris defects. Her father was said to have a similar condition.

Findings. Vision in the right eye is 20/40 and in the left 20/70 with correction. In the right eye the iris is hypoplastic throughout, and there are areas inferiorly and temporally in which only pigment epithelium remains. The pupil is eccentric

FIG. 83   and slightly displaced superiorly and nasally (Fig. 83, *A*). In the left eye the remaining iris also appears hypoplastic, but in addition there is a total loss of iris temporally almost to the angle (Fig. 83, *B*). Only about half of the sphincter remains, and that is hypoplastic. In both eyes the lenses are clear, but there is a poor macular reflex, with excessive pigmentation in the macular region. Intraocular pressure in both eyes is 20 mm. Hg (Schiøtz).

Course. The patient was lost to follow-up.

Partial aniridia

History. This 10-year-old girl with no ocular symptoms was seen because her 9-year-old sister was having headaches and was found to have partial aniridia (Fig. 83). Her brother had a similar condition, but three other siblings are normal. Her father was also said to have the same eye condition.

Findings. Vision in both eyes is 20/60. In the right eye the iris is grossly

FIG. 84   abnormal, with the entire central area devoid of iris tissue (Fig. 84, *A*). Only a small portion of the sphincter remains superiorly, with some strands stretching across the central area to a small amount of the remaining iris inferiorly. In addition, there is some pigment epithelium remaining temporally. The left eye has similar findings in the iris except that the hypoplasia is slightly less pronounced (Fig. 84, *B*). The lens is clear, but there is a poor macular reflex. Intraocular pressure is 23 mm. Hg (Schiøtz) in both eyes.

Course. The patient was lost to follow-up.

Partial aniridia

History. This 13-year-old boy was seen because his two sisters had partial aniridia (Figs. 83 and 84). The father was said to have a similar condition.

Findings. Vision in both eyes is 20/70 without correction. In the right eye there is an absence of all the iris except for a stump in some locations extending in

FIG. 85   about 1 mm. from the limbus (Fig. 85, *A*). In the left eye the iris is absent temporally; nasally there is marked hypoplasia with only pigment epithelium remain-

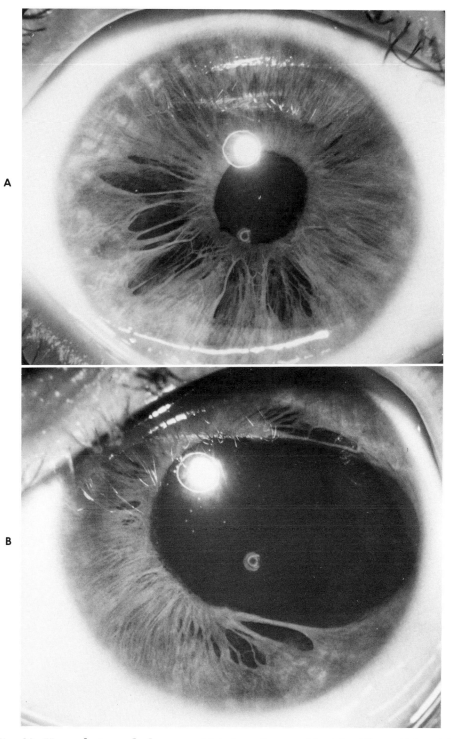

Fig. 83. *Hypoplasia and absence of iris in a 9-year-old girl with partial aniridia.*
A, In the right eye the pupil is eccentric and the iris stroma irregularly thinned.
B, In the left eye most of the temporal iris is absent, and the remaining iris is
hypoplastic. Three of the six siblings in the family have iris defects.

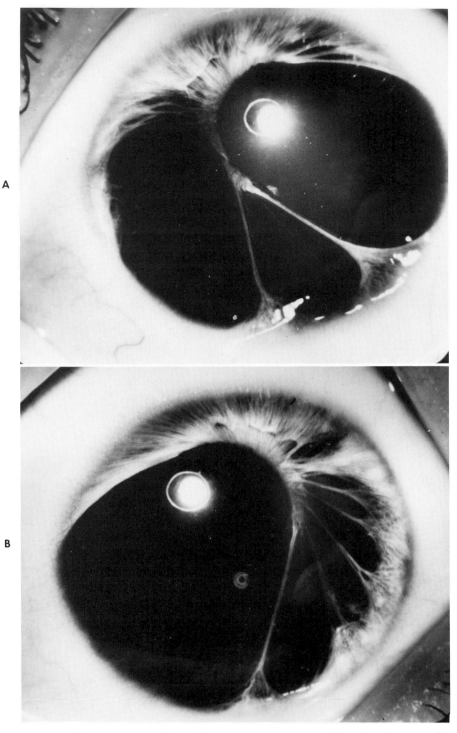

Fig. 84. *Absence of much of the iris in a 10-year-old girl with partial aniridia.* Her 9-year-old sister (Fig. 83) has less marked iris defects. **A,** In the right eye most of the iris is absent, with strands of iris tissue stretching across the central area. **B,** In the left eye some markedly hypoplastic iris remains temporally and superiorly, but elsewhere it is absent.

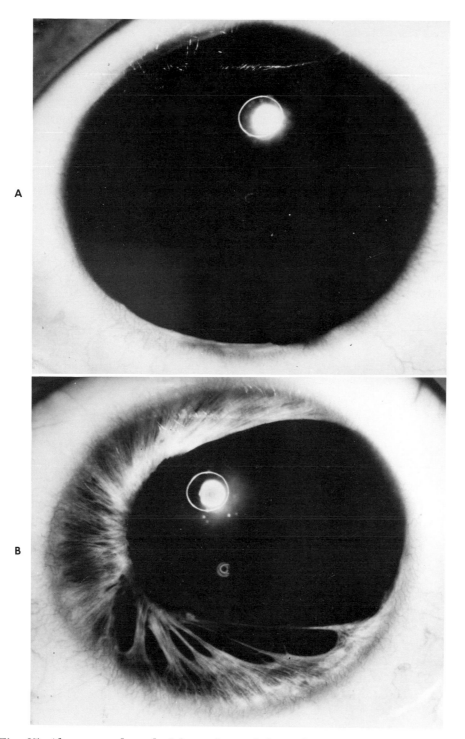

Fig. 85. *Absence and marked hypoplasia of the irides in a 13-year-old boy with partial aniridia.* His two sisters (Figs. 83 and 84) are similarly affected. **A,** In the right eye only a stump of iris is visible at the limbus in some areas. **B,** In the left eye there is absence of the iris temporally and marked hypoplasia nasally.

ing in some areas (Fig. 85, *B*). The lenses are clear, and the fundus is normal except for a poor macular reflex.

Course. The patient was lost to follow-up.

Aniridia

History. At birth this 5-year-old boy was noted to have aniridia and a convergent strabismus. About a year and a half ago he was found to be nearsighted and was given corrective lenses. There was no family history of aniridia.

Findings. Vision in both eyes is about 8/150. Both eyes show a gross pendular nystagmus in all directions of gaze, and there is a variable esotropia. A small amount of iris root is visible temporally, and the lenses are dislocated superiorly FIG. 86 so that about a third of the corneal aperture is aphakic (Fig. 86). The lenses are clear, and the fundi can be visualized with the indirect ophthalmoscope and appear to be normal.

Course. There was gradual opacification of the lens of the left eye, and a secondary galucoma developed. Subsequently, a total retinal detachment was found, and 8 years later a trabeculectomy and lens aspiration were performed on the left eye. It was planned to perform retinal detachment surgery in the near future.

Aniridia

History. At birth this 16-year-old boy was found to have aniridia identical in appearance to that of his father. Later it was found that he also had myopia and had developed a pendular nystagmus. At 9 months of age he was found to have borderline intraocular pressures, and administration of pilocarpine drops was

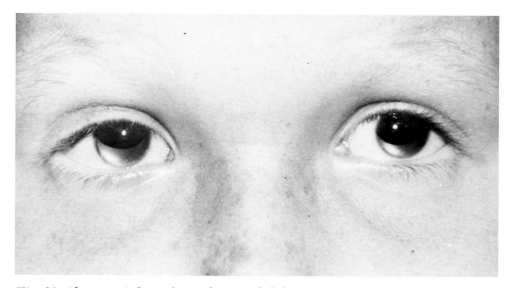

Fig. 86. *Absence of the irides and upward dislocation of the lenses in a 5-year-old boy with aniridia.* A stump of iris is visible temporally in both eyes, and the lenses are dislocated so that the lower one third of the corneal aperture is aphakic.

instituted. Since then he has continued to use drops, and intraocular tensions were no higher than the teens. Three years ago he was noted to have early cataracts.

Findings. Vision in both eyes is counting fingers at 5 feet. There is rapid pendular nystagmus in all directions of gaze. In both eyes there is no iris visible, and the lenses show posterior and some anterior subcapsular opacities as well as peripheral spokes. There also appears to be slight upward dislocation of the lens in the left eye. The right disc is normal, but the left shows moderate cupping of questionable glaucomatous type. Gonioscopy shows that there is a stump of iris remaining to a variable degree around the entire circumference of the angle, with open angle in some places (Reel IX-6). The ciliary processes are easily visible immediately beneath the stump of iris. Tension by applanation tonometry is 16 mm. Hg in both eyes.

REEL IX-6

CONGENITAL HORNER'S SYNDROME

Miosis, ptosis, ipsilateral anhidrosis, apparent enophthalmos, and heterochromia characterize congenital Horner's syndrome. Depigmentation of the iris occurs for unknown reasons and is especially prominent in deeply pigmented irides. The condition may be idiopathic or due to birth injury. Except for the depigmentation of the iris on the involved side, the syndrome is similar to that of the acquired type (p. 179). The ptosis, which is due to paralysis of Müller's muscle in the eyelids, is slight compared with that resulting from paralysis associated with third nerve involvement. In the congenital type it is sometimes almost undetectable. The miosis is maximal immediately after the sympathetic nerve has been sectioned and within a few days the enervated iris dilates slightly due to increased sensitivity to epinephrine. The pupillary reaction to epinephrine and cocaine is diagnostic (p. 180).

Congenital Horner's syndrome

History. Since birth this 3-year-old boy's left eye had a blepharoptosis and a miotic pupil. More recently it was noted that the eyes were of a different color. At birth the patient had been delivered with forceps, which resulted in a scar on the left side of his neck.

Findings. The patient appears to have good vision in both eyes. The right eye is normal, with a brown iris. In the left eye there is a slight ptosis, the iris is light blue, and the pupil is about half the size of the right pupil (Fig. 87). The remainder of the examination reveals no other abnormalities.

FIG. 87

Course. When the boy was seen 4 years later, the ocular findings were unchanged.

MICROCORIA (CONGENITAL MIOSIS)

Congenital abnormally small pupils characterize microcoria. The pupils respond slightly if at all to light and to mydriatic drugs. They do not dilate when the patient is looking at a distant object in dim illumination. The iris is lacking the normal circular contraction folds. The failure of the pupils to react to strong mydriatic drugs and the lack of other abnormalities should differentiate congenital miosis from the miosis due to a sympathetic lesion as in Horner's syndrome.

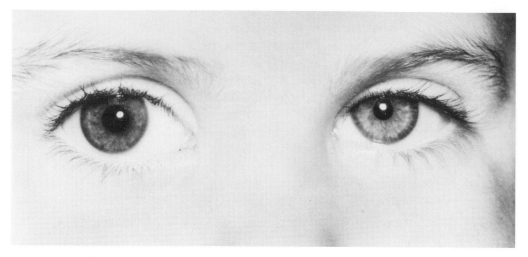

Fig. 87. *Light blue iris in the left eye of a 3-year-old boy with congenital Horner's syndrome.* In contrast to the left iris, the right iris is brown. There is a slight ptosis of the left eye, and the pupil is relatively miotic. At birth there was a forceps injury to the left side of the neck.

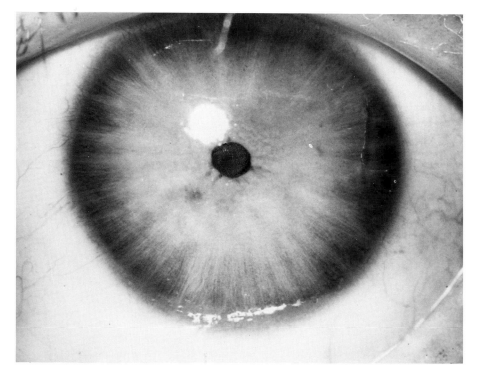

Fig. 88. *Markedly miotic pupils in a 24-year-old man with microcoria.* The pupils react slightly to light and do not dilate with instillation of cyclopentolate. Presumably he was born with this abnormality and also has cardiac lesions and congenital cervical abnormalities.

Microcoria (congenital miosis)

History. For as long as he can remember this 24-year-old man had small pupils. In addition, he was found to have a congenital fusion of the cervical vertebrae and a cardiac lesion diagnosed as fibroelastosis with heart block.

Findings. Vision is 20/30 in each eye. The eyes are normal in all respects except for the pupils, the right one being about 1 mm. and the left 0.5 mm. in size. (Fig. 88). The pupils react very slightly to light (both direct and consensual). With cyclopentolate instillation the pupils do not dilate, but the reaction to light is abolished. Neither 4% cocaine nor 1:1000 epinephrine drops produce any change in the pupils.

Course. One month later the patient died because of cardiac failure.

FIG. 88

CONGENITAL MELANOSIS OCULI AND NEVUS OF OTA

Excessive melanin pigmentation of the episclera and uvea characterizes congenital melanosis oculi. If the additional feature of periorbital skin pigmentation is present, the condition is referred to as the nevus of Ota. Usually evident at birth, these conditions may be transmitted as a weak dominant trait. By slit-lamp examination the discoloration of the bulbar conjunctiva can be seen to be deep to the conjunctiva, in the episclera. In addition, the iris on the involved side is usually a dark brown color; and when the other iris is blue, there is a marked contrast. The entire fundus also appears darker on the involved side due to the excessive choroidal pigmentation. The retina is never affected.

When the periorbital skin and occasionally the distribution of the entire first and second divisions of the trigeminal nerve are pigmented, the condition is referred to as the nevus of Ota (oculodermal melanocytosis). Both congenital melanosis oculi and the nevus of Ota are almost invariably unilateral; rare cases of bilateral involvement have been described. Congenital melanosis oculi may be confused with congenital conjunctival melanosis, which is also present at birth. The latter is characterized by brown pigmentation and can be seen by slit-lamp examination to be in the conjunctiva rather than to be the bluish discoloration deep to the conjunctiva.

Complications of congenital melanosis oculi are pigmentary glaucoma and malignant melanoma of the choroid. Although both of these conditions are relatively rare, adults having congenital melanosis oculi or nevus of Ota should be examined periodically.

Congenital melanosis oculi

History. Since birth this 42-year-old woman had a dark spot on her left eye. This did not change, and she was asymptomatic except for the presence of multiple chalazia.

Findings. The vision in both eyes is 20/20, and the right eye is normal. In the left eye there is a bluish pigmentation starting at the limbus and extending almost to the inferior cul de sac from the 4 o'clock to the 8 o'clock position (Reel IX-7). By slit-lamp biomicroscopy this is seen to be mostly deep to the conjunctiva, in the episclera. The lower half of the iris is a velvety dark brown in contrast to the upper half, which is a yellowish brown. The pupil is round and reacts normally. The posterior segment is normal.

REEL IX-7

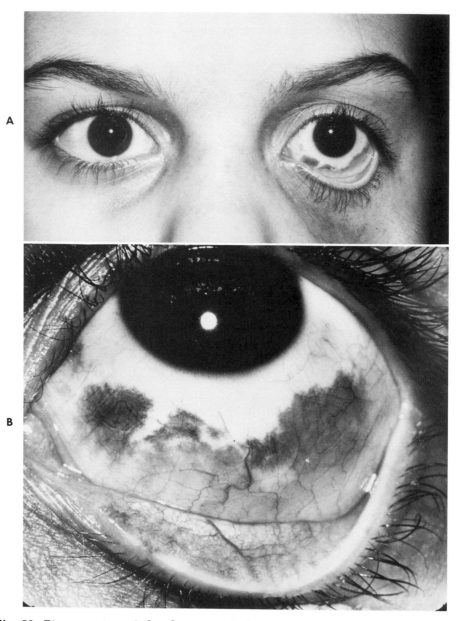

Fig. 89. *Pigmentation of the skin around the left eye, bluish discoloration of the left sclera, and a darkly pigmented left iris in an 11-year-old girl with nevus of Ota (oculodermal melanocytosis).* The abnormal pigmentation was present at birth and has not changed.

Course. Four years later the findings were identical to those seen earlier.

Nevus of Ota (oculodermal melanocytosis)

History. At birth this 11-year-old girl had spots on her left eye. At 5 years of age the lids of the left eye darkened. She was entirely asymptomatic.

Findings. The right eye is normal and has a light brown iris. The skin around the left eye is more darkly pigmented than the rest of the face (Fig. 89, *A*). FIG. 89 There is a bluish discoloration of the lower portion of the globe, which is seen best when the patient is looking upward (Fig. 89, *B*). By slit-lamp examination this irregular splotchy pigmentation is in the sclera or episclera deep to the conjunctiva. The iris is dark brown and lacks the clearly defined crypt formation seen in the right eye.

Chapter 6

Systemic diseases affecting the iris

DIABETES MELLITUS

Cataract formation and neovascularization of the iris and its complications in association with diabetes are a common finding in the anterior segment, while retinopathy is common in the posterior segment. Since significant changes in blood glucose levels affect lens hydration and refractive power, blurring of vision may be the first sign of diabetes. The usual finding is myopia. In the young diabetic patient who develops a true diabetic cataract, flocculent white "snowflake" cortical opacities are almost pathognomonic for diabetes. Rapid progression to a mature cataract is common. In the older diabetic patient the cataract is of the senile type but begins earlier in life than in the senile individual without diabetes.

Rubeosis iridis is usually associated with a preexisting diabetic retinopathy. It is characterized by a peripupillary wreath of small vessels and a similar wreath peripherally with connections between the two. A delicate vascular membrane derived from the iris stroma develops; this condition explains the later development of an ectropion uveae upon contraction of the membrane. Profuse neovascularization on the root of the iris frequently infiltrates the angle structures and results in severe glaucoma, presumably due to obliteration of the outflow channels. Occasionally these blood vessels bleed, initiating a spontaneous hyphema. Diabetic retinopathy, usually the earliest ocular finding in diabetes, is characterized by punctate hemorrhages or true microaneurysms on the venous side of the retinal capillaries. Later, hard or waxy exudates appear, and cotton wool patches, hemorrhages, and neovascularization also occur. In rare instances, the milky-appearing vessels of the lipemia retinalis may be seen without diabetic retinopathy.

Rubeosis iridis is also seen in association with retinal venous occlusion. Again, rubeosis of the trabecular meshwork occurs with a secondary glaucoma due to an impaired facility of outflow. Glaucoma usually occurs about 3 months after the occlusion. Subsequently, peripheral anterior synechias also close the angle. Sometimes preexisting open angle glaucoma is responsible for precipitation of the vein occlusion, after which the glaucoma becomes more severe. In such instances the opposite eye is also usually found to have open angle glaucoma.

Diabetic rubeosis

History. For 15 years this 39-year-old man had diabetes mellitus for which he was treated with insulin. Two and a half years ago he had "iritis" in the right eye and 2 years ago a retinal hemorrhage in the left eye. About a week ago he noted redness of the left eye without pain. Yesterday examination revealed a tension of 80 mm. Hg (Schiøtz) in the left eye, and he was treated intensively with miotics and acetazolamide.

Findings. The vision in both eyes is 20/100. In the right eye the anterior segment is normal except for early peripheral rubeosis of the iris. The media, including the vitreous, are clear; but there is marked diabetic retinopathy, with neovascularization of the disc, peripapillary hemorrhages, and multiple small retinal hemorrhages throughout the fundus. In the left eye there is moderate conjunctival injection and marked neovascularization of the entire iris, with a prominent ectropion uveae (Fig. 90). Here, too, the media are clear; but there FIG. 90 is extensive neovascularization of the disc, with multiple retinal hemorrhages

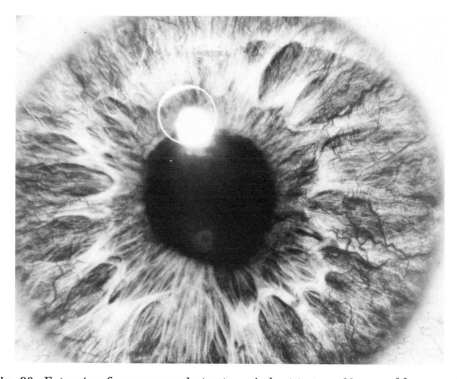

Fig. 90. *Extensive fine neovascularization of the iris in a 39-year-old man with diabetic rubeosis.* The entire iris is involved with numerous fine blood vessels. Ectropion uveae and angle neovascularization are also present. Extensive diabetic retinopathy is a prominent feature.

throughout the fundus. Gonioscopy reveals fine vascularization of the entire trabecular meshwork in an otherwise normal wide-open angle. The left eye is more extensively involved than the right, with one small peripheral anterior synechia. The intraocular pressure is 13 mm. Hg (Schiøtz) in the right eye and 20 mm. Hg (Schiøtz) in the left.

Course. Less intensive use of miotics resulted in a marked elevation of the intraocular pressure in the left eye. Subsequently, even though he was receiving miotics, the patient's intraocular pressure was uncontrolled, and bullous keratopathy developed. A vitreous hemorrhage then occurred in the right eye. A thermal cautery (Scheie) filtering procedure was performed on the left eye. Postoperatively, despite recurrent bleeding into the anterior chamber, a large filtering bleb formed. However, the filtering procedure did not control the intraocular pressure, and 6 weeks later four points of penetrating cyclodiathermy were applied to the left eye. Postoperatively the intraocular pressure remained in the teens in both eyes, but within 2 months it had risen to the 40's. Additional cyclodiathermy points were applied. Within a year there was evidence of massive vitreous retraction in the right eye, with light perception only and a markedly elevated intraocular pressure. The left eye was blind and was evidently becoming phthisical.

Diabetic rubeosis

History. Since the age of 4 this 23-year-old girl had diabetes. Recently the vision became markedly reduced in each eye due to diabetic retinopathy. The patient also developed a markedly elevated intraocular pressure in her right eye. Two months ago a cyclodiathermy procedure was carried out.

Findings. The vision in both eyes is hand movements. In the right eye the iris is uniformly infiltrated with numerous tortuous vessels, and there is an ectropion uveae extending around the entire pupillary border about ½ mm. in width. The lens is clear, but there is marked diabetic retinopathy, with extensive retinitis proliferans. Gonioscopy reveals neovascularization of the iris extending to the angle and almost total peripheral anterior synechia formation except in a few areas where there is a marked pigmentation of the trabecular REEL X-1 meshwork (Reel X-1). The intraocular pressure is 48 mm. Hg (Schiøtz). In the left eye the findings are similar to those of the right except that the rubeosis is less marked and the intraocular pressure is borderline.

Course. The patient was lost to follow-up.

Diabetic atrophy of iris pigment epithelium

History. About a year ago this 52-year-old woman noticed blurring of vision in both eyes. She then developed cellulitis in her right foot and was found to have diabetes. With treatment of her diabetes the cellulitis promptly cleared, but her visual loss persisted. Two weeks ago she was first seen by an ophthalmologist, who found an intraocular pressure of 80 mm. Hg (Schiøtz), along with marked retinal diabetic changes, in the left eye. Treatment was instituted with acetazolamide and epinephrine (1%) drops.

Findings. The vision in the right eye is 20/100 and in the left counting fingers at 6 feet. In both eyes the corneas are clear and the anterior chambers deep.

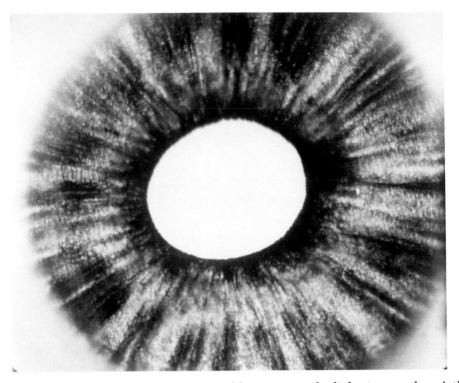

Fig. 91. *Iris translucency in a 52-year-old woman with diabetic atrophy of the iris pigment epithelium.* Transillumination of the irides reveals a number of radial red streaks in the iris due to the transmission of the red reflex of the fundus. Marked diabetic retinopathy and glaucomatous cupping are present.

Gonioscopy shows early vascularization of some of the trabecular meshwork in the right eye and total vascularization of the meshwork in the left. The pupil in the right eye is round, but the pupil in the left is ovoid. By transillumination both irides show marked loss of pigment epithelium, with radial streaks of red reflex extending from the sphincter out to the periphery of the iris (Fig. 91). FIG. 91 The fundi show neovascularization of both discs and many hemorrhages and exudates out to the equator. In the left eye there is marked cupping of the disc. The intraocular pressure in the right eye is 12 mm. Hg and in the left 23 mm. Hg (Schiøtz).

Course. A corneal trephine procedure was performed on the left eye. Postoperatively there was bleeding, and a bleb failed to form. A fibrin clot formed in the region of the operation, and it appeared that the iris was being pulled up into the trephine opening by the fibrin. Three small cryotherapeutic applications were applied to the operative area, and with massage the bleb gradually formed over the next 5 days. During the next 6 months the intraocular pressure was under fair control in both eyes with the patient receiving miotics and epinephrine drops, but the diabetic retinopathy steadily progressed. A year later the left eye was very soft, with light perception only, while vision in the right continued to be counting fingers. Three years later vision in the right eye was only hand movements, and there were extensive vitreous changes; there was no light perception in the left eye, which had a partially opaque cornea.

CYSTINOSIS

Sparkling fine crystals in the cornea, conjunctiva, and rarely in the iris and choroid represent the ocular findings in cystinosis. An inborn error of metabolism, cystinosis is usually transmitted as an autosomal recessive trait. A number of amino acids may be abnormally metabolized; but cystine, being the least soluble, is deposited in various tissues of the body, including the cornea and conjunctiva.

Such patients are dwarfed and suffer from anorexia, vomiting, and constipation. Early findings are glycosuria, aminoaciduria, and hypokalemia. Later they develop renal tubular disease with renal failure. There is no known treatment, and affected children usually die within the first decade of life.

The corneas are almost pathognomonic for cystinosis, multiple myeloma being the only other condition with a similar appearance. Grossly, the cornea exhibits a generalized clouding if extensively involved. In the earlier stages, slit-lamp biomicroscopy is necessary for the diagnosis. There are numerous, slightly angular, sparkling crystals in the anterior stroma centrally but involving all layers peripherally. The conjunctiva shows many crystals, which tend to accumulate around blood vessels under the epithelium, frequently in clumps, as opposed to the uniform distribution in the cornea. Occasionally, numerous crystals may be visible in the iris stroma and throughout the fundus, presumably in the choroid.

Cystinosis

History. At 6 months of age this 10-year-old boy was found to have anemia, and further investigation led to the diagnosis of Lignac-Fanconi syndrome (cystinosis). Except for slower than normal growth and development, he did well on treatment with vitamins and iron by mouth. His appetite was poor, and he refused to drink milk. Two years ago he became photophobic and had his first attack of tetany, for which he was treated with calcium lactate and sodium bicarbonate by mouth. About a year ago he again had tetany, and at this time he was treated with intravenous calcium gluconate. He developed cardiac failure and leg edema and was treated by digitalization. The nonprotein nitrogen level was elevated, and the blood calcium level low. A month ago he became dyspneic and was found to have hepatic enlargement, splenomegaly, and anemia.

Findings. The patient, a dwarf, has bowing of the tibias and a prominent thoracic cage. He is pale and listless and has a uremic odor. His eyelids are swollen; and because of photophobia, he keeps his eyes closed. Vision in each eye is 8/200. Slit-lamp examination shows the entire cornea and iris surface of each eye to be uniformly infiltrated with a myriad of fine, slender, shiny crystals (Reel X-2). The conjunctiva also shows the same crystalline deposits. The anterior chamber and media are normal, but fundus examination reveals the maculas to be grayish and surrounded by a pale zone.

REEL X-2

Course. The patient's right ventricular failure was treated by digitalization and his anemia by blood transfusions. The edema of the face and extremities gradually subsided. Repeated blood studies and urinalysis were consistent with cystinosis and associated renal failure. At age 11 years he died of renal failure.

SARCOIDOSIS (BOECK'S SARCOID)

Bilateral granulomatous anterior uveitis and band keratopathy are the most common ocular findings in sarcoidosis. Of unknown cause, sarcoidosis is a chronic granulomatous disease that occurs in any organ. There is widespread dissemination in the reticuloendothelial system and frequently involvement of the skin, lymph nodes, lungs, liver, spleen, bones, and eyes. The lesions are discrete, noncaseating aggregations of epithelioid cells surrounded by moderate lymphocytic infiltration. Diagnosis is sometimes difficult and may be made by exclusion; but a positive Kveim reaction, negative tuberculin skin test, and x-ray evidence of typical lung and bone lesions will usually establish the diagnosis. Exacerbations and remissions are the rule; the course is chronic, and there is occasional spontaneous and complete recovery.

The most common ocular finding is that of a bilateral anterior uveitis. The granulomatous type of mutton-fat keratic precipitates is commonly found, and the

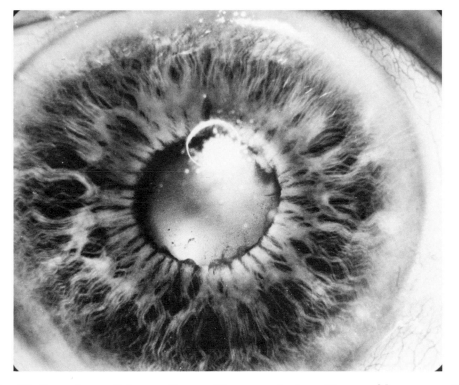

Fig. 92. *Irregular nodules on the pupillary margin in a 79-year-old woman with Koeppe nodules due to sarcoidosis.* A number of rounded nodules with a mutton-fat appearance extend into the pupillary opening. Six months ago the patient had an iritis and was found to have the typical clinical signs and laboratory findings of sarcoidosis.

presence of multiple fleshy vascularized nodules of the iris is almost pathogno-monic. Aside from the corneal involvement secondary to uveitis, band keratophy commonly results from the hypercalcemia that often accompanies sarcoidosis. When retinal involvement occurs, sarcoid nodules are seen as white perivenous infiltrates. Treatment with both topical and systemic administration of corti-costeroids is indicated for the uveitis. Systemic administration of corticosteroids is usually corrective for hypercalcemia, with resolution of the band keratopathy if it is not too advanced. Sometimes topical EDTA applications are required for the band keratopathy.

Koeppe nodules in sarcoidosis

History. About 6 months ago this 79-year-old woman developed an inflamed right eye, which on ophthalmologic examination was found to be due to an iritis. Mydriatics and topical administration of steroids were instituted, and a week later the anterior chamber reaction had subsided. A chest x-ray film showed a lobulated enlargement of the right hilum, which is compatible with sarcoid. The blood calcium level was high normal, and the sedimentation rate was elevated to 42 mm/hour. The patient had no recurrence of her iritis.

Findings. The vision in the right eye is counting fingers at 5 feet and in the left 20/40. In the right eye the anterior chamber is deep and clear, and the iris is normal except for a somewhat irregular pupil, which is fixed due to posterior synechias. At the pupillary margin are a number of small irregular nodules ex-tending into the pupillary opening (Fig. 92). Some of these have a mutton-fat appearance. An incipient cataract is present with moderate nuclear sclerosis, and fundus examination reveals a hole in the macula. In the left eye the anterior segment is normal, and there is an incipient cataract. The fundus examination reveals a pigmentary change within the macula but no hole. The intraocular pres-sure is 12 mm. Hg (Schiøtz) in both eyes.

FIG. 92

Course. Six months later there was no change in the patient's ocular status, and there were no signs of recurrent iritis.

Sarcoid uveitis

History. This 24-year-old black woman had no ocular symptoms until 5 days ago, when the left eye developed a grating sensation and became very red. Two days ago topical administration of corticosteroids and mydriatics was initiated because of iritis in the right eye. Her parotid glands were found to be enlarged.

Findings. The vision in the right eye is 20/40 and in the left 20/30. There is a moderate conjunctival injection in the right eye, and the lower half of the right cornea shows many mutton-fat keratic precipitates. The anterior chamber con-tains some cells and minimal flare. At the 5 o'clock position there is a pinkish mass extending out from the angle onto the iris, almost reaching the margin of the dilated pupil (Reel X-3). Gonioscopy shows that this mass involves the entire angle and depresses the iris posteriorly (Fig. 93). The surface of the mass is moderately pigmented. The angle is open elsewhere, and there are many nodules of exudate on the trabecular meshwork. The media are clear, and the fundus is normal. In the left eye there are a few cells and a minimal flare.

REEL X-3
FIG. 93

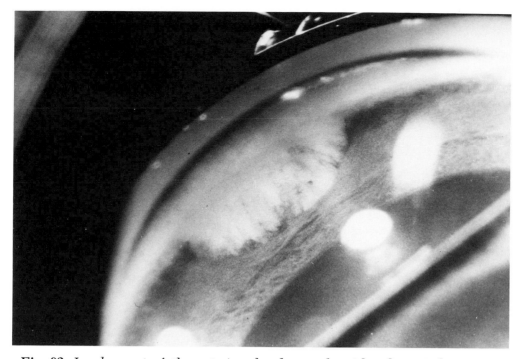

Fig. 93. *Involvement of the anterior chamber angle with a large inflammatory nodule in a 24-year-old woman with sarcoid uveitis.* By gonioscopy a pinkish mass can be seen filling the angle and extending out onto the iris, depressing it. The mass reaches almost to the pupillary margin (see Reel X-3), has a moderately pigmented surface, and is pink.

Course. The treatment was continued, and biopsy of the posterior cervical glands showed focal granulomatous disease, compatible with sarcoidosis. With systemic administration of corticosteroids the patient's ocular problems completely subsided. Chest x-ray films had shown hilar shadows, and these had also resolved. With the patient receiving corticosteroid drops daily, there were no signs of ocular difficulty 3 years later.

Sarcoid uveitis

History. About 3 years ago this 23-year-old man first noted decreased vision in his left eye and about 6 months later in his right. This was associated with some redness and pain in the eyes. Some treatment, the details of which are unknown, was carried out. Two years ago a biopsied node in his neck showed sarcoidosis. Corticosteroid drops were then instituted, with relief of his pain and redness. In the past 2 months the patient's vision became so poor that he was unable to work.

Findings. The vision in the right eye is hand movements and in the left light perception. In the right eye there is moderate conjunctival injection and an early band keratopathy. There are some mutton-type keratic precipitates, but the anterior chamber is clear. Complete posterior synechia formation (occluded pupil) and some neovascularization of the iris are present (Fig. 94). The an- FIG. 94

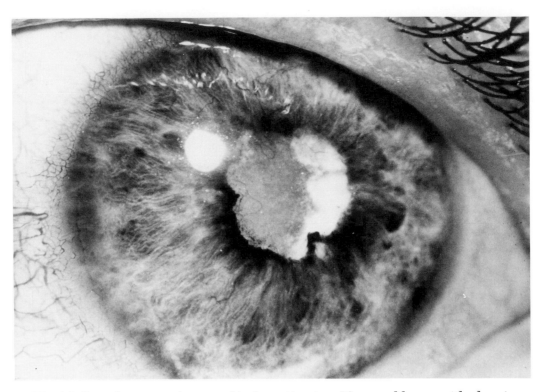

Fig. 94. *Complete posterior synechia formation in a 23-year-old man with chronic sarcoid uveitis.* The pupillary margin is completely adherent to the anterior capsule, producing an irregular pupillary opening. The lens is cataractous.

terior chamber is shallow, and there is a suggestion of iris bombé. The lens cortex is almost completely opacified, and only a dull fundus red reflex can be obtained. Findings in the left eye are similar to those in the right except for the absence of band keratopathy in the left eye. Gonioscopy reveals numerous peripheral anterior synechias and excessive vascularization of the angle. Intraocular pressure in the right eye is 16 mm. Hg (Schiøtz), and the left eye is extremely soft (phthisical).

Course. Chest x-ray films showed hilar adenopathy and nodular infiltrates typical of sarcoidosis. The patient was also found to have cervical adenopathy, and the tuberculin skin test 1:100 was negative. Six months later there were no signs of active uveitis, and an intracapsular cataract extraction was performed on the right eye. In spite of postoperative systemic administration of corticosteroids and ACTH, the anterior chamber filled with fibrin, which gradually resolved, leaving only a thin pupillary membrane through which a hazy vitreous could be seen. Three weeks postoperatively the patient had 20/200 vision, and he returned to his home in Canada. Three years later he returned with a dense pupillary membrane in the right eye. A discission was performed, which resulted in a hyphema that nearly filled the anterior chamber. The patient then returned to Canada and was lost to follow-up.

Iris nodules in Boeck's sarcoid

History. About a month ago this 38-year-old woman noticed blurring of vision in her right eye. She also noticed three "lumps" on her iris. There was no pain in the eye, and only slight redness was present. The patient's general health is good.

Findings. The vision in the right eye is 20/30 and in the left 20/20. A few mutton-fat keratic precipitates are seen in the central portion of the cornea. Three pink masses are visible at the periphery of the iris, the largest extending from the 9 o'clock to the 11 o'clock position (Reel X-4). These masses are covered   REEL X-4 with fine vessels, are irregularly rounded, and appear to push the iris backward rather than infiltrate it. By indirect ophthalmoscopy white exudates can be seen at the extreme periphery of the fundus in both eyes, but the exudates are more marked in the right. X-ray films of the chest show typical sarcoidosis of the lungs. The tuberculin skin test is negative.

Course. Examination 1 year later showed a complete resolution of the masses, with only minimal atrophy of the iris in the area of the largest nodule.

RHEUMATOID ARTHRITIS

Chronic anterior uveitis, keratoconjunctivitis sicca, and scleromalacia perforans are the important ocular conditions associated with rheumatoid arthritis. The most common of the collagen disorders, rheumatoid arthritis is a chronic systemic disease of unknown cause affecting women almost twice as often as men. Major manifestations involve many of the joints, with changes in synovial membranes, periarticular structures, cartilage, skeletal muscles, and perineural sheaths. The onset of symptoms may be insidious or abrupt, and pain in the joints of the fingers, wrists, knees, and feet is most characteristic. Exacerbations and remissions are the rule, followed by progressive permanent deformity. Chronic anterior uveitis is seen occasionally in rheumatoid arthritis, more frequently in Still's disease (chronic polyarthritis in children), and most commonly in ankylosing spondylitis (Marie-Strümpell disease). Typically, it is a recurrent iritis with a relatively mild reaction and a nongranulomatous appearance and is commonly accompanied by cataracts and band keratopathy as a late complication.

Scleromalacia perforans is a rare and serious condition associated with rheumatoid arthritis. It is always associated with long-standing rheumatoid arthritis, usually in older women, is frequently bilateral, and has a slow, gradual evolution in which subconjunctival nodules are later followed by necrosis, thinning of the anterior sclera, and finally the development of bluish ectatic areas. There is no pain or inflammatory reaction, and occasionally perforation occurs. Chronic iridocyclitis or secondary infection with endophthalmitis is rarely seen, and sometimes the eye becomes phthisical.

The least serious and the most common ocular condition associated with rheumatoid arthritis is keratoconjunctivitis sicca seen in Sjögren's syndrome. This is associated with a decrease in lacrimal and salivary secretion, with the ocular signs of photophobia, and with foreign body sensation. Shredding of the corneal epithelium and a positive Schirmer test are diagnostic. Staining of the cornea with rose bengal also shows the corneal abnormalities, in contrast to fluorescein, which does not.

Iritis with rheumatoid arthritis

History. Since she was 28 years old this 51-year-old woman had episodes of polyarticular pain, which initially lasted only a few days, leaving no joint difficulty until she was 36. For the past 15 years, however, there has been almost constant joint stiffness. Gold injections were given about 7 years ago, and the results were good. Intermittently for the past 10 years she has taken corticosteroids systemically in small amounts. About 20 years ago she had acute iritis in the right eye, lasting several months; the iritis recurred 5 years later. Response to topical administration of corticosteroids was good. About 4 years ago typical posterior subcapsular cataracts of the steroid type were observed. Two weeks ago she had another recurrence of iritis in the left eye, which responded promptly to topical administration of corticosteroids and mydriatics.

Findings. Vision in the right eye is 20/30 and in the left 20/200. The right eye is normal, but in the left there are numerous flat keratic precipitates scattered FIG. 95 throughout the lower two thirds of the cornea (Fig. 95). The anterior chamber has a minimal number of cells and a moderate flare. The pupil is widely dilated due to mydriatics. In the posterior subcapsular region of the lens is a granular discrete cataract. The fundus is normal. Intraocular pressure in the right eye is 18 mm. Hg and in the left 14 mm. Hg (Schiøtz).

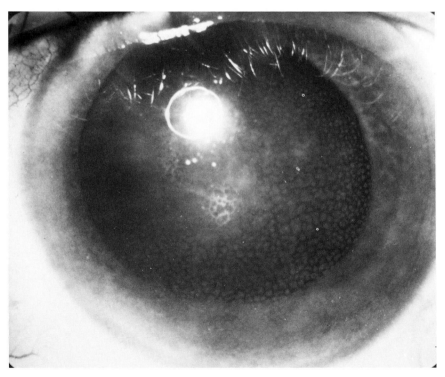

Fig. 95. *Numerous flat keratic precipitates in a 51-year-old woman with rheumatoid arthritis and iritis.* The lower two thirds of the posterior surface of the cornea is covered with keratic precipitates, with only a minimal number of cells and a moderate flare in the anterior chamber. She has had rheumatoid arthritis for 23 years, and her first attack of iritis occurred 20 years ago.

Course. Over the next 2 months there was a gradual resolution of the iritis in the left eye. The topical administration of corticosteroids was gradually discontinued. A week later there was a recurrence of a low-grade iritis, which lasted another 6 months, requiring topical administration of corticosteroids in small amounts. The patient moved to Arizona to see if a dry climate would help her arthritis.

Iritis with rheumatoid arthritis

History. Six months ago this 44-year-old woman developed a red painful left eye with decreased vision. She was treated for a week, and the eye was normal until 3 days ago, when she had a recurrence of the same symptoms, associated with a stiff neck.

Findings. Vision in the right eye is 20/20 and in the left 20/50. The right eye is normal, but the left eye has a moderate conjunctival injection and a prominent ciliary flush. The anterior chamber contains two fibrin masses, one in the pupillary area and another in the lower third of the chamber (Fig. 96). The FIG. 96 pupil is fixed by posterior synechias. The anterior chamber contains many cells and a marked flare. The posterior segment cannot be visualized. The intraocular

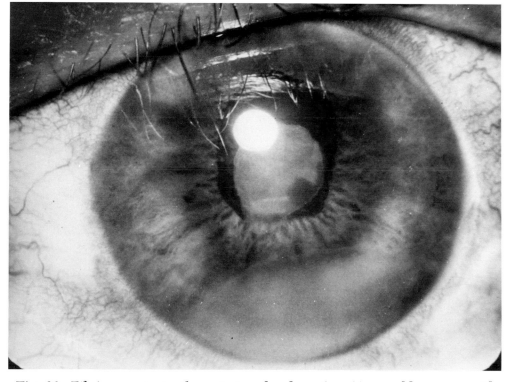

Fig. 96. *Fibrin masses in the anterior chamber of a 44-year-old woman with rheumatoid arthritis and iritis.* One mass of fibrin lies in the pupillary area and the other in the lower third of the anterior chamber. Three days ago she had a recurrence of her iritis with the development of the fibrin in the anterior chamber. Subsequently, after intensive treatment the fibrin completely absorbed.

167

pressure in the right eye is 22 mm. Hg (Schiøtz) and in the left 12 mm. Hg (Schiøtz).

Course. Mydriatic solution was injected subconjunctivally, dilating a small upper portion of the pupil. Topical administration of corticosteroids and mydriatics was instituted, and 10 days later the fibrin completely absorbed, leaving the anterior chamber clear. A history was then obtained of pain and swelling of the knees 3 months previously and a similar episode involving the hips a year ago. Following a thorough work-up, a diagnosis of rheumatoid arthritis was made. Treatment with aspirin gave the patient considerable relief, but she continued to have difficulty in various joints, with severe stiffness on awakening in the morning. Six months later she had another recurrence of the iritis in her right eye. This again responded to mydriatics and topical administration of steroids. Over a period of the next 2 years she continued to have further progression of her arthritic process, with stiffness of her knees and hips. There was no recurrence of her ocular problems.

NEUROFIBROMATOSIS (VON RECKLINGHAUSEN'S DISEASE)

Tumors of the skin and nerve sheaths, pigmentation (cafe au lait spots), bony lesions, buphthalmos, and other developmental defects characterize neurofibromatosis, a congenital disease. Almost every tissue in the eye can be involved by the tumors found in neurofibromatosis. The sites of ocular involvement in order of frequency are the eyelids, optic nerve, orbit, retina, iris, cornea, and tarsal and bulbar conjunctiva. Congenital glaucoma occurs as a complication, due usually to the obstruction of the outflow channels by neurofibromatous tissue. The majority of these cases have multiple neurofibromas or plexiform neurofibroma of the lid, and it is reported that 50% of the cases with lid involvement have congenital glaucoma as a complication. Neurofibromatosis may also cause proptosis, and central lesions produce optic atrophy, papilledema, and palsy of the ocular muscles. Gliomas of the optic nerve are frequently associated, and any child with unexplained visual loss should be carefully examined for cafe au lait spots on the skin.

Neurofibromatous nodules on the iris are a frequent occurrence and are rarely associated with glaucoma. Typically, a number of brownish or yellowish nodules varying from less than 1 mm. in size to 2 mm. in diameter are seen on the iris. The number and prominence of neurofibromas of the iris appear to be greater in the older patient, indicating that they develop with age.

Treatment depends on the portion of the eye involved and whether the lesion is symptomatic. Neurofibromatous iris nodules apparently cause no harm, but in congenital glaucoma associated with neurofibromatosis, with abnormal tissue visible gonioscopically, goniosurgery is probably indicated.

Iris nodules in neurofibromatosis

History. Three years ago shortly after developing sharp shooting pains in the back of his head, this 29-year-old man was found to have neurofibromatosis. Soon after, he experienced loss of vision in his left eye and was discovered to have papilledema with vision reduced to 20/200. A lumbar puncture showed a pressure of 300 mm. H₂O and a protein level of 70 mg/100 ml. Further studies indicated a left frontal intracranial tumor, for which a left frontal lobectomy was performed. Histopathologic diagnosis was glioblastoma multiforme. Postoperatively, radiation treatment was given to this area. In the past month the patient had a recurrence of his occipital headaches and excessive fatigue.

Findings. Vision in both eyes is 20/20. The anterior segments are normal except for the irides, which have many elevated brown nodules distributed at random over the surface (Reel X-5 and Fig. 97). Most of these nodules are less than 1 mm. in size, and a number of them involve the sphincter region. They do not seem to invade the underlying blue stroma of the iris, and they do not affect the pupillary action. Gonioscopy shows no involvement of the angle. Fundus examination shows that the disc margins are blurred, more in the left eye than the right, and that there is a venous pulsation only in the right eye. The intraocular pressure is 16 mm. Hg (Schiøtz) in both eyes.

REEL X-5
FIG. 97

Course. A pneumoencephalogram showed a communicating type of hydrocephalus, with enlargement of the ventricles, particularly on the left. There was no evidence of recurrence of the tumor. A year later the headaches worsened, and the patient stopped work. It was thought that the tumor had recurred. He was referred to another hospital and was lost to follow-up.

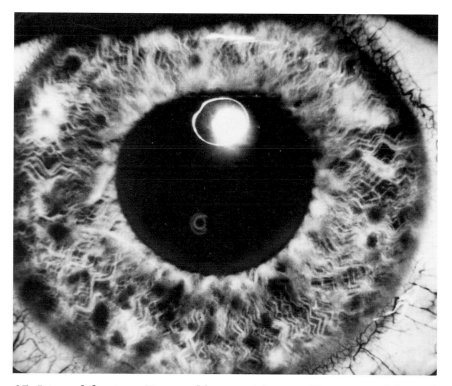

Fig. 97. *Iris nodules in a 29-year-old-man with neurofibromatosis.* Many elevated light brown nodules are distributed at random over the surface of both irides (see Reel X-5). Most are less than a millimeter in size and do not invade the underlying stroma.

Neurofibromatosis

History. Since birth this 15-year-old boy had proptosis and ptosis of the upper lid of the left eye. By 7 months of age there was pendular nystagmus confined to that eye. X-ray films showed the left orbit to be larger than the right and the optic canal to be enlarged. Further investigation showed a left optic atrophy and dark pigmented spots suggestive of cafe au lait spots on the body skin. X-ray films taken after air injection in the left orbit showed a mass in the apex that was not attached to the globe. By age 2 there was very little progression of the exophthalmos, but it was apparent that the vision in the eye was markedly reduced. Hertel exophthalmometry showed an exophthalmos of 5 mm., and 2 years later this had remained the same. X-ray films now showed dysplasia of the greater wing of the left sphenoid and depression of the floor of the sella on the left. A diagnosis of neurofibromatosis with congenital dysplasia of the greater wing of the sphenoid was made. Vision was found to be 20/30 in the right eye and 20/300 in the left. The patient was then lost to follow-up until a week ago.

FIG. 98   *Findings.* Vision in the right eye is 20/25 and in the left counting fingers at 1 foot. The right eye is normal except for numerous brown nodules varying from 0.1 mm. to 2 mm. in size on the surface of the iris (Fig. 98, *A*). The pupil reacts normally. In the left eye there is a pulsating exophthalmos and a prominent ptosis of the upper lid (Fig. 98, *B*). The corneal diameter is 12.5 mm., and the limbal region is opacified and vascularized. The anterior chamber is deep. The iris contains a number of large nodules similar to those seen in the right eye. The pupil is dilated (6 mm.) and does not react. There is a prominent ectropion uveae extending onto the iris, in some places more than 1 mm. The lens is clear, and the vitreous contains many vitreous opacities. A highly myopic fundus and cupped atrophic disc can be visualized. Applanation tonometry shows tensions of 9 mm. Hg in the right eye and 30 mm. Hg in the left. By gonioscopy the angle of the right eye is normal, but in the left the anterior chamber is unusually deep and there are a number of broad tentlike peripheral anterior synechias. Field examination shows the right eye to be normal except for a questionably enlarged blind spot and the left to have only an inferior temporal field remaining. The patient's skin has numerous cafe au lait spots (Fig. 98, *C*).

Course. Pilocarpine drops were instituted in the left eye, and 6 months later the intraocular pressure was normal.

VOGT-KOYANAGI-HARADA SYNDROME (UVEOMENINGITIC SYNDROME)

Exudative iridocyclitis and choroiditis associated with patchy depigmentation of the skin and hair characterize Vogt-Koyanagi syndrome. Other frequently associated findings are deafness and tinnitus, loss of hair, and whitening of the eyelashes and eyebrows. Pleocytosis of the cerebrospinal fluid in association with exudative detachment of the retina has been called Harada's syndrome. However, it is now believed that Harada's syndrome is only a variation of the syndrome described by Vogt and by Koyanagi.

The disease occurs most frequently in young men of the more pigmented

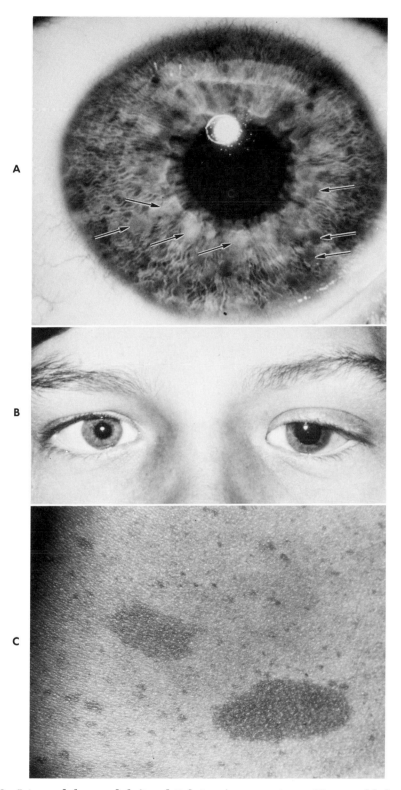

Fig. 98. *Iris nodules and left orbital involvement in a 15-year-old boy with neurofibromatosis.* **A,** In the right eye there are numerous brown nodules up to 2 mm. in size on the surface of the iris. **B,** The left eye has a ptosis and a pulsating exophthalmos. **C,** The skin has numerous cafe-au-lait spots.

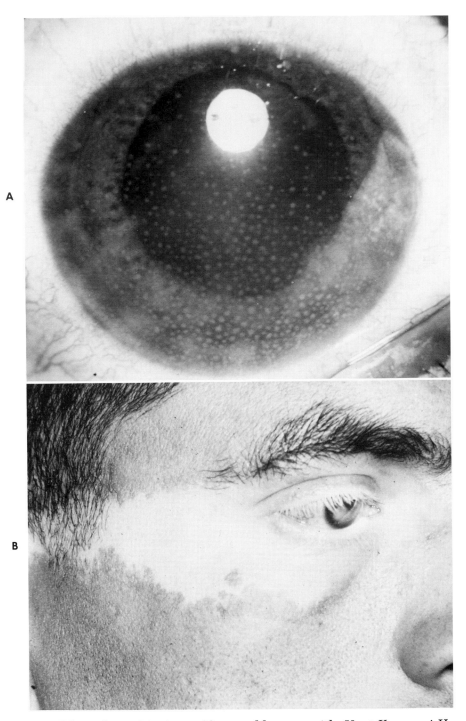

Fig. 99. *Bilateral uveitis in a 30-year-old man with Vogt-Koyanagi-Harada syndrome.* **A,** Numerous keratic precipitates in the right eye are associated with a severe uveitis and lymphocytes in the spinal fluid. **B,** Poliosis of the eyelashes and periorbital vitiligo extending back to the ear developed 6 months after the bilateral uveitis. The patient then developed secondary glaucoma and bullous keratopathy.

races and is most common in Japan. The cause is unknown, but the work of Japanese investigators tends to implicate a virus as a causative agent. Others have favored an allergic origin. The microscopic picture is similar to that of sympathetic ophthalmia, but a relationship between these two conditions has not yet been established. The syndrome frequently runs a long course of recurrent iridocyclitis leading to complete blindness. Treatment with steroids is thought to have benefited some patients.

Vogt-Koyanagi-Harada syndrome

History. This 30-year-old man noticed "puffy" eyelids and an aching above both eyes for 2 years. The eyes were inflamed, and the vision was slightly decreased. Six weeks later there was a sudden almost complete loss of vision overnight. Examination at that time revealed bilateral anterior and posterior uveitis of a severe degree (Fig. 99, *A*). Lymphocytes were found in the spinal FIG. 99 fluid on two occasions, but subsequently none were present. Depigmentation of the skin around the eyes developed about 6 months after the onset of the disease. Because of an uncontrollable intraocular tension, paracentesis was performed on both eyes, followed by an iridectomy on the right eye. Despite therapy, which included ACTH and systemic administration of corticosteroids, the intraocular tension remained elevated, and there was little change in the visual acuity and the uveitis. Recently the patient was troubled with excessive tearing.

Findings. Vision is limited to hand movements in the right eye and is 10/200 in the left. Both corneas are somewhat opaque, the right more than the left. Some pigment disturbance can be visualized in the retina of the left eye. The skin around the eyes is completely depigmented back to the ears, and there is poliosis of all the eyelashes (Fig. 99, *B*). The intraocular pressure is 30 mm. Hg (Schiøtz) in the right eye and 43 mm. Hg (Schiøtz) in the left.

Course. The patient developed bullous keratopathy in both eyes. Neurectomy of the greater and lesser petrosal nerves resulted in a reduction of the excessive tearing and improvement of the bullous keratopathy. The patient's condition gradually improved, and there was no further evidence of active inflamation. Twelve years later the intraocular pressures in both cycs wcrc normal, and the vision in the right eye was light perception but in the left 20/30 with correction.

BEHÇET'S SYNDROME

Recurrent uveitis usually with hypopyon and retinal vasculitis comprises the ocular findings characteristic of Behçet's disease. Typically, recurrent aphthous lesions of the mouth and ulcers of the genitalia occur; various other lesions, such as phlebitis, arthritis, colitis, and meningitis, may be associated. A viral cause has been suspected, but others have thought the origin to be allergic or have considered the condition to be a collagen disease. Some have proposed bacterial infections, such as hypersensitivity to an avirulent bacterium, a viridans streptococcus infection, or a *Staphylococcus albus* infection.

The uveitis, which is both anterior and posterior, is bilateral and occurs in crises at intervals of several months. Frequently it does not occur in both eyes simultaneously. The retinal vasculitis often causes infarcts and hemorrhages and

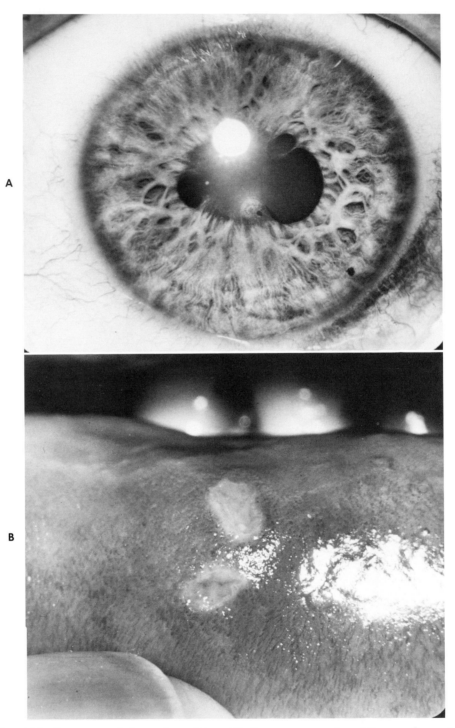

Fig. 100. *Recurrent bilateral uveitis with hypopyon and aphthous ulcers in a 41-year-old man with Behçet's syndrome.* **A,** Irregular pupillary opening due to dense posterior synechias resulted from recurrent attacks of hypopyon uveitis. **B,** Aphthous-type ulcers occurred on the lower lip. The patient also had vesicular lesions on the corona penis.

is most commonly the cause of severe loss of vision. Occasionally conjunctivitis and keratitis occur. Treatment with corticosteroids has been reported to be both beneficial and deleterious. Recently, the immunosuppressive drugs chlorambucil and azathioprine (Imuran) have been reported to be effective. Long-term therapy is usually required.

Behçet's syndrome

History. Three months ago this 41-year-old man, who had lived in Turkey all his life, developed pain and photophobia in the left eye. Corticosteroids were given topically, but there was little improvement. Several weeks ago he became worse, and he was found to have uveitis in both eyes and a hypopyon in the left eye. A spontaneous remission of his symptoms followed.

Findings. Vision in the right eye is 20/20 and in the left counting fingers. In the right eye there is minimal injection of the conjunctiva, the cornea and anterior chamber are clear, and the pupil is round. Pigment is attached to the anterior capsule in the pupillary area, but the lens is otherwise clear. Fundus examination shows that the superior nasal vein is sheathed and that in this distribution are many retinal hemorrhages typical of a vein occlusion. Near the ora are some round inflammatory exudates. Gonioscopy reveals that the angle is open and normal except for pigment clumps inferiorly. In the left eye there is moderate conjunctival injection, a clear cornea, and a clear anterior chamber of normal depth. The pupillary opening is irregular, and more than half of its margin is involved with dense posterior synechias (Fig. 100, A). The portion FIG. 100 of the lens that can be visualized is normal, and the fundus has no gross abnormalities. Gonioscopy shows a normal angle except for excessive pigment clumping inferiorly. On the lower lip are several aphthous-type ulcers (Fig. 100, B). The patient also has genital lesions in the form of erythematous and vesicular lesions on the corona penis.

Course. Although inpatient studies and consultation with various services revealed no important abnormalities, there was general agreement that Behçet's syndrome was the most likely diagnosis. The patient then returned to Turkey and was lost to follow-up.

JUVENILE XANTHOGRANULOMA (NEVOXANTHOENDOTHELIOMA)

Spontaneous hemorrhage in an infant, followed by residual tumor tissue on the iris, is typical of juvenile xanthogranuloma. This ocular complication may occur before the typical skin changes, which consist of multiple reddish yellow benign xanthomatous papules. These may be seen at birth or within the first 6 months; the papules have a predilection for the head and scalp, occurring in successive crops, finally with a spontaneous remission. The hyphema, which is not uncommonly the presenting symptom, clears, and typically there is an infiltration of the iris by salmon-colored lesions. These extend into the angle, embarrass the outflow channels, often with an increased ocular pressure. As a result of the secondary glaucoma, the cornea may become enlarged, and the condition may be confused with congenital glaucoma. Except for permanent damage from the glaucoma, juvenile xanthogranuloma is benign and is not associated with the systemic manifestations found in Letterer-Siwe and Hand-Schüller-Christian diseases.

Juvenile xanthogranuloma

History. Four months ago this 11-month-old child developed a spontaneous hyphema in the left eye, which resolved in 10 days, with no residual defect in the eye. About a week ago a second hyphema occurred; and as this absorbed, a tumor was visible in the inferior angle. There was no trauma associated with either episode of hyphema, and the child appeared to be otherwise entirely normal.

Findings. The right eye is normal in all respects. In the left there is mild conjunctival injection, a clear cornea, and an anterior chamber of normal depth. In the inferior portion of the anterior chamber involving the angle from the 5 o'clock to the 7 o'clock position is an irregular light brownish mass of REEL X-6 tissue, with some small vessels extending from the iris into its base (Reel X-6). General examination of the patient reveals no abnormal findings except for a number of pinpoint erythematous lesions on both arms.

Course. Gonioscopy with the child under general anesthesia revealed the

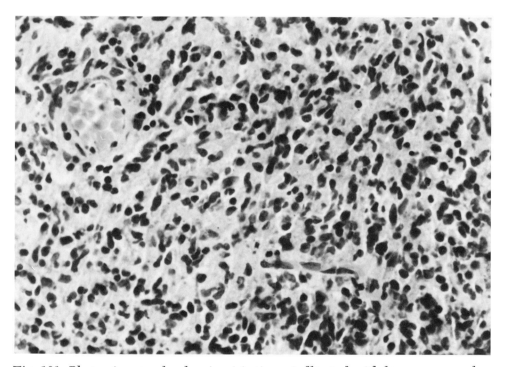

Fig. 101. *Photomicrographs showing iris tissue infiltrated with large mononuclear cells in an 11-year-old child with juvenile xanthogranuloma.* Following two episodes of spontaneous hyphema in the left eye, an irregular light brownish mass of tissue (see Reel X-6) was found in the inferior portion of the anterior chamber. An iridectomy that included the tumor mass provided the pathologic specimen showing tissues typical of juvenile xanthogranuloma. (H & E stain; ×1600.)

tumor to involve the angle and arise from the surface of the iris. Examination of the fundus showed no abnormalities. Results of laboratory studies, including x-ray films of the chest and thymus and an I.V. pyelogram were all normal. A month later a third hemorrhage occurred, but this absorbed in about 2 days, and an iridectomy involving all of the tumor mass was then performed. The postoperative course was uneventful. Histopathologically, the iris tissue was infiltrated with large mononuclear cells typical of juvenile xanthogranuloma (Fig. 101). Two years later there had been no further bleeding or signs of recurrence of the tumor. The patient was then lost to follow-up.   FIG. 101

HODGKIN'S DISEASE

Painless progressive enlargement of lymphoid tissue, with lymphadenopathy and frequently with splenomegaly, is characteristic of Hodgkin's disease. It more commonly affects the younger age group. Enlargement of the cervical lymph nodes is usually the first symptom. The course of the disease may be rapid, or the disease may run a chronic course for many years. From an ocular standpoint, the finding of infiltration of the uveal tract that produces a picture like that of uveitis has been reported, although this is apparently rare.

Plastic iritis with Hodgkin's disease

History. About 5 months ago this 17-year-old girl developed a red, photophobic left eye, with blurring of vision. About 3 months ago her right eye became red, and she had a bilateral iritis. In spite of mydriatics and hot compresses, there was a gradual progression of the inflammation. After I.V. typhoid fever therapy totalling 500 million units there was gradual improvement. However, a month ago her iritis worsened, and beginning posterior subcapsular cataracts were noted. High doses of vitamin C given parenterally for several weeks produced no improvement.

Findings. Vision in both eyes is 5/200. There is moderate conjunctival injection in both eyes, and the anterior chambers contain numerous cells and a heavy flare. Bilateral posterior synechias are more marked in the left eye than in the right. In addition, the left eye has a 1-mm. hypopyon and a number of yellowish keratic precipitates in the lower portion of the cornea (Fig. 102, A). In both eyes   FIG. 102
are anterior capsular opacities with prominent posterior subcapsular cataracts. The fundus cannot be visualized. Repeated *Brucella* and tuberculin skin tests are negative. Results of the general physical examination and the routine laboratory studies are normal.

Course. A retrobulbar injection of corticosteroid was given in the left eye; and 1 week later the hypopyon had cleared, and the anterior chamber cells and flare had decreased considerably. The right eye remained the same. Over the next month repeated subconjunctival injections of cortisone acetate were given in the left eye, resulting in gradual decrease in the inflammation and a slight increase in visual acuity. At this time subconjunctival injections of cortisone acetate were also given in the right eye and at weekly intervals for the next several months, after which cortisone drops were used instead. There was gradual improvement of the vision in both eyes and a lessening of the inflammatory signs. Finally, it was possible to visualize the fundus of the right eye, and

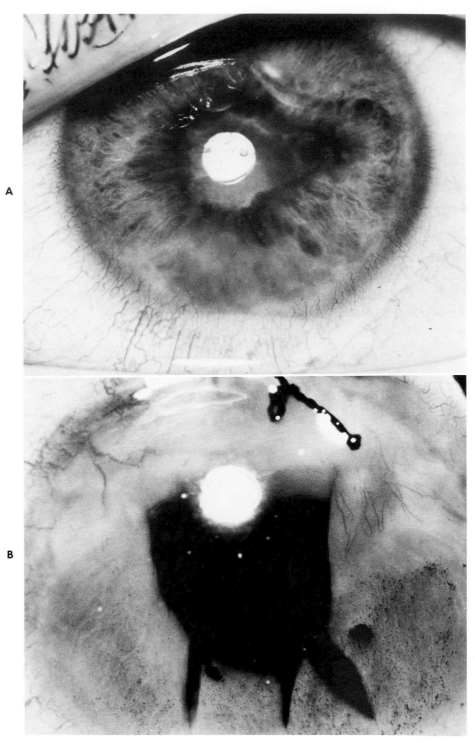

Fig. 102. *Severe bilateral iritis and secondary cataracts in a 17-year-old girl with Hodgkin's disease.* **A,** Marked anterior chamber reaction is present with a small hypopyon and multiple posterior synechias due to an iritis of 3 months' duration. **B,** Following an intracapsular cataract extraction there was gradual development of a dense pupillary membrane for which a discission was subsequently performed. Postoperatively the vision was correctable to 20/70.

there was definite macular edema, with some vitreous exudation and possible organization. The left fundus could not be visualized due to the small occluded pupil. In another 6 months the patient developed cervical lymphadenopathy, and a lymph node biopsy showed Hodgkin's disease with mediastinal and axillary involvement. There was gradual increase in the size of the cervical nodes, and triethylamine therapy was begun. With the patient receiving topical administration of cortisone and mydriatics there was a slow improvement and an increase in vision to 20/100 in the left eye. Also, it appeared that with triethylamine therapy there was definite improvement of her general disease. For the next year there were no signs of ocular inflammation, but the posterior subcapsular changes gradually increased until mature cataracts developed in both eyes. An intracapsular cataract extraction was performed on the left eye, and the postoperative course was uneventful. With correction 20/200 vision was obtained, but a pupillary membrane gradually developed over the next 2 years. The patient was then struck in the left eye and developed a total hyphema followed by hematogenous pigmentation of the cornea. Two years later the hematogenous pigmentation had cleared, but there was a dense pupillary membrane. A discission of the pupillary membrane was performed in an attempt to improve her vision over the present hand movements. A very heavy membrane was encountered, and a piece was removed superiorly and cuts made into the drawn-up pupil (Fig. 102, B). Postoperatively, there were no complications, and her vision was correctable to 20/70. X-ray treatment was instituted for the glandular involvement with the Hodgkin's disease; she did quite well for another year, at which time she had a severe exacerbation of Hodgkin's disease, with hepatosplenomegaly, anemia, and generalized lymphadenopathy. Treatment was instituted with nitrogen mustard, and the response was good. In another year vision declined in the left eye until she could only count fingers at 1 foot. There were no signs of inflammation; but there was a marked band-shaped keratopathy, and the eye appeared to be developing phthisis bulbi. Over the next 3 years there was little change in her ocular status, but she experienced gradually increasing disability from Hodgkin's disease. Chlorambucil was instituted but could not be used in very large doses, because it induced nausea. Systemic administration of corticosteroids decreased a pleural effusion and pain. The patient then developed lymphomatous infiltration of the skin of the abdomen, for which radiation was given. There was a gradual downhill course, with icterus; she finally died 8 years after the diagnosis of her systemic disease had been made. The autopsy findings showed malignant lymphoma of the Hodgkin type.

HORNER'S SYNDROME

Relative miosis, ptosis, apparent enophthalmos, and ipsilateral anhidrosis characterize Horner's syndrome. When the condition is congenital, there is also a heterochromia due to failure of iris pigment formation on the involved side. The condition is due to paralysis of the sympathetic nerve supply either from lesions in the sympathetic pathways within the central nervous system or from lesions in the neck. Removal of the superior cervical ganglion or section of the lower cervical or upper thoracic nerve roots can cause Horner's syndrome. Within the central nervous system Horner's syndrome may result from occlusion of the posterior cerebellar arteries or basilar artery or may be associated with multiple sclerosis and with tumors of the cervical cord. Outside the central nervous system some of the more common lesions that may cause the condition are apical pulmonary disease, mediastinal tumor, aortic aneurysm, trauma, and cervical lymphadenopathy.

In Horner's syndrome there is a hypersensitivity of the pupil to epinephrine and a decreased sensitivity to mydriatic drugs such as atropine and cocaine. Thus several instillations of 1:100,000 epinephrine cause mydriasis and lid retraction in the involved eye but no reaction in the normal side. Conversely, cocaine (4%) instilled in the involved eye shows a reduced effect but produces a well-dilated pupil in the normal eye.

Horner's syndrome with lateral medullary syndrome

History. About a week ago this 41-year-old man noted a tingling of the right hand. Two days ago he developed numbness of the left side of his face, and the next morning he had ataxia of the left arm and an episode of vomiting and vertigo. He then noted diplopia. The patient had been in good health except for hypertension.

Findings. There is a moderate ptosis of the left upper lid. The left pupil is relatively miotic. There is hypesthesia of the left cornea, decreased sweating of the left side of the face, and dilatation of the conjunctival vessels of the left eye. Investigation of the extraocular movements shows a skew deviation, with a right hypertropia of 8° in all fields of gaze. There is also a weakness of the left lateral rectus, which is detectable only with a red glass. There is a horizontal

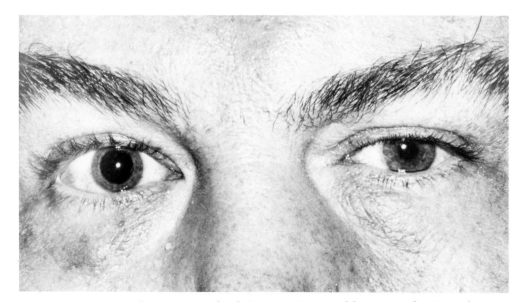

Fig. 103. *Ptosis and miosis on the left in a 41-year-old man with Horner's syndrome.* The patient developed a skew deviation and typical findings of Horner's syndrome in association with a left lateral medullary syndrome.

nystagmus on lateral gaze and vertical and rotary nystagmus on upward gaze. The fundi are normal and the visual fields full.

Course. Cocaine (10%) instilled in both eyes caused a prompt dilatation of the right pupil, with no effect on the left (Fig. 103). There was gradual improve- FIG. 103 ment of the ataxia and a decrease in the diplopia, particularly on upward gaze during the next week. The blood pressure ranged between 180/120 and 170/110 mm. Hg. Results of all laboratory studies were normal, and no cause for occlusion of the posterior inferior cerebellar artery on the left could be determined. The patient was then lost to follow-up.

Acquired Horner's syndrome

History. This 32-year-old woman is said to have first had the signs of Horner's syndrome on the right side at age 7. This followed the lancing of an abscessed gland in the right neck region and the subsequent ligation of the carotid artery. The only eye complaints at the present are a difficulty in focussing when the patient is reading.

Findings. The vision in both eyes is 20/20. There is a slight droop of the right eyelid. The right iris is hazel, while the left is brown; the size of the right pupil is 2½ mm., while the left is 4 mm. (Fig. 104). There is also a decrease in FIG. 104 sweating of the right side of the face, with some pallor of the skin. The remainder of the anterior and posterior segments of both eyes are entirely normal. With phenylephrine (10%) drops the dilatation of the right eye is greater than that of the left. Intraocular tensions in both eyes are 14 mm. Hg (applanation tonometry).

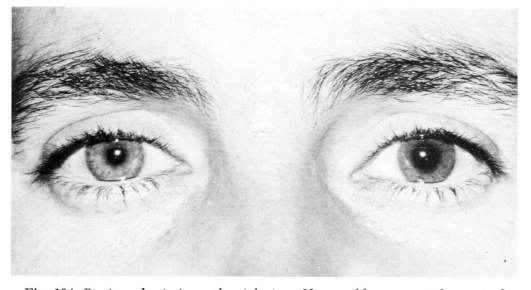

Fig. 104. *Ptosis and miosis on the right in a 32-year-old woman with acquired Horner's syndrome.* At age 7 she had an abscessed gland in the right neck region lanced and a ligation of the carotid artery. Horner's syndrome occurred at the time this procedure was done.

Course. Over the next three years there was no change in the patient's ocular status, but she developed essential hypertension.

TONIC PUPIL (ADIE'S SYNDROME)

Absent or retarded constriction of the pupil in reaction to light but normal reaction to the near stimulus characterizes the tonic pupil. Once the pupil has constricted, it dilates more slowly than normal in the dark or when the person is looking into the distance. Frequently the pupil responds to the near reflex completely, although somewhat slowly, and to light only minimally. Accommodation of the lens is sometimes affected, and the individual has difficulty in reading. While the condition is usually unilateral, occasionally both eyes are affected, but the effect in each eye is different in degree and in time of onset. The condition generally occurs in young women and is associated with absent ankle and knee reflexes. In some instances it is familial. It usually is present throughout life, without serious neurologic abnormality. Vermiform movements of the sphincter muscle may be seen biomicroscopically. Also diagnostic is the hypersensitivity of the pupil to methacholine chloride (Mecholyl); a few drops of 2.5% solution instilled in the conjunctival sac result in prompt and intense miosis of the tonic pupil, in contrast to absence of reaction of a normal pupil. This reaction is apparently due to denervation hypersensitivity that indicates involvement of the final postganglionic nerve fiber to the iris sphincter arising in the ciliary ganglion.

Bilateral myotonic (Adie's) pupil

History. About 15 years ago this 47-year-old woman was noted to have different-sized pupils. At that time the left pupil was larger than the right and did not constrict in bright illumination. Recently the right pupil tended to be larger than the left. Also, the patient said she had some difficulty in focussing at near objects. Since her childhood the left eye was nearsighted, but because she had a good right eye the nearsightedness of the left eye was never corrected with glasses.

Findings. Vision in the right eye is 20/30 with correction and in the left 20/400. Except for the pupils, the eyes seem to be normal. The pupil of the right

FIG. 105   eye is about 7 mm. in size and of the left 4 mm. (Fig. 105, *A*). There is no reaction to either direct or consensual light; but when the patient is placed in the dark, the pupils gradually dilate to 9 mm. in the right and 7 mm. in the left. When the patient fixates on a near object, the pupils promptly constrict to 3 mm. in the right and 2 mm. in the left (Fig. 105, *B*). There is then a slow return of the pupils to their previous size. One drop of 2.5% methacholine instilled into both conjunctival sacs produces a slow constriction of the pupils to 4 mm. in the right and 3 mm. in the left. By slit-lamp examination there is an unusual vermiform movement of the iris as the bright light gradually causes a slow and incomplete constriction of the pupils. The range of accommodation in her right eye is somewhat reduced but probably normal for her age. She has decreased ankle jerks bilaterally.

Course. Three years later there was no appreciable change in the patient's ocular status.

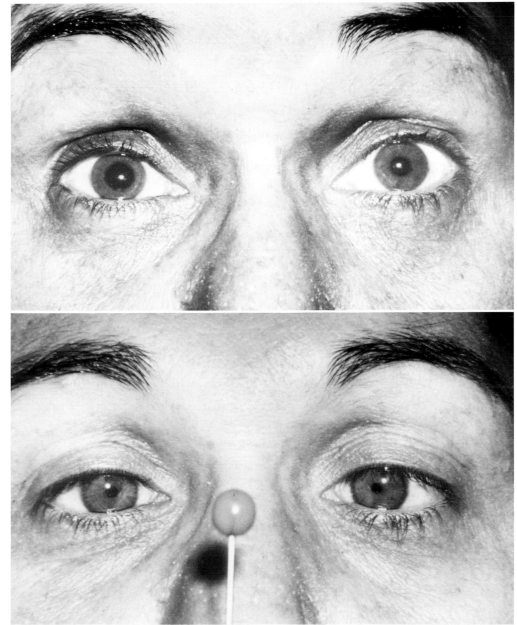

Fig. 105. *Bilateral semidilated pupils with little reaction to light but normal reaction to accommodation in a 47-year-old-woman with bilateral myotonic pupils.* **A,** The right pupil is moderately dilated and the left slightly dilated in bright light. **B,** Fixation on a close object produces prompt constriction of both pupils. The patient has decreased ankle jerk reflexes bilaterally. Methacholine chloride (2.5%) produces constriction of both pupils.

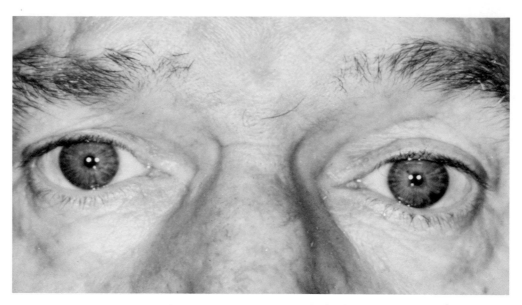

Fig. 106. *Miotic pupils that are nonreactive to light but constrict with accommodation in a 58-year-old man with Argyll-Roberston pupils.* The patient apparently acquired lues 6 years ago and now has a positive reaction to serologic tests.

ARGYLL-ROBERTSON PUPIL

Absent or sluggish pupillary reaction to light, with a normal reaction to the near stimulus, characterizes the Argyll-Robertson pupil. Pupils are typically miotic in both eyes, frequently of slightly different size and irregular. The importance of the finding of an Argyll-Robertson pupil lies in the frequency of its association with neurosyphilis. At one time it was thought to be pathognomonic for syphilis of the central nervous system, but other lesions in the region of the tectum, such as encephalitis, pinealomas, vascular lesions of the mesencephalon, and thalamic lesions, can produce the typical pupillary findings. The frequency of an associated paresis of upward gaze and of convergence in lesions of the mesencephalon are important differential points. Patients with diabetes mellitus, chronic alcoholism, and multiple sclerosis also can develop an Argyll-Robertson pupil.

Argyll-Robertson pupils

History. About 6 years ago this 58-year-old man, a chronic alcoholic, had a penile lesion for which he had an uncertain number of injections, possibly of penicillin, for treatment. Recently he became confused, forgetful, and somewhat disoriented. He also developed a cerebellar ataxia.

Findings. Vision in both eyes is 20/30. Both eyes are normal in all respects FIG. 106 except for the pupils, which are miotic, between 1.5 and 2 mm. in size (Fig. 106). There is practically no response to bright illumination or to the slit-lamp beam, but both pupils react well to accommodation. The ocular motility is full, and visual fields are normal.

Course. Cortical function tests showed mental retardation, with recent memory loss and visual motor function and common sense judgment defects. Cervical spine x-ray films showed no abnormalities to explain his ataxia. Reaction of the patient's serum to the Hinton serologic test was positive to two dilutions. The diagnosis was central nervous system lues. The patient was then lost to follow-up.

Chapter 7

Inflammatory conditions of the iris

EXOGENOUS BACTERIAL UVEITIS

A suppurative uveitis usually occurs when bacteria invade the uveal tract. Frequently a purulent panophthalmitis is associated, but in some instances only an exudative iritis occurs. Sources of such infections are ulcerations of the cornea, perforating wounds, postoperative infections, and infected filtering blebs. The most common organism, *Staphylococcus,* typically produces a gelatinous coagulum in the anterior chamber from toxins elaborated by the organism. A severe staphylococcal conjunctivitis can produce such a reaction. Intensive antibiotic therapy will usually be successful if initiated at a sufficiently early stage. Streptococcal uveitis produces a virulent purulent uveitis and also may lead to loss of the eye. In contrast, *Pneumococcus* appears to produce its iritic reaction by diffusion of its exotoxin through the cornea from a pneumococcic corneal ulcer. A sterile hypopyon is typical. Unless perforation of the ulcer occurs, there is usually no residual uveal damage. In ulcers due to *Pseudomonas aeruginosa* (pyocyanic ulcer) the rapid development of a large hypopyon is classical. Despite intensive antibiotic therapy the eye is frequently lost.

The *Proteus* group of bacilli are commonly found in the conjunctival sac and are usually innocuous. However, if introduced into the eye either by perforation of a corneal ulcer or during surgery, panophthalmitis may result. In contrast, gonorrheal uveitis occurs with nonperforating corneal involvement, with a large hypopyon. With perforation, the eye may be lost; but if treatment is adequate, there are no permanent sequelae in the uveal tract. Ophthalmia neonatorum, now rare, is due to gonococcal keratoconjunctivitis in the newborn; it frequently led to marked loss of vision and even to a disorganized globe.

Although generally an endogenous disease, uveitis associated with *Treponema pallidum* can accompany primary syphilitic scleroconjunctivitis. In acquired syphilis, iridocyclitis occurs at the onset of the secondary stage; a more generalized uveitis occurs in the late tertiary stage, with a diffuse chorioretinitis.

Iritis occurring in the late secondary stage of infection produces a diffuse congestion of the iris with, in some cases, the development of pink nodules near the pupillary margin (microscopic gummas). In tertiary syphilis, iritis is granulomatous, similar to that seen in tuberculous disease.

Uveitis secondary to corneal ulcer

History. Three weeks ago this 67-year-old woman underwent a scleral buckling on the left eye for an extensive retinal detachment. The postoperative course was uneventful. A week ago she developed pain in the left eye and was found to have a central denuded area of her cornea, with an infiltrate superiorly and a small hypopyon. Chloramphenicol (Chloromycetin) and mydriatics were given topically, and lincomycin hydrochloride (Lincocin) was given parenterally. In 4 days the hypopyon had become worse, and the culture was still negative. Oxacillin sodium (Prostaphlin) was substituted for the lincomycin, and methicillin sodium (Staphcillin) given topically was used alternately with the chloramphenicol drops. In another 2 days there was still further increase in the hypopyon, and corticosteriods were given systemically. Two days later a second culture showed coagulase-positive hemolytic *Staphylococcus aureus* sensitive to methicillin. The hypopyon remained the same for the past several days, and the corneal infiltrates were stationary.

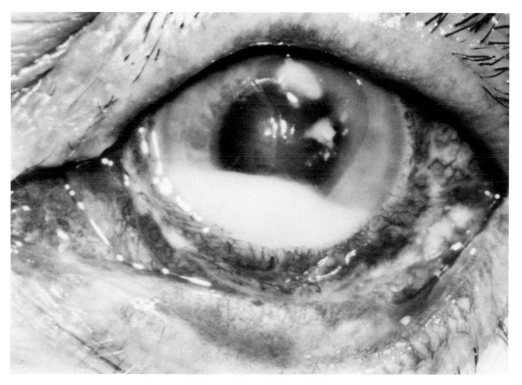

Fig. 107. *Deep stromal infiltrates in the left eye of a 67-year-old woman with a uveitis secondary to a corneal ulcer.* Cultures of the ulcer showed hemolytic *Staphylococcus aureus,* and the infection slowly subsided when she received subconjunctival methicillin and retrobulbar injections of corticosteroids.

FIG. 107

Findings. Vision in the right eye is 20/20 and in the left hand movements only. The right eye is normal. In the left eye there is marked conjunctival injection, and the cornea is diffusely edematous and has a central epithelial defect (Fig. 107). In the pupillary area there are two deep stromal infiltrates, and there is a hypopyon that fills about one third of the chamber. The pupil is semidilated, and the iris contains dilated blood vessels. The posterior segment is difficult to visualize.

Course. Methicillin was injected subconjunctivally and repeated in 2 days. Methylprednisolone acetate (Depo-Medrol) was also administered to the retrobulbar region. There was a definite improvement following these medications. Ten days later the epithelial defect had decreased and the hypopyon resolved. Six weeks later the cornea was hazy, with some increase in thickness, and there were no signs of active infection. The patient was then lost to follow-up.

Delayed postoperative bacterial endophthalmitis

History. Ten years ago this 62-year-old woman was discovered to have advanced open angle glaucoma in both eyes. Despite maximum medical treatment, there was gradual increase in the field defects over a period of 5 years. She then had two trephine procedures performed in the right eye and one in the left. Following these procedures, with maximum medical medication her intraocular pressure remained normal. Six months ago she was found to have an advancing cataract in the left eye, and an extracapsular cataract extraction was performed. Postoperative vision was 20/200 with correction. Six weeks ago she was readmitted, and an intracapsular cataract extraction was performed on the right eye. There were no postoperative complications. An inferior approach was used to avoid involving the bleb superiorly. This morning she awoke with pain and decreased vision in her right eye.

FIG. 108

Findings. Vision in the right eye is light perception and in the left 20/70 with correction. In the right eye there is a moderate lid edema and marked diffuse conjunctival injection, with a prominent ciliary flush. The bleb superiorly is elevated and white. The anterior chamber contains white strands of fibrin and a small hypopyon (Fig. 108, *A*). The left eye is aphakic and is normal except for the deep glaucomatous cupping.

Course. The conjunctiva and fluid from an anterior chamber paracentesis were cultured. Smears showed numerous polymorphonuclear leukocytes and a few small gram-positive cocci. Intensive topical, systemic, and subconjunctival treatment with antibiotics was initiated, and corticosteroids were given systemically. The anterior chamber progressively filled with fibrin and white cells. Two days later a second anterior chamber tap was performed, but the smears gave no further information than the first tap. Four days later the culture finally showed alpha hemolytic *Streptococcus,* which was sensitive to oxacillin, the antibiotic, which, among others, had been given systemically. During the next week there was no appreciable change in the eye except for a flat anterior chamber and iris and pupillary area filled with a whitish membrane (Fig. 108, *B*). A posterior sclerotomy produced large amounts of clear yellow fluid, and the anterior chamber re-formed after lysis of the pupillary membrane. Four days later it was clear that the left eye had no light perception, and finally a few days later it was

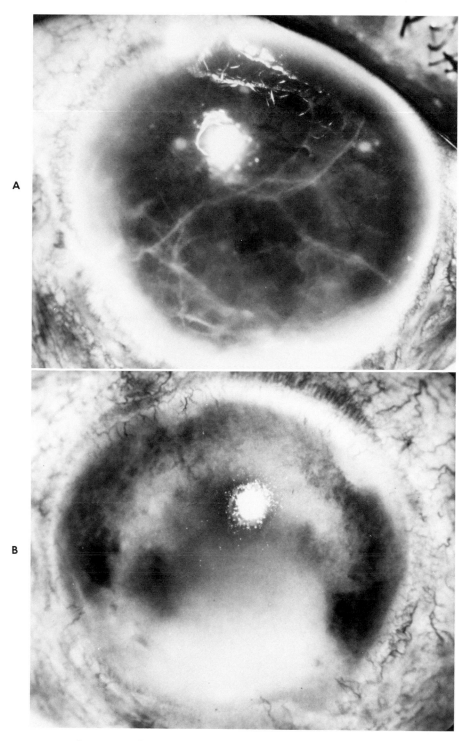

Fig. 108. *Fibrin strands in the anterior chamber and hypopyon in the right eye of a 62-year-old woman with a postoperative bacterial endophthalmitis.* **A,** Six weeks ago she had a cataract extraction, and there were no problems until the sudden onset of a fibrinous iritis. **B,** The anterior chamber tap showed alpha hemolytic *Streptococcus;* but despite intensive antibiotic therapy, the anterior chamber became flat, and a dense white pupillary membrane developed. Subsequently, the eye became blind and was enucleated.

enucleated. The postoperative course was uneventful, and the histopathologic diagnosis was bacterial endophthalmitis, with destruction of the retinal elements and the posterior pole.

Iritis secondary to bacterial ulcer

History. Four years ago this 75-year-old woman was found to have a neglected angle closure glaucoma in the left eye, with corneal edema and an intraocular pressure of 79 mm. Hg (Schiøtz). A peripheral iridectomy was performed on the left eye, followed by a prophylactic peripheral iridectomy on the right eye. Postoperatively, most of the angle of the left eye remained closed. There was gradual return of vision in the left eye, and the intraocular pressure was borderline with the patient receiving maximum medical treatment. A year later she had an acute attack of iritis in the left eye, with epithelial edema. When the patient was seen a year later, her eye had no light perception, and the intraocular tension was markedly elevated. The patient returned today with a red and sore left eye.

Findings. It is impossible to determine the vision in either eye due to poor cooperation. The right eye has an iridectomy superiorly, and there is no gross abnormality. The left eye has a central ulceration that involves most of the

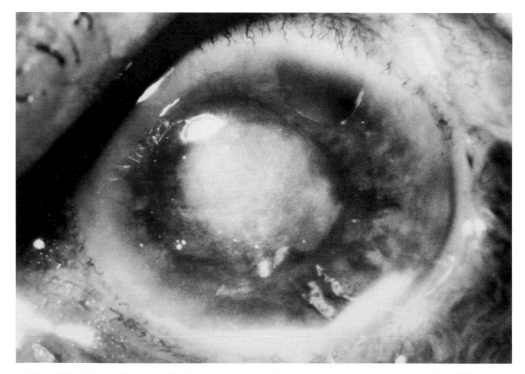

Fig. 109. *Central corneal ulceration and hypopyon in the left eye of a 75-year-old woman with a bacterial corneal ulcer and secondary iritis.* The eye, which is blind due to angle closure glaucoma, recently developed a central ulcer that a culture showed to be caused by *Pneumococcus*. Intensive antibiotic and mydriatic therapy promptly produced healing of the ulcer.

thickness of the cornea. The anterior chamber contains many cells and a 2-mm. hypopyon (Fig. 109). There is a peripheral iridectomy superiorly, and the iris FIG. 109 contains numerous blood vessels, particularly around the sphincter.

Course. A culture showed *Pneumococcus*, and the patient was treated with penicillin subconjunctivally and with mydriatics. In a week the eye was clear, and the ulcer healed. The patient was lost to follow-up.

Uveitis associated with a *Pseudomonas* corneal ulcer

History. Many years ago this 74-year-old woman had peripheral iridectomies performed in both eyes for glaucoma. Subsequently an intracapsular cataract extraction was performed on the right eye, and bullous keratopathy developed due to vitreous contact with the cornea. This condition persisted, resulting in very poor vision in this eye. Three years ago an intracapsular cataract extraction was performed on the left eye, and the visual result was good. For more than a year the patient had been treated with echothiophate in the right eye for mild glaucoma. About 1 month ago she developed pain in the right eye and was found to have a central corneal ulcer with a hypopyon. Cultures showed

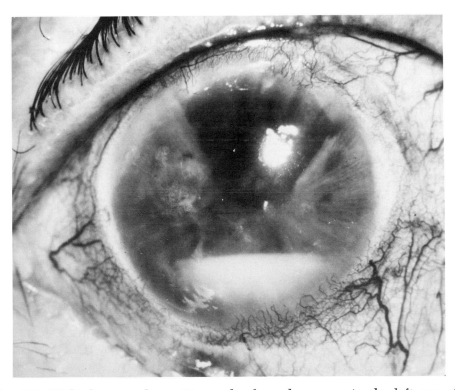

Fig. 110. *Multiple corneal opacities and a large hypopyon in the left eye of a 74-year-old woman with a uveitis secondary to a* Pseudomonas *corneal ulcer. The patient had a bullous keratopathy associated with vitreous contact with the cornea following a cataract extraction. The bullae became secondarily infected with* Pseudomonas, *which responded to treatment with gentamicin administered subconjunctivally and topically.*

this to be caused by *Pseudomonas,* and intensive treatment was given with various antibiotics, including gentamicin sulfate (Garamycin), both subconjunctivally and in the form of drops. There was gradual clearing of the hypopyon and ulcer over a period of 10 days, but yesterday the condition became worse with recurrence of the hypopyon.

FIG. 110

Findings. Vision in the right eye is 20/50 and in the left counting fingers at 1 foot. There is marked conjunctival injection in the right eye, a diffusely hazy cornea, and several localized areas of leukoma (Fig. 110). There is a 4-mm. hypopyon, and the anterior chamber is unusually shallow. It is difficult to evaluate the condition of lens, and the fundus cannot be visualized. There is a surgical aphakia of the left eye and signs of macular degeneration. Intraocular pressure in the right eye is 37 mm. Hg (Schiøtz) and 12 mm. Hg (Schiøtz) in the left eye.

Course. With the patient receiving large doses of acetazolamide, the intraocular pressure promptly became normal. Gentamicin drops were continued, and in 3 days the cornea was healed and the hypopyon was resolving.

Proteus uveitis

History. One week ago this 5-year-old boy was struck in the left eye with the point of a compass. For several days the eye seemed normal; but then it became painful, and a hypopyon developed. Penicillin was given systemically

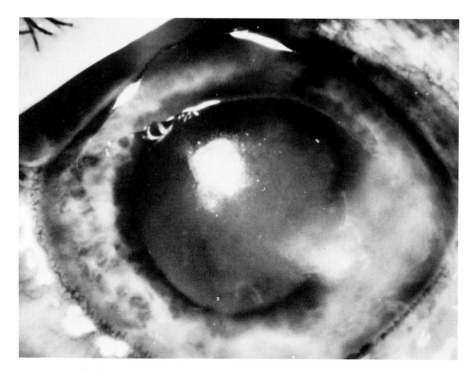

Fig. 111. *Healed corneal perforation in the left eye of a 5-year-old boy with uveitis due to* Proteus *infection.* The accident occurred 1 week ago and responded to subconjunctival colistin treatment. Subsequently, a mass of yellowish material formed in the lens or vitreous, and the eye became blind.

and subconjunctivally, but his condition gradually became worse. The next day the culture showed a mixed infection of *Staphylococcus aureus* and *Proteus*. Colistin was given subconjunctivally, and the signs of anterior chamber involvement markedly improved. The treatment was repeated the next day. In 3 more days there was a good pupillary response, but a cataract was now visible.

Findings. The right eye appears to be normal in all respects. In the left eye there is a marked conjunctival chemosis, and the cornea is diffusely hazy, with a healed corneal perforation in the 4 o'clock position (Fig. 111). The anterior chamber contains many cells, but there is no hypopyon. The pupil reacts sluggishly, and there is some posterior synechia formation inferiorly. The lens is diffusely cloudy.   FIG. 111

Course. There seemed to be some improvement over the next week; but then the eye bcame more irritable, and a mass of yellowish material could be visualized either in the lens or vitreous, and the eye became blind. One month later enucleation was performed; the histopathologic diagnosis was endophthalmitis, cyclitic membrane, and reaction to lens cortex. The postoperative course was uneventful.

Endophthalmitis from infected filtering bleb

History. Thirteen years ago this 58-year-old woman had a filtering operation performed on her left eye for chronic open angle glaucoma. At that time the right eye was almost blind due to glaucomatous damage. Over the years the filtering bleb in her left eye performed well but was noted to be very thin. Three days ago she developed tearing and irritation in the left eye, with some blurring of vision a day later and severe loss of vision yesterday.

Findings. The vision in the right eye is counting fingers at 3 feet and in the left counting fingers at 1 foot. The anterior segment of the right eye is normal, with a miotic pupil. The lens shows some posterior subcapsular opacities, which makes visualization of the fundus difficult. However, the disc is seen to be markedly cupped and atrophic, which is typical of glaucoma damage. In the left eye there is marked conjunctival injection and a slightly elevated area at the limbus at the 2 o'clock position, which appears to be the infected filtering bleb. The cornea is edematous and thickened; there are numerous cells and some fibrin in the anterior chamber, and there is a 2-mm. hypopyon (Reel X-7). The lens   REEL X-7 is difficult to evaluate, and the fundus cannot be visualized. The intraocular pressure is 20 mm. Hg (Schiøtz) in the right eye and 7 mm. Hg (Schiøtz) in the left.

Course. Cultures and smears were taken of the conjunctiva, and aqueous was obtained from an anterior chamber aspiration. The smears were negative for bacteria. Intensive therapy was initiated with lincomycin, chloramphenicol, and corticosteroids systemically and gentamicin by sub-Tenon's injection. There was prompt improvement of the anterior chamber reaction, with complete clearing in 3 days. However, the vitreous contained numerous yellow floaters, which made visualization of the fundus impossible. Two days later the vitreous cleared sufficiently so that a number of scattered hemorrhages in the posterior pole could be visualized. Cultures continued to be negative. However, the vision improved only to counting fingers at 2 feet. Despite continued resolution of the vitreous opacities, 4 days later the patient could see only hand movements. The hemorrhages, which could not explain the marked loss of vision, remained about the same; but it became evident that the disc was pale, and there was some constriction of the retinal arterioles. In a few more days the vision dropped to light perception only, and an electroretinogram (ERG) showed normal cone function but grossly abnormal visually evoked response (VER) consistent with marked optic nerve damage. A month later the vision in the left eye remained at light perception only; the retinal hemorrhages had almost totally absorbed, and the vitreous was entirely clear. The optic nerve head showed increased atrophy. Five months later the vision had returned to 20/60; tension revealed by applanation tonometry was 19 mm. Hg, and the disc remained pale. There was stippling of pigment in the macular area, but fluorescein angiography showed no abnormalities.

Luetic iritis

History. Nine years ago this 42-year-old man had his first attack of iritis in the left eye. At that time he was found on two occasions to have a positive reaction to the Hinton test. He had had a chancre 2½ years previously, which was treated with arsenic and bismuth. He was in the process of having a course of penicillin injections. The iritis in the left eye responded to intravenous typhoid fever therapy. Five years ago he had another attack of iritis in his left eye, and 4 days ago his third attack began. Mydriatics and topical administration of corticosteroids were initiated 2 days ago.

Findings. The vision in the right eye is 20/30 and in the left 20/40. The right eye is normal, but in the left there is marked conjunctival injection, with a prominent ciliary flush (Reel XI-1). The cornea is clear except for many fine keratic precipitates, and the anterior chamber contains many cells and a marked flare. Inferiorly there are several masses of fibrin and hemorrhage filling the angle. The pupil is moderately dilated, with posterior synechia formation inferiorly. There are many fine tortuous vessels involving most of the surface of the iris. On the anterior capsule of the lens are pigment clumps from old posterior synechias. The posterior segment appears normal.

REEL XI-1

Course. Over a period of 2 weeks there was some improvement, and then the patient's iritis recurred despite continuation of treatment. Secondary glaucoma developed, which required acetazalamide and epinephrine drops for its control. A low-grade uveitis persisted for 9 months before his left eye finally was free from any inflammation. Another attack 2 years later was successfully treated with corticosteroids given systemically. On this occasion mutton-fat keratic precipitates were seen. Two years later the intraocular pressure was found to be 68 mm. Hg (Schiøtz), and there was an iris bombé. Again, there was prominent neovascularization of the entire iris and extensive posterior synechia formation. After the attack of iritis resolved, a peripheral iridectomy was performed. The patient was then lost to follow-up.

Luetic iritis

History. Seven years ago this 45-year-old woman had "iritis" in the left eye and 2 years ago was found to have a positive reaction to the Hinton test. Four months ago she developed halos, redness, and blurring of vision in the right eye. Two weeks later she was found to have an intraocular pressure of 65 mm. Hg (Schiøtz) in the right eye and was treated with pilocarpine and acetazolamide, which only partially controlled her elevated intraocular pressure. A short time ago she stopped going to her ophthalmologist when he insisted that she needed an operation.

Findings. Vision in the right eye is 20/40 and in the left 20/25 with correction. The right eye shows mild ciliary injection and a small pupil that reacts sluggishly to light. The anterior chamber contains occasional cells and some flare, and inferiorly there are a number of large nonpigmented keratic precipitates on the corneal endothelium. The media are clear, and the optic nerve head shows definite glaucomatous cupping. Gonioscopic examination of the right eye shows large exudates on the peripheral iris and along the meshwork (Reel XI-2). REEL XI-2 Large dilated vessels are visible in the angle, and on the posterior surface of the cornea a number of large keratic precipitates can be seen. A few exudates on the trabeculum appear to be touching the cornea, with early peripheral anterior synechia formation. Gonioscopy of the left eye shows a few peripheral anterior synechias inferiorly. There are no other abnormalities of the left eye. The intraocular pressure in the right eye is 45 mm. Hg (Schiøtz) and in the left 17 mm. Hg (Schiøtz).

Course. Mydriatics and corticosteroid drops were instituted, along with epinephrine (1%) drops and acetazolamide. Two days later the intraocular pressure in the right eye had been reduced to high normal, and the patient's reaction to a Hinton test was reported as positive. Four days later the intraocular tensions were normal, and there was no injection of the right eye. Reaction to a quantitative Hinton test was positive in a 1:8 dilution, and the patient was considered to have latent syphilis. She refused to have a lumbar puncture. A series of fifteen penicillin injections was given, and in another month there was no sign of inflammation in her right eye. When examined 10 years later, she had had no further ocular complaints, although she was found to have developed mild diabetes.

Old gonococcal ophthalmia

History. At birth this 18-year-old girl had marked purulent discharge from both eyes. Over a period of 8 months she was treated with irrigations day and night every half hour with methylcellulose solution, along with zinc sulfate drops, atropine drops, and boric acid ointment applied to the lids. On several occasions smears showed gram-negative extracellular diplococci. Whereas the right cornea had a relatively small superficial ulcer, the left cornea was involved by an extensive and deep ulcer. A conjunctival flap was performed on this eye, but a week later the cornea perforated and on healing produced a large adherent leukoma inferiorly. Eventually, there was no further staining of the corneas, and the cultures were negative. There was no recurrence of inflammation of the eyes thereafter.

Findings. Vision in the right eye is 20/30 and in the left hand movements. In the right eye there is a small leukoma in the lower third of the cornea, but the pupillary area is clear and the iris normal. There is a small anterior subcapsular

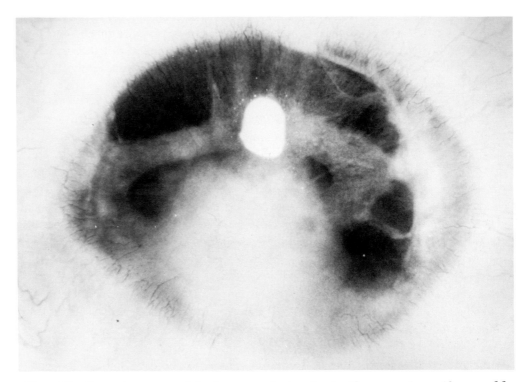

Fig. 112. *Extensive corneal leukoma and atrophy in the eye of an 18-year-old girl with an old gonococcal ophthalmia.* At birth the patient had a marked purulent discharge bilaterally lasting 8 months. Smears showed gram-negative extracellular diplococci.

FIG. 112 cataract, and the fundus is normal. In the left eye there is extensive leukoma formation of the lower half of the cornea, with a shallow anterior chamber and multiple atrophic areas of the iris (Fig. 112). The pupil is markedly distorted and oval in shape. The lens appears to be clear, but no fundus detail can be visualized. There is a fine horizontal nystagmus in all directions of gaze. The intraocular pressure is 24 mm. Hg (Schiøtz) in the right eye and 28 mm. Hg in the left.

Course. The use of pilocarpine drops in both eyes was instituted, although there was some uncertainty as to whether this treatment was required. The patient was then lost to follow-up.

VIRAL UVEITIS

Uveitis caused by various viruses is usually low grade, often transient, and exudative. However, in herpes simplex, herpes zoster, and varicella, the process may be prolonged and recurrent. Influenza is probably the most common cause of mild bilateral viral uveitis, while variola, vaccinia, mumps, lymphogranuloma venereum, and cytomeglic inclusion disease are occasional causes. On rare occasions infectious hepatitis, dengue, pappataci fever, psittacosis, foot and mouth disease, and verrucae also produce uveitis.

Herpes simplex is known to cause an iridocyclitis in the absence of herpetic keratitis; cultures of the virus have been obtained from smears from the iris and ciliary body. Sometimes the iritis is violent and occasionally hemorrhagic. The same trigger mechanism for development of keratitis may also reactivate the iridocyclitis. However, the keratitis may be minimal or absent. It is well known that the herpes simplex virus may spread from one eye to the other via the optic nerve, the second or sympathizing eye being involved a week or two after the first eye, sometimes with evidence of encephalitis.

A serious complication of herpes zoster ophthalmicus is severe anterior iridocyclitis, which generally occurs late in the course of the disease but may rarely be seen even before the cutaneous eruption. It is said that uveitis does not occur unless the nasociliary nerve is affected (Hutchinson's law), but this is not always true. The most common involvement of the iris is a diffuse exudative type of iritis, which may vary from a mild to a severe process with many keratic precipitates, sometimes fibrinous deposits, and a hypopyon. Secondary glaucoma may develop; but a hypotony, which may finally lead to phthisis bulbi, is frequently seen. Diffuse or segmental iris atrophy is a common end result if the eye is not lost.

A rare type of involvement in herpes zoster is the eruptive lesions of the iris resembling those of the skin and cornea. These are characterized by swollen areas and vascular dilatation of the iris, frequently with secondary bleeding. The pain of the iritis is usually severe, and the process may take many months to clear.

Treatment of herpes simplex iritis is difficult, but small amounts of topically administered corticosteroids are usually effective when used cautiously in combination with idoxuridine to avoid secondary corneal involvement. In herpes zoster, iridocyclitis is responsive to corticosteroids, particularly if given systemically. Injections of convalescent serum early in the disease have been reported to be effective.

Herpes zoster uveitis

History. Five days ago this 62-year-old woman developed vesicles on the right side of her forehead and nose. A few days later the right eye became red and painful.

Findings. There are several large vesicles on the right forehead and nose, with multiple erythematous areas involving the right side of her nose and forehead (Fig. 113, A). The vision is 20/20 in each eye. In the right eye there is swelling of the upper lid and marked injection of the bulbar conjunctiva. There are a number of small areas of fluorescein staining of the corneal epithelium, but the anterior chamber contains no cells or flare. The left eye is normal. Intraocular pressure in the right eye is 30 mm. Hg and in the left 24 mm. Hg (Schiøtz). FIG. 113

Course. Acetazolamide was given because of the elevated tension in the right eye. When the patient was seen 3 days later, the skin lesions were regressing, and she had developed blurring of vision in the right eye. The corneal epithelial defects were more prominent, and there was now a central striate keratopathy and diffuse corneal edema (Fig. 113, B). By slit-lamp biomicroscopy a moderate flare was visible, but because of the corneal opacification it could not be determined whether there were cells. The left eye was entirely normal. The intraocular pressure was 27 mm. Hg (Schiøtz) in the right eye and 18 mm. Hg (Schiøtz) in the left. Corticosteroid drops were used at frequent intervals, along with mydriatics and idoxuridine (IDU) ointment. Three days later the striate keratopathy was somewhat more marked, and numerous fine keratic precipitates could be seen on the posterior surface of the cornea. The intraocular pressure was now normal. In another 2 weeks there was some improvement in the corneal edema,

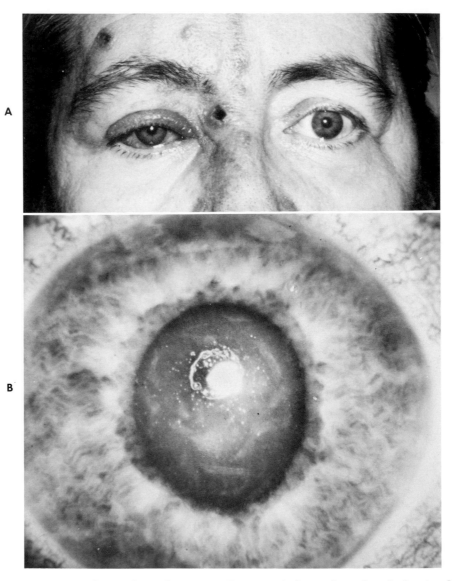

Fig. 113. *Vesicular and erythematous lesions of the right side of the forehead and nose, with iritis and striate keratopathy in the right eye in a 62-year-old woman with herpes zoster uveitis.* **A,** Regressing skin lesions typical of herpes zoster ophthalmicus involve the right nose and forehead region. **B,** The right cornea is diffusely edematous, and there is a central striate keratopathy; by slit-lamp examination there is an aqueous flare. Subsequently, keratic precipitates and a secondary glaucoma developed.

and no cells or flare could be seen. There was also a definite improvement in the patient's vision. Corticosteroid drops were discontinued; but when she was seen in 2 more weeks, she had marked loss of vision, with an intraocular pressure of 52 mm. Hg by applanation tonometry. There was marked corneal epithelial edema and punctate staining, with marked keratic precipitate formation. The pupil was irregular, and there were a number of posterior synechias. Mydriatics and corticosteroid drops were reinstituted, and glycerol was given parenterally, reducing the intraocular pressure to 27 mm. Hg by applanation tonometry. In another week the cornea had cleared; but there were still many keratic precipitates, and the pupil was fixed, due to posterior synechias. The intraocular pressure was normal. There continued to be some epithelial staining of the cornea and moderate cells and flare in the anterior chamber. This condition persisted intermittently for the next 3 months. The patient was then lost to follow-up; but she returned 6 years later, when she was found to have a low-grade anterior uveitis in both eyes. Her vision was now reduced to 20/400 in the right eye and 20/50 in the left. Corticosteroids and mydriatics were again used, and the uveitis completely resolved in about 3 months.

MYCOTIC AND PROTOZOAN UVEITIS

Antibiotic and steroid therapy have both been responsible for the increase in fungal infections, especially mycotic keratitis. If the fungal ulcer does not perforate, the iritis is relatively low grade. Treatment, if successful, results in complete clearing of the uveal inflammation. In the acute stages hypopyon is common. When the fungus is introduced into the eye or when the cornea perforates, vitreous involvement results in multiple slowly progressive "snowballs," with eventual loss of the eye. Any of the pathogenic fungi, including *Cryptococcus, Mucor, Blastomyces, Aspergillus, Coccidiodes,* and *Candida,* may be involved. Treatment is difficult and prolonged. Antibiotics, particularly streptomycin and the tetracyclines, and all corticosteroid therapy must be discontinued. Antifungal agents such as nystatin, amphotericin B, 5-fluorocystine (Ancobon), and Pimaricin may be effective.

The only protozoan of consequence to affect the eye is *Toxoplasma gondii.* Choroiditis from this organism is common. Both congenital and acquired forms are well known. In the presence of active posterior uveal involvement, an anterior uveitis of the granulomatous type may also occur; mutton-fat keratic precipitates, peripheral anterior synechias, and Koeppe nodules may be seen. Treatment of ocular toxoplasmosis is not always successful, but pyrimethamine (Daraprim), sulfonamides, and corticosteroids given systemically may be effective, with folinic acid to avoid thrombocytopenia and leukopenia. The course of the disease may be prolonged despite intensive therapy.

Iritis secondary to fungal keratitis

History. About a month ago this 75-year-old man developed an irritated right eye, which went untreated for 2 weeks. A smear of a corneal ulcer was then taken and a culture made; antibiotics (chloramphenicol and neomycin) given topically and cycloplegics were initiated. Despite intensive therapy for a week, there was gradual increase in the size of the ulcer, with progression of an anterior uveitis. Gentamicin administered subconjunctivally and topically was then substituted, with apparent temporary improvement; but 5 days later there was increased corneal involvement, and the anterior chamber filled with fibrin and white blood cells. The cause was thought to be fungal, and amphotericin B drops were begun; but the vision was reduced to light perception only, and the eye was very painful.

Findings. The vision in the right eye is light perception only and in the left 20/60. The lids of the right eye are swollen; the conjunctiva is markedly injected and chemotic. The cornea is diffusely cloudy, with a large central and

FIG. 114   nasal infiltrate involving more than half the cornea (Fig. 114, *A*). The corneal periphery is infiltrated with numerous superficial vessels. The anterior chamber is about two thirds filled with pus, and the pupil is not visible. The left eye is normal except for moderate nuclear sclerosis of the lens.

Course. Enucleation was performed, and the postoperative course was uneventful. Histopathologic examination showed the cornea to be filled with hyphae typical of mucormycosis (Fig. 114, *B*). The anterior chamber contained numerous white blood cells, fibrin, and a number of multinucleated giant cells (Fig. 114, *C*).

Fungal endophthalmitis

History. Seven weeks ago this 77-year-old woman had an uneventful cataract extraction. Three weeks postoperatively she developed anterior uveitis, which was treated with systemic administration of corticosteroids, and 5 weeks postoperatively she was noted to have a corneal infiltrate and a hypopyon. Culture of the corneal infiltrate showed coagulase-positive *Staphylococcus aureus*, and intensive antibiotic therapy with penicillin was instituted. With no improvement in 4 more days, drug therapy was changed to administration of cephalothin (Keflin) both systemically and subconjunctivally. The patient developed a cushingoid response to the systemic use of corticosteroids and a steroid-induced diabetes. There was no response to the intensive antibiotic treatment, and scrapings of the ulcer did not show any bacteria. Because of the possibility that a fungus infection had been enhanced by the corticosteroids, she was given amphotericin B subconjunctivally, but there was no improvement; in a few days the anterior chamber became filled with masses of white material and exudate.

Findings. The vision in the right eye is questionable light perception. The conjunctiva of the right eye is markedly chemotic, and the cornea is thickened,

---

Fig. 114. *Large corneal infiltrates and hypopyon in the right eye of a 75-year-old man with fungal keratitis and secondary iritis.* The patient had an irritated eye for 2 weeks, after which he was treated with intensive antibiotics for another 2 weeks, with gradual worsening of his keratitis. **A,** The anterior chamber was almost filled with pus. **B,** Photomicrograph of cornea showing hyphae typical of mucormycosis. (PAS stain; ×1000.) **C,** Photomicrograph of anterior chamber containing numerous white blood cells, fibrin, and multinucleated giant cells. (PAS stain; ×1000.)

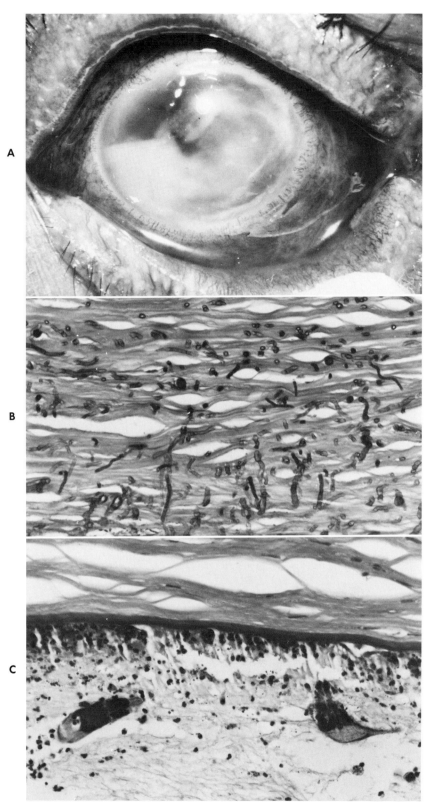

Fig. 114. For legend see opposite page.

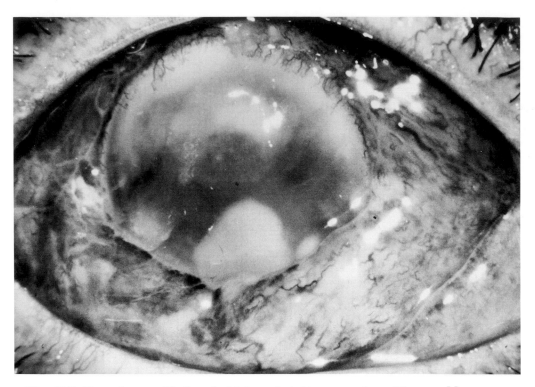

Fig. 115. *Densely opacified and thickened right cornea in a 77-year-old woman with a fungal endophthalmitis.* Seven weeks ago the patient had a cataract extraction, and 3 weeks postoperatively she developed an anterior uveitis, which was treated by systemic administration of corticosteroids. Two weeks later there were corneal infiltrates and a hypopyon. Subsequently, amphotericin B was given subconjunctivally, but the eye became blind and was enucleated.

FIG. 115 with the entire upper half densely opacified (Fig. 115). The anterior chamber contains a large mass of white fluffy material inferiorly, and elsewhere it is filled with fibrin and purulent material. Visualization of the iris and pupil is not possible.

Course. Two days later the patient agreed to enucleation, which was performed. The postoperative course was uneventful. Histopathologic examination showed an endophthalmitis, both fungal and bacterial; and both by culture and by histopathologic findings the fungus was proved to be *Mucor.*

"Toxoplasmic" uveitis and episcleritis

History. Since childhood this 43-year-old woman had poor vision in her right eye, which tended to be sensitive to bright light and which deviated outward. Six months ago the eye first developed severe pain and redness. Her local physician treated this condition with various pills, and in a short time she became asymptomatic. About 3 months ago the pain in her eye recurred, and this time it was treated with topical administration of corticosteroids; the condition gradually improved. A week ago the pain and redness in the right eye returned;

202

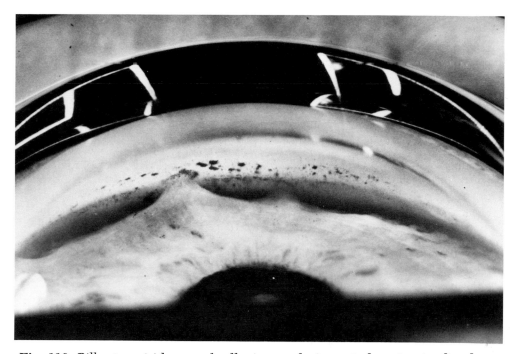

Fig. 116. *Pillar-type iridocorneal adhesions and pigment clumping in the chamber angle in a 43-year-old woman with "toxoplasmic" uveitis and episcleritis.* Since childhood the patient had poor vision in her right eye and recently developed episcleritis and low-grade iritis. Gonioscopy showed old peripheral anterior synechias, and the fundus had numerous chorioretinal heavily pigmented lesions typical of toxoplasmosis. Pyrimethamine and triple sulfas produced gradual improvement of her condition.

the patient was again treated with topical administration of corticosteroids and mydriatics.

Findings. The vision in the right eye is counting fingers at 1 foot and in the left 20/15. In the right eye there is a large patch of purplish red discoloration of the episclera extending from the 10 o'clock to the 1 o'clock position and involving the limbus. The remainder of the conjunctival vessels are somewhat dilated and tortuous. The lower third of the cornea is involved by a uniform whitish opacification of the posterior surface of the cornea. The remainder of the cornea is clear except for occasional pigmented keratic precipitates. The anterior chamber contains a small number of cells and a minimal flare. The pupil is normal, and there are a number of pigment deposits on the anterior capsule of the lens, which is otherwise normal. There is cellular invasion of the anterior vitreous. The eye is highly myopic, and there are numerous chorioretinal lesions that have heavy pigmented borders and atrophic centers. None of the lesions appear to be actively inflamed. In the left eye the anterior segment is normal. Fundus examination reveals many small healed and apparently inactive chorioretinal lesions especially temporally and inferior to the disc. In-

FIG. 116 traocular pressure is 18 mm. Hg (Schiøtz) in both eyes. By gonioscopy the angle of the anterior chamber in the right eye exhibits a number of large pillar-type iridocorneal adhesions (Fig. 116). There are many clumps of dark pigment on the peripheral cornea and trabecular meshwork. Where the angle is not involved with synechias, it is wide open.

Course. A tuberculin skin test in the highest dilution was positive, although the chest x-ray film was normal. All medications were discontinued, and streptomycin and isoniazid were given systemically for 1 week, at which time there was an increase in the pain and redness in the patient's right eye. A paracentesis was performed on the anterior chamber of the right eye. The precipitin test of the aqueous humor was positive for *Toxoplasma*. A *Toxoplasma* dye test titer of the patient's serum was found to be positive in 1:1024 dilution. Accordingly, pyrimethamine (Daraprim) and triple sulfas were initiated. This treatment was continued for 2 months, during which there was definite improvement of the pain and redness in the right eye. However, a month later there was an exacerbation of the pain, which was treated with topical and systemic administration of corticosteroids. The episcleritis and anterior uveitis promptly improved. The patient was asymptomatic until 11 years later, when she again had an attack of anterior uveitis and mild episcleritis. The signs and symptoms again resolved in about 2 months with the patient receiving topical administration of corticosteroids and mydriatics. Two years later she developed leg lesions and a fluctuant node in the right cervical area. An aspirate of the node grew *Mycobacterium tuberculosis*, and a biopsy of the legs confirmed erytherma nodosum. Treatment with isoniazid (INH), and para-aminosalicylic acid (PAS), ethambutol was continued for a year; by then the patient had become asymptomatic and was considered cured.

Toxoplasmic uveitis

History. About 3 years ago for several weeks this 23-year-old woman saw black spots before her left eye and was told that she had scars on the back of her left eye. Until a month ago she had no further difficulty, but at that time she noted sudden loss of vision and recurrence of her previous symptoms. Her general health was good.

Findings. Vision in the right eye is 20/20 and in the left eye hand movements only. The right eye is normal, including findings of the fundus examination by indirect ophthalmoscopy. In the left eye there is moderate ciliary injection, and the cornea is clear except for multiple large mutton-fat keratic

FIG. 117 precipitates involving the lower two thirds (Fig. 117). When the pupil, which is somewhat irregular, is dilated, a marked flare and many cells can be seen. Brown pigment is on the anterior capsule of the lens, and the vitreous is filled with many cells and strands. Visualization of the fundus is difficult, but several large areas of chrioretinitis can be visualized.

Course. X-ray films of the chest were normal; routine blood studies were within normal limits; and reactions to blood serologic tests were negative. Tuberculin and histoplasmin skin tests were negative. The laboratory lost a blood sample for a Sabin-Feldman dye test. Treatment was instituted with large doses of systemically and topically administered corticosteroids. A week later keratic

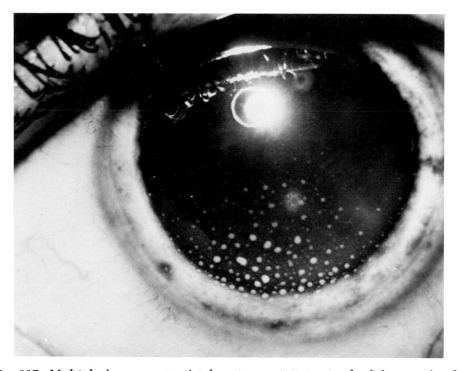

Fig. 117. *Multiple large mutton-fat keratic precipitates in the left eye of a 23-year-old woman with toxoplasmic uveitis.* A month ago the patient had sudden loss of vision and now has an active anterior uveitis and several large areas of chorioretinitis. Corticosteroids, pyrimethamine, and sulfonamide therapy produced a regression of the uveitis and chorioretinic lesions.

precipitates had disappeared, and there was only minimal flare and cells in the anterior chamber. Although the vitreous was still cloudy, indirect ophthalmoscopy revealed a large chorioretinitic scar, with a peripheral yellow mass, which appeared to be active chorioretinitis. Because of the classic lesions of the retina, pyrimethamine and sulfonamide therapy was begun. The patient developed a reactive depression, which was presumably steroid induced; the systemic administration of steroids was reduced, and retrobulbar corticosteroid injections were given instead. A month later the active chorioretinitis lesion was resolving, and beginning pigmentation was observed. In another month minimal activity remained, and 4 months later there were no signs of activity. The patient's vision improved to only 20/50.

SYMPATHETIC OPHTHALMITIS

Bilateral inflammation of the entire uveal tract following a perforating wound involving uveal tissue, with a latent period of at least 2 weeks, characterizes sympathetic ophthalmitis. Both eyes are affected simultaneously with a granulomatous uveitis of insidious onset and progressive course. The exact cause is unknown, but a hypersensitivity (autoimmune) reaction to uveal pigment seems to be the likely explanation. The injured eye (exciting eye) almost invariably has been involved with an injury with prolapse of the iris or ciliary body. The condition may follow a surgical procedure such as an iris inclusion glaucoma operation (iridencleisis); but far more commonly it follows injuries with uveal trauma, especially when treatment is not prompt or adequate. Enucleation of the injured eye performed within 2 weeks provides almost complete protection against the condition. Sympathetic uveitis almost never occurs in an eye in which there is suppuration. Delayed or incomplete healing of a wound involving uveal tissue appears to be the most likely causative situation. The older literature indicates that about 2% of perforating wounds resulted in sympathetic ophthalmitis, in contrast to no cases in 2,300 eyes wounded during World War II.

The appearance of a low-grade uveitis in the sympathizing eye is the first sign. Often the injured, or exciting, eye already has a low-grade uveitis associated with the injury. Once the process has begun in the sympathizing eye, enucleation of the exciting eye is ineffective. The uveitis is granulomatous with heavy mutton-fat keratic precipitates, anterior and posterior synechias, and some posterior uveal tract involvement. The sympathizing eye may end up with poorer vision than the exciting eye. Corticosteroids, administered systemically and topically, have a remarkably favorable effect on the disease, especially if they are instituted early.

Histopathologically, there is a diffuse and often massive infiltration of the uveal tract with lymphocytes, epithelioid cells, and giant cells. Small hemispherical accumulations of epithelioid cells with scattered pigment cells occur in the pigment epithelium of the retina (Dalen-Fuchs nodules).

Sympathetic uveitis

History. About 3 months ago while watching a truck dumping tin cans, this 13-year-old boy felt something strike his right eye. His local physician gave him eye drops, but the right eye continued to be blurred and slightly painful. About 2 weeks ago he was seen for the first time by an ophthalmologist, who found bilateral iritis and a healed corneal perforation of the right eye. Vision in each eye consisted of counting fingers at a few feet. High doses of ACTH and topically administered corticosteroids and mydriatics were given. A secondary glaucoma present in the left eye improved after a few days. In 2 weeks both eyes became white.

Findings. Vision in the right eye is 20/70 and in the left 20/30. In the right eye the conjunctiva has only minimal injection except at the limbus inferiorly. A large adherent leukoma involves the inferior temporal quadrant, FIG. 118 and a number of pigmented keratic precipitates are visible (Fig. 118). There is moderate flare and a few cells in the anterior chamber. The pupil is oval, and dense posterior synechias involve the entire pupillary border. Although the lens appears clear, the fundus cannot be visualized. In the left eye there is minimal conjunctival injection, and the cornea is clear except for a number of REEL XI-3 mutton-fat keratic precipitates in the central and inferior portion (Reel XI-3). There is a moderate flare in the anterior chamber, and the pupillary border is irregular due to multiple posterior synechias. The lens is clear and the fundus normal. The intraocular tension is 10 mm. Hg (Schiøtz) in both eyes.

Course. There was continued clinical improvement until a few months later

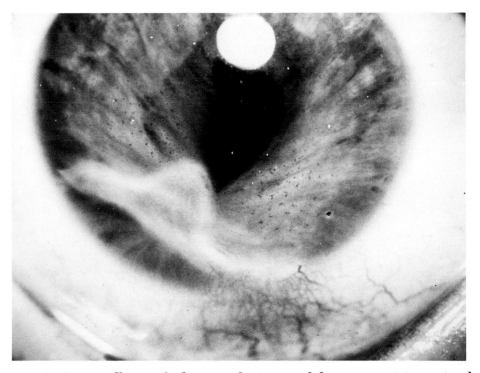

Fig. 118. *Large adherent leukoma and pigmented keratic precipitates in the right eye of a 13-year-old boy with sympathetic uveitis.* Three months ago the patient had a corneal perforation and 2 weeks ago was found to have bilateral iritis. Intensive corticosteroid, ACTH, and mydriatic therapy resulted in a marked improvement. In the left eye (see Reel XI-3) there are a number of mutton-fat keratic precipitates centrally and inferiorly. Subsequently, there were recurrences of the uveitis in both eyes and a marked secondary glaucoma in the left eye.

when the patient developed pain and redness in the left eye with an intra-ocular pressure of 67 mm. Hg (Schiøtz). Iris bombé was present; and a basal iridectomy was performed, followed by systemic corticosteroid treatment. A week later the intraocular tension again rose; it was discovered that the iridectomy was not basal, and numerous peripheral anterior synechias were seen gonio-scopically. Several recurrences of the uveitis in both eyes were controlled with systemic and topical administration of corticosteroids, and the intraocular pressure in the left eye required diisopropyl fluorophosphate (DFP) drops. Despite intermittently elevated tensions in the left eye, 2 years later there was no glau-comatous cupping, and the visual fields were normal. Five years after the accident the patient's vision was 20/40 in the right eye and 20/25 in the left.

PHAKOANAPHYLACTIC UVEITIS

Generalized uveitis following traumatic or operative perforation of the lens characterizes phakoanaphylactic uveitis (endophthalmitis phakoanaphylactica). The process has a latent period varying from 24 hours to 2 weeks and may be associated with an extracapsular cataract extraction, discission, lens trauma, or a spontaneous rupture of the lens capsule. A more common situation is the development of the reaction after an extracapsular cataract extraction has been performed in one eye and the other eye develops a mature lens with leakage of the cortical material into the anterior chamber. The reaction may be so violent and generalized that the eye may require enucleation when the course is prolonged, with permanent changes in the cornea, iris, anterior chamber, angle, and pupil. Sometimes the reaction is so severe that an endophthalmitis of other cause is seriously considered. Circulating antibodies to lens proteins can be found, and it is clear that an allergic response to lens protein has been produced that is similar to the allergic response to uveal tissue in sympathetic ophthalmitis. Histopathologically, the lens tissue is found to be invaded by polymorphonuclear leukocytes and mononuclear phagocytes; giant cells surround the lens material. Keratic precipitates are commonly found, and there is almost always a pupillary cyclitic membrane. As in phakolytic glaucoma, the posterior segment is usually unaffected unless long-standing glaucoma has produced optic disc changes.

Treatment consists of removal of excessive cortical material in either eye, if possible, along with mydriatics and corticosteroids given topically and systemically. In the event of a leaking hypermature cataract in the second eye, intracapsular cataract extraction is usually curative. Secondary glaucoma may occur and should be treated to avoid optic nerve damage. If phthisis bulbi occurs, enucleation may be required.

Phakoanaphylactic uveitis

History. For several years this 65-year-old woman noted gradual loss of vision in both eyes until 9 months ago she was almost totally incapacitated. She was found to have almost mature cataracts in both eyes, and a planned extracapsular cataract extraction was performed on the more mature cataract in the left eye. Postoperatively there was some reaction, but only a minimal amount of cortex remained. One month postoperatively she developed ciliary injection, cells and flare in the anterior chamber, and keratic precipitates in the right eye. Topical administration of corticosteroids and mydriatics was initiated, but she did not return for any follow-up visits until today when the pain became so severe that she could not stand it any longer.

Findings. Vision in the right eye is light perception only and in the left 20/30 with correction. In the right eye there is a marked ciliary injection and many fine keratic precipitates on the endothelium. The anterior chamber is about half REEL XI-4 filled with purulent and fibrinous material (Reel XI-4). The pupillary area is completely filled with a white membrane. In the left eye there is a complete surgical coloboma superiorly and some capsular remnants in the pupillary area. The vitreous and fundus are normal.

Course. Systemic and topical administration of corticosteroids and mydriatics was initiated for treatment of the uveitis in the right eye. In 2 days there was little change, and an unplanned extracapsular cataract extraction was performed. Postoperatively the anterior chamber contained many cells and some cortical material. Resolution was slow, and a membrane formed on the vitreous face. A week later the anterior chamber became flat, and it was evident that the patient had a complete pupillary block. An iridectomy and posterior sclerotomy were

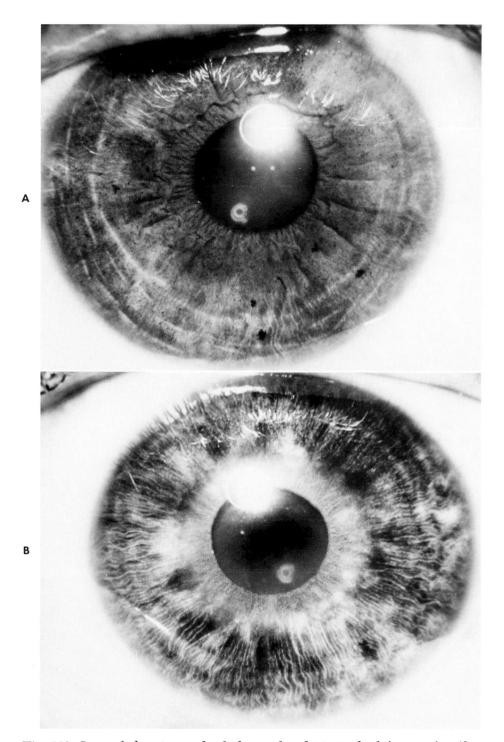

Fig. 119. *Stromal thinning and a lighter colored iris in the left eye of a 42-year-old woman with heterochromic iridocyclitis.* Recently the patient noticed that vision in her left eye was blurred and that her irides were a different color. **A,** The right iris is brown and is normal, with prominent contraction furrows. **B,** The left iris is a light greenish color, and the stroma is irregularly thinned. Keratic precipitates, a minimal anterior chamber reaction, and a posterior subcapsular cataract are present. With the patient receiving corticosteroid and mydriatic therapy the iritis subsided, but the cataract continued to progress.

209

carried out on the right eye. Postoperatively she had a hyphema and a marked striate keratitis. During the next 6 months the cornea became opacified and the anterior chamber shallow. The eye gradually developed phthisis bulbi. Eight years later there was a marked band keratopathy and an extremely soft eye, while the left eye continued to have good vision.

HETEROCHROMIC IRIDOCYCLITIS (FUCHS'S SYNDROME)

Unilateral heterochromia, keratic precipitates, and secondary glaucoma characterize heterochromic iridocyclitis. The cause of this rare condition is a complete mystery. The condition appears to be congenital, slowly progressively, with lens changes not occurring until early adult life. No cause has ever been found for the iridocyclitis, which is apparently the primary condition. The keratic precipitates are fine and nonpigmented. There is usually an aqueous flare, and often the vitreous contains dustlike opacities. The iris gradually becomes pigmented and atrophic. As atrophy progresses, the iris becomes lighter in color and translucent, due to degeneration of the iris pigment epithelium. In some patients there is sympathetic paralysis, and rarely unilateral nerve deafness. The posterior segment is not involved. The condition is unusual in that it appears to be congenital but requires years to run its course. There is no pain and little redness in the eye, but the iris heterochromia is apparent early in life.

Cataract extraction, often uneventful, is usually required. The most serious complication of Fuchs's syndrome is secondary glaucoma.

Heterochromic iridocyclitis

History. For at least a year this 42-year-old woman was noted to have different-colored irides and blurring of vision in her left eye. For 9 months she was given corticosteroids systemically for an iritis in her left eye. Some improvement occurred, but a psoriatic skin condition became worse. Several subconjunctival injections of corticosteroids were given, as well as intensive administration of corticosteroids and mydriatics topically. Recently there was marked reduction in the activity, including resolution of a number of large keratic precipitates.

FIG. 119 *Findings.* Vision in the right eye is 20/20 and in the left 20/30. The right eye is normal, including a brown iris with prominent contraction furrows (Fig. 119, A). In the left eye there are a few nonpigmented keratic precipitates in the lower portion of the cornea and a minimal number of cells and flare in the anterior chamber. The iris is lighter than that of the right eye and has a greenish color. Stromal thinning and loss of sphincter tissue permits visualization of iris pigment epithelium in a number of areas (Fig. 119, B). In the posterior subcapsular region of the lens are a number of granular opacities. The vitreous contains cellular debris, and the fundus is normal. Intraocular pressure is 20 mm. Hg (Schiøtz) in both eyes.

Course. During the next year slit-lamp biomicroscopic examination continued to reveal some cells in the anterior chamber. For another 4 months the patient had no signs of inflammation, but the cataract formation gradually progressed until the vision had decreased to 20/200 in the left eye. She was then lost to follow-up.

Chapter 8

Degenerative and atrophic conditions of the iris

IRIS ATROPHY IN SENILITY AND MYOPIA

Thinning of the iris stroma especially in the pupillary area, with increased visibility of the sphincter muscle, is typical of senile atrophy of the iris. Early in adult life the entire iris stroma begins to thin, with a decrease in saturation in the color of the iris. The crypts gradually disappear, and the sphincter muscle becomes visible as a brown circular structure contrasting with the lighter iris surrounding it. Iris vessels become more easily visible, and some are converted to white lines containing no blood. The pigment frill at the margin of the iris frequently becomes transparent, producing an irregular moth-eaten appearance of the pupillary margin. Peripherally, atrophy of the stroma may be sufficient so that pigment epithelium, dark brown in color, can be visualized between the remaining stromal fibers. Depigmentation of the pigment epithelium also occurs so that transillumination shows translucency of the iris in a high percentage of individuals in their 70's and 80's. Sometimes there is pigment dispersion, giving a salt-and-pepper appearance to the stroma when examined by slit-lamp biomicroscopy.

Occasionally in a highly myopic eye a reverse type of degenerative change may occur in which there is proliferation of pigment epithelium in the form of an extensive ectropion uvea. The iris stroma may be unaffected except that it becomes covered to a variable extent by a sheet of pigment epithelium that can extend from the pupillary margin the entire width of the iris to the angle recess. By the time these marked changes occur, the eye is usually blind; and an associated retinal detachment is a common occurrence. The common type of iris atrophy associated with myopia is very similar to the senile type.

Senile iris atrophy

History. For about 5 years this 78-year-old man had gradual failing of vision, and in the past 6 months this became much more marked. Moreover, he noted halos in both eyes at night.

Findings. The vision in both eyes is counting fingers at about 4 feet. In both eyes the corneas are clear except for a posterior embryotoxon (Axenfeld's anomaly) seen only temporally and nasally because of a superior and inferior arcus senilis. The anterior chambers are deep and clear. The iris is markedly atrophic around the irregular pupil, and there is a prominent gray ring represent-ing the sphincter and much thinning of the iris stroma to the extent that pigment

FIG. 120   epithelium is easly visible everywhere (Fig. 120). Almost mature cortical cataracts are present, and only a dull red fundus reflex can be obtained. Intra-ocular tension in both eyes is 37 mm. Hg (Schiøtz).

Course. Because of the elevated intraocular pressures, tonography was per-formed about 5 hours later. Intraocular tensions at this time were 17 mm. Hg (Schiøtz) in both eyes. Tonography showed a marked decrease in the facility of outflow and a low rate of aqueous formation. Gonioscopy showed an open angle except for iris stromal attachments to Schwalbe's line, which bridged the

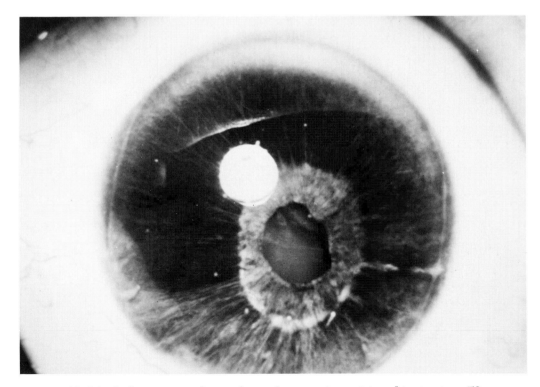

Fig. 120. *Marked iris stromal atrophy and a prominent iris sphincter in a 78-year-old man with senile iris atrophy.* The stroma is so thin that pigment epithelium is visible and the outline of the sphincter muscle easily discernible. Advanced cortical cataracts are also present in both eyes.

meshwork (a finding that is consistent with Axenfeld's anomaly). Pilocarpine (4%) drops were initiated in both eyes, and the intraocular pressure remained well within normal limits. A planned extracapsular cataract extraction was performed on the left eye. Considerable difficulty was encountered when an iridectomy was attempted, because the iris had no substance except in the pupillary area. Postoperatively there were no complications. An intracapsular cataract extraction was performed on the right eye, and again there were no postoperative complications. Six weeks later refraction of the patient showed his vision to be 20/40 in the right eye and 20/100 in the left. He was then lost to follow-up.

Iris degeneration in high myopia

History. This 19-year-old boy had been born 7 weeks prematurely. At age 5 he was found to have a vision of 3/200 in his right eye and 20/30 in his left eye, with a marked esotropia. The right eye exhibited a high myopia and a posterior staphyloma and dragged disc. Five years ago he was found to have an almost total retinal detachment in the right eye, but no operative procedure was undertaken. Two years ago he developed a mature cataract and an unusual iris pigmentation. Subsequently, the anterior lens capsule became wrinkled, and a year ago the anterior chamber was found to contain crystals.

Findings. The right eye is blind, and the vision in the left eye is 20/30 with correction. In the right eye the cornea is clear, and the anterior chamber is deep. The pupil is semidilated, and the iris has a most unusual appearance because the iris pigment epithelium has proliferated over the anterior surface of the iris extending to the angle in many places (Reel XI-5). Light blue areas   REEL XI-5 that represent normal iris stroma where not completely covered by the pigment epithelium are visible in the peripheral iris. In the pupil can be seen a mature cataract with a wrinkled anterior capsule and some posterior synechias. Visualization of the posterior segment is impossible. Except for mild myopia, the left eye is normal.

Course. Six months later the right eye remained unchanged.

ESSENTIAL IRIS ATROPHY

Unilateral progressive iris atrophy, peripheral anterior synechia formation, and glaucoma characterize essential iris atrophy, most commonly seen in women between the ages of 30 and 40 years. Slow and insidious in onset, the first sign is an oval or displaced pupil. An area of iris atrophy develops and progresses to total loss of stromal tissue and pigment epithelium, with displacement of the pupil away from the atrophic area and with broad and usually truncated synechias extending well onto the cornea in an otherwise open angle. In some patients a fine beaten silver appearance (not as coarse as that seen in typical endothelial dystrophy) may be visible in the endothelium. In those patients who have endothelial changes, intermittent halos may result from corneal edema in the presence of even normal or only slightly elevated intraocular pressures. As the disease progresses with more synechial involvement, the tension becomes elevated, requiring medical and finally surgical treatment. The tension may remain normal for years, especially if the synechias bridge the trabecular meshwork. Rarely, essential iris atrophy occurs bilaterally; generally it is seen only in young men, and some cases have been reported to be X-linked recessive.

Progressive iris atrophy without pigment epithelial involvement but with multiple snyechia formation and marked endothelial dystrophy characterizes Chandler's syndrome, which is probably a form of essential iris atrophy. Early iris atrophy is not a prominent feature. In fact, the peripheral anterior synechias may precede atrophy in some cases. While the presenting symptoms in classical essential iris atrophy are distortion of the pupil and pseudopolycoria, in Chandler's syndrome the initial complaints are halos and blurring of vision from corneal edema. Intraocular pressures may be as low as the middle or high teens. Because of the lesser degree of iris involvement, the pupil is not markedly displaced and may even be perfectly round. The synechias involve the trabecular meshwork and extend well onto the cornea, in contrast to the bridging that occurs in the classical essential iris atrophy. The corneal edema in Chandler's syndrome is partially controlled by a lowering of the intraocular pressure with miotics and carbonic anhydrase inhibitors. Hypertonic ointments and drops may be of help, but eventually filtering procedures, such as trephination, may be necessary to keep the pressure sufficiently low. Nevertheless, bullous keratopathy may still ensue, with loss of useful vision, requiring penetrating keratoplasty.

Of the two types, Chandler's syndrome may be the more common. Because the iris atrophy is not as evident and because corneal edema is such a prominent feature, the condition is not always recognized. If corneal edema and bullous keratopathy are sufficiently severe, detection of peripheral anterior synechias and iris atrophy may be impossible.

The cause of both types is obscure. Vascular occlusive disease has been suggested, but neither the occurrence in only one eye nor the endothelial changes can be explained on this basis. A congenital anomaly has been proposed to explain the endothelial changes, but the unilaterality again is evidence against this hypothesis. Both types must be classified as an abiotrophy of the iris.

The differential diagnosis involves such congenital conditions as corectopia, coloboma, and polycoria, none of which is progressive. Although senile iris atrophy and iridoschisis are progressive, they do not ordinarily result in peripheral anterior synechia formations, and they are usually bilateral. Rieger's syndrome is occasionally progressive in early life and thus could be confused with a juvenile bilateral essential iris atrophy. However, the dominant inheritance found in Rieger's syndrome should easily differentiate the two conditions (p. 143).

Essential iris atrophy

History. About 3 years ago this 38-year-old woman noticed that the pupil of her left eye had become pulled to one side. About a year ago she noticed that a hole had appeared in her iris.

Findings. The vision in the right eye is 20/15 and in the left 20/20. Examination of the right eye, including the iris, shows no abnormalities. In the left eye the pupil is displaced superiorly and temporally so that its lower nasal border FIG. 121 is at the center of the eye (Fig. 121, A). Nasally and inferiorly there is a marked iris atrophy that includes the pigment epithelium. Gonioscopy reveals that extensive peripheral anterior synechias, particularly adjacent to the dis-

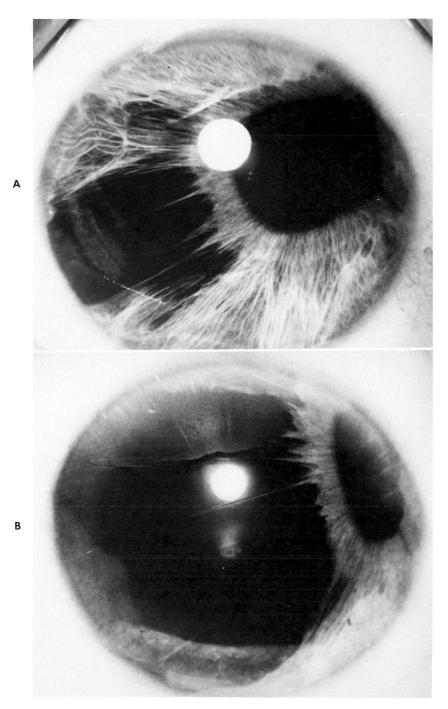

Fig. 121. *Marked progressive iris atrophy and displacement of the pupil in the left eye of a 38-year-old woman with essential iris atrophy.* **A,** The pupil is displaced superiorly and temporally, and a large hole through the iris has appeared inferiorly and nasally. The patient noticed the pupillary defect about 3 years ago. **B,** Eight years later there was gradual progression of the iris atrophy, with further displacement of the pupil and total atrophy of most of the iris. Gonioscopy (see Reel XI-6) reveals multiple broad synechias, many of which appear to bridge the trabecular meshwork. A mild glaucoma was controlled with pilocarpine drops.

placed pupil and the area of maximal iris atrophy, are present. The sphincter of the iris is intact and reacts to light. The intraocular pressure is 17 mm. Hg (Schiøtz) in both eyes.

Course. Over a period of 8 years there was gradual progression of the atrophic process in only the left eye until the pupil was markedly displaced and the patient was seeing through a large hole in the iris (Fig. 121, *B*). It appeared that less than a fifth of the original iris tissue remained, but the sphincter could still be identified. Multiple broad synechias were visible by gonioscopy, REEL XI-6 and many appeared to bridge the trabecular meshwork (Reel XI-6). In some places the atrophy was so extensive that no iris tissue remained to involve the angle structures. Because the intraocular tension had become somewhat elevated in recent months, pilocarpine drops were given, bringing the intraocular pressure to within normal limits. The vision remained at 20/20, and the right eye was normal with 20/15 vision. The visual fields of the right eye were normal, but in the left there was slight enlargement of the blind spot.

Essential iris atrophy

History. For about a year this 55-year-old man had noted blurring of vision in the right eye. About 6 months ago he was found to have an intraocular tension of 50 mm. Hg (Schiøtz) in the right eye; medical therapy was initiated, and the tension returned to normal.

Findings. Vision in the right eye is 20/40 and in the left 20/20. There is mild injection of the conjunctiva of the right eye, and the cornea shows a fine guttate appearance of the endothelium by specular reflection. The iris is grossly FIG. 122 abnormal, with the pupil displaced superiorly and temporally (Fig. 122, *A*). In the central portion of the iris the stroma is markedly thinned, and in a number of places the pigment epithelium is also absent. On the remaining iris are many small dark brown masses that have the appearance of iris nevi. Bordering the eccentric pupil is a prominent ectropion uveae. Peripheral anterior synechia formation is present almost everywhere (Fig. 122, *B*) except from the 12 o'clock to the 2 o'clock position. The posterior segment is normal. The left eye, including the intraocular tension, is normal.

Course. Despite maximal medical glaucoma therapy, the intraocular tension gradually became elevated and finally reached the mid 30's with an associated corneal edema. A posterior sclerectomy filtering procedure was performed, along with the removal superiorly of about half of the iris. Immediately postoperatively the patient developed a persistent bullous keratopathy, and a cataract developed shortly thereafter. The patient was found to have carcinoma of the lung, from which he died about a year later.

Essential iris atrophy (Chandler's type)

History. About 7 months ago this 43-year-old woman noticed that her right pupil was irregular. Since then the pupil has remained about the same.

Findings. The vision in both eyes is 20/20. In the right eye by slit-lamp biomicroscopy the cornea is seen to have a fine endothelial beaten silver appearance. The anterior chamber centrally is of normal depth, and the pupil is oval FIG. 123 shaped due to traction toward the 2 and 7 o'cock positions (Fig. 123, *A*).

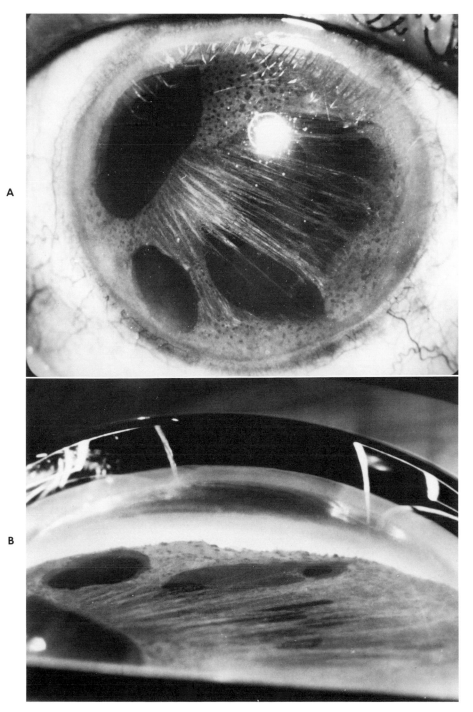

Fig. 122. *Displacement of the pupil and irregular atrophy of the iris stroma and pigment epithelium in the right eye of a 55-year-old man with essential iris atrophy.* **A,** The pupil is displaced superiorly and temporally, and much of the iris is thinned or absent. Slit-lamp examination shows a fine guttate defect of the endothelium. **B,** Gonioscopy reveals that almost the entire angle is involved with peripheral anterior synechia formation. There is marked elevation in tension, which is controlled by medical therapy. However, subsequently the tension could not be controlled, and a filtering procedure was performed, followed by persistent bullous keratopathy and cataract formation.

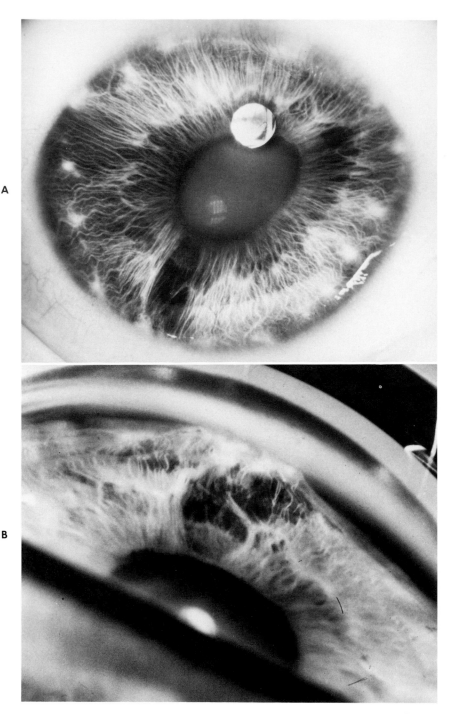

Fig. 123. *Localized iris stromal thinning and peripheral anterior synechias in the right eye of a 43-year-old woman with Chandler's type of essential iris atrophy.* **A,** The pupil is ovoid, and at the 2 o'clock and the 7 o'clock positions there is stromal thinning. Slit-lamp biomicroscopy shows a fine endothelial beaten silver appearance. **B,** Gonioscopy reveals a broad iridocorneal adhesion at the 7 o'clock position. Similar smaller synechias are at the 2 o'clock and the 10 o'clock positions. Subsequently, the patient developed blurring of vision associated with mild elevation of intraocular pressure. Finally, a trephine procedure was required, and 14 years later she was asymptomatic.

At the 7 o'clock position and to a lesser extent at the 2 o'clock there is thinning of the stroma and tenting of the peripheral iris. By gonioscopy a large truncated peripheral synechia is revealed at the 7 o'clock position (Fig. 123, *B*), and a similar synechia is seen at the 2 o'clock position. An early synechia formation is also visible at the 10 o'clock position. The posterior segment is normal. The left eye has no abnormality in the corneal endothelium. The pupil is round, and there is no atrophy of the iris. The posterior segment is also normal. Intraocular pressures are normal and equal in both eyes.

Course. Six months later a new synechia was noted to have formed at the 4 o'clock position, and there was further iris stromal thinning, with the resultant relaxation of the traction on the pupil, which resumed a round contour. Pilocarpine drops were now instituted on a prophylactic basis in the right eye. Four years later while still using pilocarpine drops the patient began to experience episodes of blurring of vision in the right eye, and her intraocular pressure was found to be elevated to 30 mm. Hg (Schiøtz). Temporarily the addition of epinephrine (2%) drops lowered the intraocular pressure; but it again became elevated, and a month later a trephine filtering procedure was performed in which a large sector of iris was excised, producing a coloboma from the 11 o'clock to the 2:30 position. Subsequently, an excellent filtering bleb developed. Fourteen years later the intraocular pressure remained around 10 mm. Hg (Schiøtz), and the patient was asymptomatic.

Essential iris atrophy (Chandler's type)

History. This 26-year-old woman had recurrent episodes of blurring in her left eye, which recently increased. She began to see halos through this eye at all times.

Findings. The vision in both eyes is 20/25. The right eye is normal. The left eye has minimal conjunctival injection, with slight corneal haze. Slit-lamp examination reveals a fine beaten silver appearance of the endothelium and peripheral shallowing of the anterior chamber. The pupil is slightly irregular, and the iris has areas of slight stromal thinning (Fig. 124, *A*). Gonioscopy reveals three broad peripheral anterior synechias; the most prominent ones are at the 11 and 2 o'clock positions (Fig. 124, *B*). The posterior segment is normal. The intraocular tension in the right eye is 15 mm. Hg and in the left 28 mm. Hg. by applanation tonometry.

FIG. 124

Course. Over the next 1½ years there was further progression of the corneal edema, peripheral anterior synechias, and iris atrophy (Fig. 124, *C*). The intraocular pressures steadily rose to the 40's and 50's while the patient was receiving maximal medical therapy. Following a trephine procedure and peripheral iridectomy a large diffuse bleb developed that involved two thirds of the circumference of the globe. This produced a hypotony of 0 to 4 mm. Hg (Schiøtz) and caused macular edema, which reduced the vision to 20/60. Over the next year there was gradual reduction of the bleb and return of vision to 20/25. Two years later the bleb suddenly became flat and the eye extremely soft. A small leak was observed in the bleb, which spontaneously resealed promptly without therapy, and the intraocular tension gradually returned to its previous level of 15 mm. Hg as revealed by applanation tonometry.

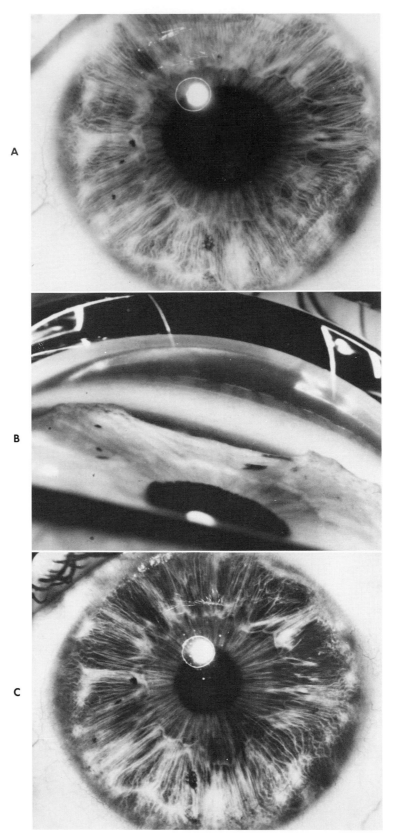

Fig. 124. For legend see opposite page.

Essential iris atrophy (Chandler's type)

History. This 41-year-old woman has been treated by her private ophthalmologist for several years for iris atrophy of her right eye. For the past 6 years she has been aware of a peculiar triangle-shaped pupil. Her primary problem was episodic corneal edema and pain, which was treated successfully with methylcellulose eye drops.

Findings. Visual acuity in the right eye is 20/25 and in the left 20/20. Schiøtz tonometry reveals an intraocular pressure of 18 mm. Hg in both eyes. Examination reveals that the cornea is clear, with a shallow anterior chamber especially superiorly. Examination with the slit lamp reveals a general thinning of the iris. The most striking part of the examination is the peculiar atrophy of the iris superiorly, with an eversion of the iris borders and apparent traction drawing the iris into the angle at the 1, 6, and 10 o'clock positions (Fig. 125). FIG. 125 The lens and the posterior segment of the right eye are normal. The left eye is normal.

Course. Over the next month the intraocular pressures became uncontrollable even though the patient was receiving maximal medication, and a trephine procedure was performed on the right eye. The postoperative course was uneventful. The pressure was well controlled over the next several years, first with the patient receiving only massage and later pilocarpine (2%). Eight years later the addition of acetazolamide and epinephrine (2%) was necessary for adequate control of intraocular tension. The visual fields of the right eye became constricted, and the vision fell to 20/70 with correction. Eight years later when the vision fell to perceiving hand movements and the pressures again were uncontrollable, and the patient was severely uncomfortable, a combined procedure was done in which an immature cataract was extracted and a scleral lip cautery filtering procedure was performed. One year later the vision was still perceiving hand movements, as the cornea remained edematous despite a functioning bleb and intraocular tensions of 20 mm. Hg by applanation tonometry and with the patient using epinephrine drops. The patient, however, was quite happy, since her pain had disappeared.

Essential iris atrophy (Chandler's type)

History. Three years ago this 48-year-old woman was discovered to have essential iris atrophy in the right eye. Two years ago and again a year ago she

---

Fig. 124. *Stromal thinning and multiple peripheral anterior synechias in the left eye of a 26-year-old woman with Chandler's type of essential iris atrophy.* **A,** The iris has several areas of mild thinning, and the pupil is slightly irregular. Slit-lamp examination reveals a fine beaten silver appearance of the endothelium. **B,** Gonioscopy shows broad peripheral anterior synechias. **C,** Gradual progression of the iris atrophy, with more synechial formation, occurred in 1½ years. The patient's initial symptom was halos due to corneal edema; this worsened, with an increase in her intraocular pressure despite maximal medical therapy. A filtering procedure was then required.

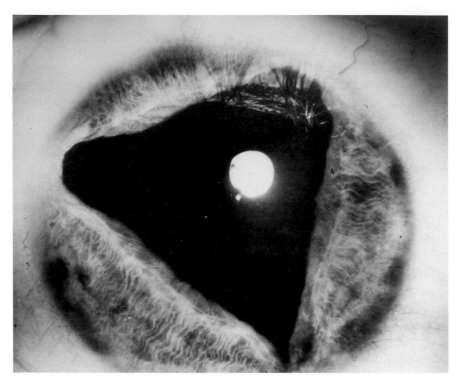

Fig. 125. *Triangular-shaped pupil, thinning of the iris, and iridocorneal adhesions in the right eye of a 41-year-old woman with Chandler's type of essential iris atrophy.* The pupillary abnormality has been present for 6 years, and her major complaint is on the basis of episodic corneal edema. Subsequently, she developed elevated intraocular pressures, which required a filtering procedure.

had cyclodiathermy procedures performed on the right eye to control the markedly elevated intraocular pressures. However, the tensions again became elevated, and the eye was almost blind. Three weeks ago she underwent a retro-orbital injection of alcohol, but there was no relief of her severe pain.

Findings. The vision in the right eye is light perception only and in the left 20/25. In the right eye there is mild conjunctival injection. The corneal epithelium is edematous and bedewed, and there is an irregularity to the endothelium. The anterior chamber is clear and of normal depth. The iris has multiple FIG. 126 areas of stromal thinning, which are most marked at the 3 o'clock position (Fig. 126, *A*). The pupil is eccentric, being displaced superiorly. There is slight nuclear sclerosis of the lens, and the fundus shows almost total glaucomatous cupping of the disc. Gonioscopy reveals about 75% of the angle to be involved with broad peripheral anterior synechias that attach anterior to Schwalbe's line. These are particularly prominent and dense in areas adjacent to the iris atrophy. The left eye, including findings revealed by gonioscopic examination, is normal.

Course. The right eye was enucleated, and there was a gross pathologic finding of multiple scars of the ciliary body and pars plana associated with the cyclodiathermy applications (Fig. 126, *B*). Histopathologic diagnosis was es-

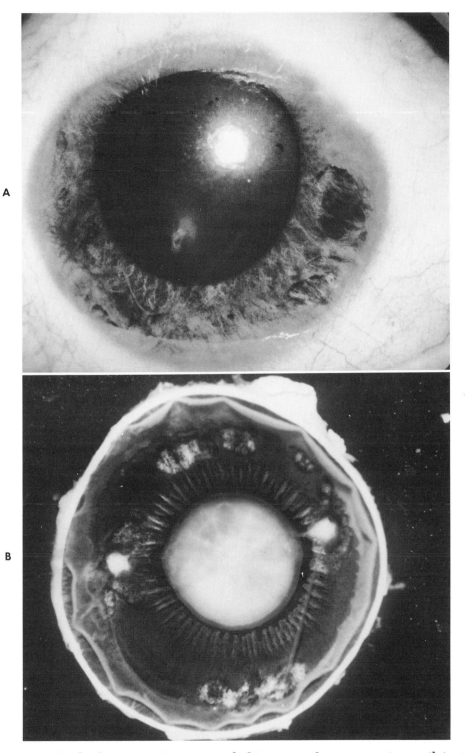

Fig. 126. *Multiple areas of iris stromal thinning and an eccentric pupil in the right eye of a 48-year-old woman with essential iris atrophy.* **A,** The iris stroma is thinned especially at the 3 o'clock position. The pupil is semidilated and displaced superiorly. Gonioscopy reveals marked peripheral anterior synechia formation. **B,** Gross pathologic specimen shows multiple scars of the ciliary body and pars plana due to cyclodiathermy applications for glaucoma.

sential iris atrophy with secondary glaucoma and optic atrophy in a glaucomatous cupped disc. Multiple areas of necrosis of the ciliary body were also present.

Essential iris atrophy (Chandler's type)

History. For about 2 years this 25-year-old woman had episodes of blurred vision in the right eye that were more noticeable at night, particularly when she was driving. Nine months ago she developed pain, redness, and tearing in the right eye, and her intraocular tension was found to be 55 mm. Hg (Schiøtz). Examination showed that she had multiple areas of iris atrophy, with large peripheral anterior synechias and glaucomatous cupping. A 10-day trial of intensive glaucomatous medical treatment failed to control the tension, and a trephine procedure was carried out. Postoperatively the intraocular pressure was low.

FIG. 127   *Findings.* The vision in the right eye is 20/20 and in the left 20/15. In the right eye there is a large succulent filtering bleb at the 12 o'clock position (Fig. 127). The cornea is clear except for broad anterior synechias at the 4 and 7 o'clock positions. There is also iris stromal thinning adjacent to the synechias.

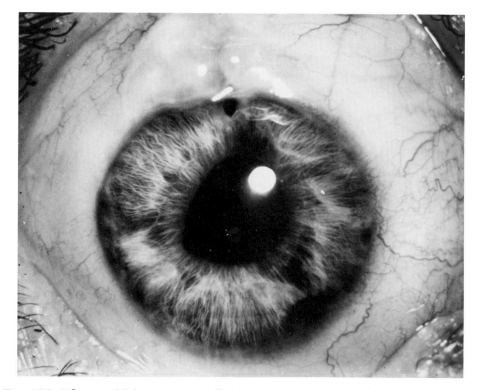

Fig. 127. *Filtering blebs, iris stromal thinning, and peripheral anterior synechias in the right eye of a 25-year-old woman with Chandler's type of essential iris atrophy.* Her intraocular tension became markedly elevated, and a trephine filtering procedure was required. The tension remained low for 5 years, when she developed corneal edema despite pressures in the low 20's. Another filtering procedure was required.

The pupil is ovoid, being pulled toward the 7 o'clock position. The media are clear, but the disc is atrophic and shows early glaucomatous cupping. Gonioscopy reveals an open angle except in the region of the extensive peripheral anterior synechias. The left eye is normal.

Course. For the next 5 years the pressure in the right eye remained in the teens without medication. The patient was then found to have corneal edema, even though her intraocular pressure was only 22 mm. Hg by applanation tonometry. The corneal edema in the right eye persisted, and a Scheie filtering procedure was performed in an attempt to lower her pressure further and avoid the corneal edema. Ten years later her vision was 20/50 in the right eye and 20/20 in the left, and the intraocular pressures were 16 mm. Hg (Schiøtz) in both eyes. The filtering bleb was functional, and there was no evidence of new peripheral anterior synechia formation. Fundus examination revealed deep glaucomatous cupping of the disc.

IRIDOSCHISIS

Localized splitting of the anterior layers of the iris stroma, with fragmentation of the fibrils, which may then float freely into the anterior chamber, characterizes iridoschisis. It is rare, is usually bilateral, and its occurrence is almost invariably restricted to the aged. Although commonly seen in eyes without other disease, it is sometimes associated with chronic open angle glaucoma. Some patients with iridoschisis develop acute angle closure glaucoma; however, except for aging, there is no relationship between the two conditions. Iridoschisis may develop following an attack of acute glaucoma (p. 34). No sex predilection or familial tendency has been found.

Although the picture of iridoschisis varies considerably, typically only the inferior portion of the iris is involved. At first there is separation of the anterior leaf of the iris stroma and fragmentation or rupture of the peripheral end of the fibers so that the entire leaf floats forward into the anterior chamber with slow progression over a number of years. There is further fragmentation of the iris into separate fibrils, which break and float centrally to cover variable amounts of the pupil. In some instances the fibrils float anteriorly and touch the cornea and may damage the corneal endothelium, with resulting corneal edema. Sometimes the process is most marked over the sphincter region, and the fibrils break near the pupillary margin and float toward the periphery of the iris. Evidently the angle is never sufficiently involved to produce glaucoma; thus the occasionally occurring corneal edema is the only direct complication. Histopathologically, the iris stroma shows marked atrophy, but there is circumscribed thickening and cellular accumulations in the dilator muscle. Iridoschisis is considered to be a senile atrophic change of the iris in which the anterior stroma separates from the posterior muscular portion due to constant pupillary dilatation and contraction.

Iridoschisis

History. Recently this 79-year-old woman noted a decrease in vision in her previously better right eye. She was otherwise asymptomatic.

Findings. Vision in the right eye is counting fingers at 3 feet and in the left 20/100. The anterior segments are normal except for the irides. In the right eye there is an area of fragmentation of the iris between the 5 and 7 o'clock positions, with iris stromal fibrils extending out into the anterior chamber. There is an almost mature cataract, with only a red reflex visible on fundus examination. In the left eye there is more extensive fragmentation of the iris, extending REEL XI-7 from the 4 o'clock to the 8 o'clock position (Reel XI-7). The iris stromal fibrils are broken and floating forward in the anterior chamber, with several almost touching the cornea. The pigment epithelium of the iris is visible due to the

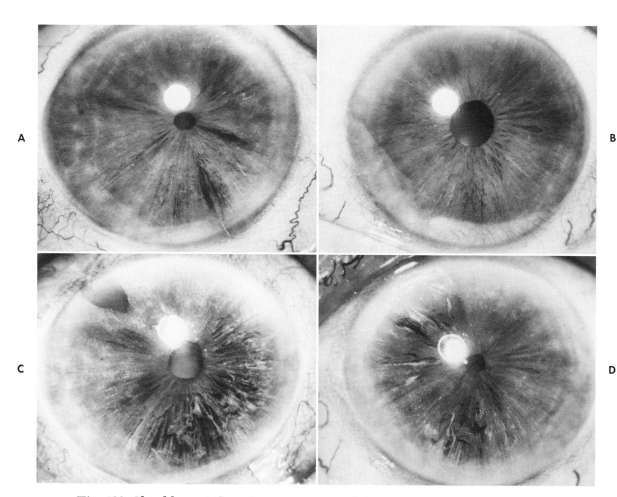

Fig. 128. *Shredding of the inferior iris stroma bilaterally in a 71-year-old woman with iridoschisis.* **A,** In the right eye the stromal fibers are separated and floating forward into the anterior chamber. **B,** In the left eye the shredding is limited to a small area inferiorly. **C,** Ten years later the right eye showed a marked increase in the shredding of the iris stroma, with visualization of the pigment epithelium in some areas. A year before, the patient had a peripheral iridectomy following an attack of acute angle closure glaucoma. **D,** The shredding and atrophy of the iris in the left eye 10 years later had progressed to involve the inferior and nasal iris.

atrophy of the stromal tissue. An immature cataract allows the visualization of a normal fundus. The intraocular tensions are normal.

Course. The patient was told to return for follow-up but was not seen again.

Iridoschisis

History. Three years ago this 71-year-old woman was found to have glaucoma in both eyes; the condition was treated with pilocarpine (4%) drops.

Findings. The vision in both eyes is 20/25. Both eyes are white. There is a prominent arcus senilis, and the anterior chambers are shallow. In the right eye the iris stroma inferiorly is shredded, and portions of it float forward into the anterior chamber, especially in one area at the 5 o'clock position, where the stroma is so thin that the pigment epithelium can be visualized (Fig. 128, *A*). In the left FIG. 128 eye there is a similar appearance, except that the entire iris from the 4 o'clock to the 6 o'clock position is shredded into fine filaments (Figs. 128, *B*). Results of the remainder of the ocular examination are normal.

Course. For 9 years the patient, receiving pilocarpine drops, remained asymptomatic, and intraocular tensions were normal. She then developed an acute attack of glaucoma in the right eye. Her intraocular pressure was 79 mm. Hg (Schiøtz) when she was seen 12 hours after the acute episode. Mannitol administered intravenously brought the tension to normal limits within a few hours, and a peripheral iridectomy was performed. Postoperatively there were no complications, and the angle was appreciably deeper. Examination of the left eye indicated that the angles were still open. A year later the iridoschisis had progressively increased so that now there was marked fragmentation of the iris stroma from the 2 o'clock to the 7 o'clock position in the right eye (Fig. 128, *C*). A peripheral iridectomy was also visible at the 10 o'clock position. In the left eye the iridoschisis had also changed markedly, with areas of fragmentation of the iris from the 6 o'clock to the 9 o'clock position (Fig. 128, *D*). Some of the iris stroma had floated forward so that it was almost touching the cornea at the 7 o'clock position. A cataract had now developed in the left eye, reducing the vision to 20/200, and an intracapsular cataract extraction was performed without complication. Corrected vision a few months later was 20/30 and remained at this level until her death from myocardial infarction a year later. The right eye had remained normotensive with the patient using pilocarpine (2%).

Iridoschisis

History. About 3 years ago this 77-year-old woman developed poor vision and pain in the left eye, and 2 weeks later iridencleisis was performed because of a markedly elevated intraocular tension. At that time abnormal iris strands were noted in the right eye. In both eyes the tension was initially within normal limits; but gradually the pressure rose, and pilocarpine drops were required. The vision remained very poor in the left eye. As time went on, the strands of iris tissue increasingly occluded the pupillary area.

Findings. Vision in the right eye is 20/70 and in the left light perception. The cornea of the right eye is normal except for a prominent arcus senilis, and the anterior chamber is shallow. The inferior half of the iris is shredded, and the iris stroma extends forward and upward into the anterior chamber, almost

FIG. 129 touching the cornea and occluding at least half of the pupil (Fig. 129). The pigment epithelial layer of the iris is intact. Visualization of the fundus is impossible due to the small pupillary area. In the left eye the cornea is edematous, and it is impossible to visualize the remainder of the eye. The intraocular tension in the right eye is 31 mm. Hg (Schiøtz) and in the left 55 mm. Hg (Schiøtz). Field examination of the right eye shows it to be constricted, with an inferior nasal step and baring of the blind spot.

Course. Over the next 2 years the vision remained about the same despite the increase in the iris strands floating up into the pupillary area.

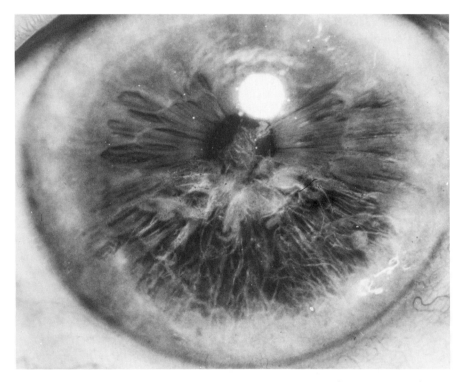

Fig. 129. *Shredding of the iris stroma inferiorly in the right eye of a 77-year-old woman with iridoschisis.* Fibrils of iris stroma extend forward to almost touch the cornea and also occlude at least half of the pupil. The intraocular pressure is somewhat elevated despite pilocarpine drops; the left eye has absolute glaucoma.

Fig. 130. *Shredding of the inferior iris stroma bilaterally and endothelial damage in the right eye in a 70-year-old man with iridoschisis.* **A,** In the right eye large clumps of iris stroma are in contact with the corneal endothelium inferiorly, with resulting stromal edema. **B,** In the left eye the process is less extensive without corneal involvement. **C,** By gonioscopy strands can be seen attached to the cornea in the right eye.

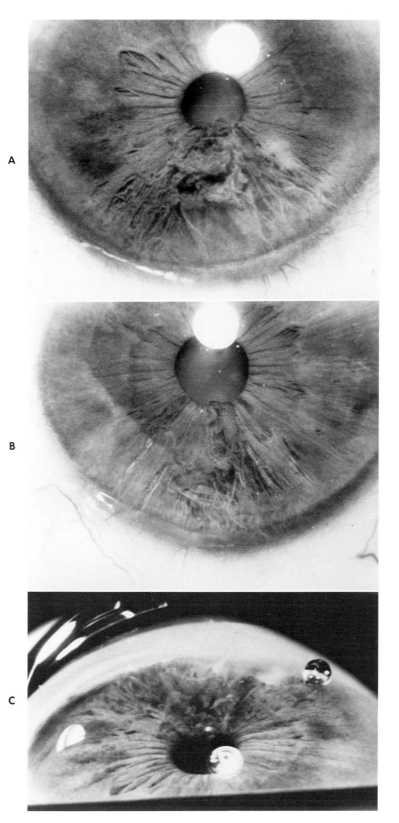

Fig. 130. For legend see opposite page.

Degenerative and atrophic conditions of the iris

Iridoschisis

History. This 70-year-old man has been blind in the left eye for at least 5 years and has had gradual loss of vision in the right eye for the past 3 to 4 years.

Findings. Vision in the right eye is counting fingers at 18 feet and in the left light perception. Externally both eyes are normal except for abnormalities of the iris. In the right eye at the 4 o'clock position there is a shredding of the iris stroma, with loose ends projecting into the anterior chamber. In the left eye (Reel XII-1) the process is more extensive, involving the iris from the 5 o'clock to the 10 o'clock position. The fibers near the sphincter are disrupted so that some of the iris tissue floats into the pupil. In places the process is so marked that iris pigment epithelium is visible behind the stromal fibers. In the right eye an apparently normal fundus is seen through an immature cataract. In the left eye an immature cataract prevents a view of the fundus. The intraocular pressures are normal in both eyes.

Course. With a myopic correction the patient's vision in the right eye was improved to 20/40. He was advised that a cataract extraction in the left eye could be performed at any time. The patient was then lost to follow-up.

Iridoschisis

History. A routine eye examination of this 70-year-old man revealed abnormal irides. He was given pilocarpine drops "prophylactically."

Findings. Vision in the right eye is 20/30 and in the left 20/40. Both eyes are normal except for the irides, which show shredding of the iris inferiorly, with large clumps of iris stroma floating in the anterior chamber. The right eye is more affected, and several of the pieces of loose iris tissue are in contact with the endothelium, resulting in diffuse stromal edema (Fig. 130, A). In the left eye the shredding is limited mostly to the midzone of the iris (Fig. 130, B). By gonioscopy it is obvious that the strands are actually attached to the cornea in the right eye (Fig. 130, C). Intraocular tensions are about 10 mm. Hg in both eyes by applanation tonometry.

FIG. 130

Course. The patient was lost to follow-up.

RUBEOSIS IRIDIS

Noninflammatory neovascularization of the iris is referred to as rubeosis iridis. The most common cause is diabetes with extensive diabetic retinopathy. Central retinal vein thrombosis is another common cause. Rubeosis iridis may also be associated with intraocular tumors, central retinal artery occlusion, Eales's disease, long-standing retinal detachment, and absolute glaucoma from any cause. Chronic iridocyclitis, especially heterochromic iridocyclitis, and extraocular arteriovenous fistulas are also known to produce rubeosis iridis. Frequently, the involved eye is blind, and the exact cause of the rubeosis may be impossible to determine. The extent and distribution of neovascularization vary with the duration of the process. Neovascular glaucoma almost invariably follows, due to neovascularization of the chamber angle. However, sometimes the glaucoma precedes the neovascularization, undoubtedly due to the development of a transparent fibrous tissue (cuticular membrane), which is visible histopathologically but not through the slit-lamp biomicroscope. The earliest stages of rubeosis iridis are usually manifested by newly formed vessels on the iris surface in the sphincter region. In contrast to normal iris vessels, which are radial, these course in all directions. Initially, they are visible only with the slit-lamp biomicroscope. New vessel formation is then apparent at the root of the iris, soon extending into the trabecular meshwork, sometimes with formation of a fibrovascular membrane with severe glaucoma. Later, the entire iris becomes infiltrated with superficial vessels that become dilated and sometimes even sinusoid. Recurrent hyphemas are common, and absolute glaucoma is universal. Finally, the neovascular tissue may lead to extensive peripheral anterior synechia formation, with closure of the angle. The stimulus for neovascularization is probably anoxia. It has been hypothesized that necrotoxins are produced and that these are responsible for the formation of new vessels.

There is no uniformly effective treatment. Surgical procedures usually lead to severe bleeding. On occasion, cyclodiathermy is effective, but cyclocryotherapy is probably more frequently so.

Rubeosis iridis

History. About 2 years ago this 55-year-old man's left eye became painful, and his vision was blurred. Recently he was given pilocarpine (2%) drops.

Findings. Vision in the right eye is 20/40 and in the left no light perception. The right eye is normal except for a diffuse lenticular haziness. In the left eye

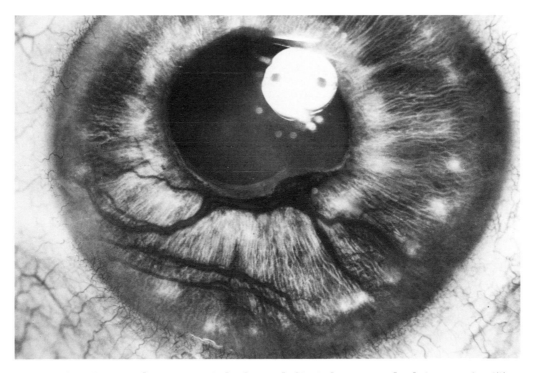

Fig. 131. *Neovascularization of the lower half of the iris in the left eye of a 55-year-old man with rubeosis iridis.* The intraocular pressure is markedly elevated, and the eye is blind. The vessels are large and sinusoid.

FIG. 131 there is moderate conjunctival injection and bedewing of the corneal epithelium. The anterior chamber is of normal depth. The pupil is irregular and fixed, with a total posterior synechia involving the lower half of the pupillary margin. Much of the iris contains neovascularization, but the vessels are sinusoid in the lower half of the iris (Fig. 131). There is a marked opacification of the lens, and the fundus is not visible. The intraocular pressure is 24 mm. Hg (Schiøtz) in the right eye and 87 mm. Hg (Schiøtz) in the left. Field examination shows the right eye to have a nasal step and a small upper Bjerrum scotoma.

Course. The patient had no pain in the right eye, and administration of pilocarpine drops was continued in both eyes. Over the next 2 years the intraocular pressure remained normal in the right eye and markedly elevated in the left. Refraction of the right eye showed that the vision had increased to 20/25. The patient was then lost to follow-up.

Rubeosis iridis

History. About 2 years ago this 79-year-old man lost all his vision in the right eye; there was no pain or halos. About a year ago examination of the right eye showed marked glaucomatous cupping, with neovascularization and attenuation of the retinal vessels. His intraocular pressure was markedly elevated in the right

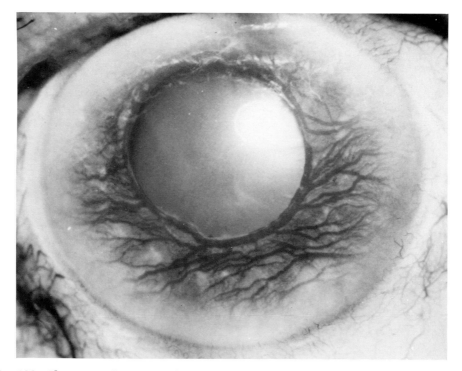

Fig. 132. *Almost total neovascularization with ectropion uveae in the right eye of a 79-year-old man with rubeosis iridis.* Recently the right eye was found to be glaucomatous, with cupping of the disc, and blind. Gonioscopy shows a marked rubeosis of the angle and peripheral anterior synechias.

eye and borderline in the left. Tonography indicated a borderline facility of outflow, and epinephrine (1%) drops were initiated. Intraocular pressure in the left eye was controlled for a while, but pilocarpine had to be added.

Findings. The right eye is blind, and the vision in the left is 20/50. In the right eye there is moderate conjunctival injection and corneal epithelial edema. The anterior chamber is clear, and the pupil is semidilated and fixed. The iris is almost totally neovascularized (rubeosis iridis), and there is an ectropion uveae at the pupillary margin (Fig. 132). There is a moderate nuclear sclerosis and a FIG. 132 dense posterior subcapsular cataract, which makes visualization of the fundus impossible. The left eye is normal except for a mild nuclear sclerosis and some posterior subcapsular opacification of the lens, which permits visualization of a normal disc. Tension revealed by applanation tonometry is 58 mm. Hg in the right eye and 24 mm. Hg in the left. Gonioscopy shows a marked rubeosis of the angle and numerous peripheral anterior synechias in the right eye and normal angle structures in the left.

Course. Two years later the intraocular pressure in the left eye was under good control with the patient taking the same medication, and the vision was 20/30 without correction. The patient was then lost to follow-up.

SECONDARY IRIS ATROPHY

Iris atrophy associated with inflammatory processes, glaucoma, trauma, and ischemia is referred to as secondary iris atrophy. Probably the most common occurrence of the condition is that following iritis. It may be diffuse, as in heterochromia iridis (Chapter 7, p. 210); or, more commonly, it may be a focal process, with thinning of the iris stroma and loss of pigment epithelium. An area of iris translucency demonstrated by scleral transillumination is a diagnostic feature. In the area of atrophy the iris and pupillary margin may be distorted. White vessels may be visible. Segmental iris atrophy is almost pathognomonic of herpes zoster infection as an aftermath of herpes zoster ophthalmicus. In this condition an entire segment, varying in width, will be involved extending from the periphery of the iris to the pupillary margin. Sometimes the atrophy is less well defined. Paralytic mydriasis is usually not due to atrophy but is a partial third nerve paralysis. Occasionally, heterochromia may develop as a manifestation of diffuse iris atrophy.

In glaucomatous iris atrophy following a primary attack of acute glaucoma the pupil is irregular and dilated and reacts poorly to light, due to sphincter damage. The entire iris stroma may be thinned by atrophy, or it may involve localized areas, particularly the sphincter. Occasionally, iridoschisis is produced (Chapter 2, p. 34). In chronic glaucoma, particularly when it is congenital, the iris stroma is uniformly thinned, and the pigment epithelium is often disturbed, with translucency of the iris and excessive liberation of pigment. This pigment is deposited in the remaining iris stroma and in the angle of the anterior chamber, resulting in heavy pigmentation of the trabecular meshwork. Sometimes fibrosis of the iris stroma results in ectropion uveae.

Traumatic atrophy of the iris depends on the type and severity of trauma. Localized atrophy is common and probably results from ischemia and necrosis.

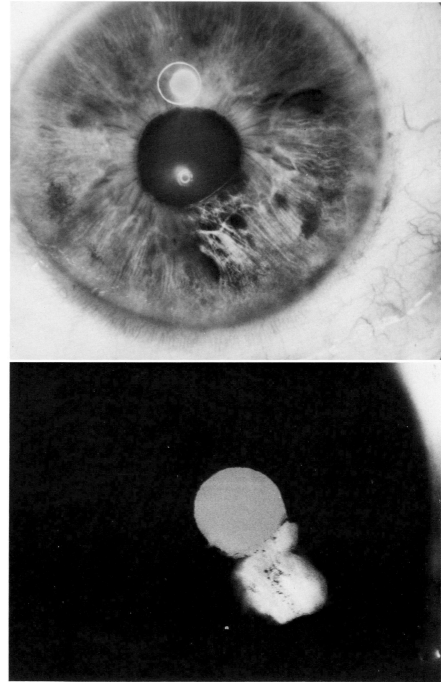

Fig. 133. *Localized iris atrophy associated with recurrent iritis in the left eye of a 56-year-old woman with focal iris atrophy.* **A,** Between the 4 and 5 o'clock positions there is an area of stromal thinning, with atrophy of the pupillary margin. **B,** By retroillumination the fundus red reflex is visible in this area, indicating atrophy of the pigment epithelium.

Focal iris atrophy with iritis

History. Nine years ago this 56-year-old woman developed blurred vision and pain in the left eye and was found to have a granulomatous iritis with secondary glaucoma. With the patient receiving mydriatics, topical administration of corticosteroids, and acetazolamide, the iritis gradually resolved in about a month. An area of iris atrophy involving the pupillary margin was noted. Over the next few months this was found to increase. Four months later she had a mild recurrence of iritis, which responded to topical administration of corticosteroids, but with no appreciable change in the iris atrophy. Other than a mild recurrence 8 months later there has been no anterior chamber activity for the past 7 years. Chest x-ray films have shown no signs of active or inactive sarcoid.

Findings. Vision in both eyes is 20/15. Both eyes are normal in all respects except for an area of atrophy in the iris of the left eye between the 4 and 5 o'clock positions. The pupillary margin is completely atrophic, along with the sphincter in an area extending two thirds of the way to the angle. The normal brown pigmentation is missing in this area, and the remaining stromal fibers are light blue, with granules of pigment on the surface (Fig. 133, A). By retro- FIG. 133 illumination a patch of red reflex can be seen through the iris somewhat larger than the atrophic-appearing iris stroma (Fig. 133, B). The flecks of pigmentation are clearly seen in the central area of abnormal transillumination. The intraocular pressure in both eyes is normal.

Course. Subsequently, the patient developed severe throbbing pain in the right temple, but the eyes showed no change. She was considered to have migraine headaches.

Focal iris atrophy secondary to recurrent iritis

History. For 32 years this 53-year-old woman had recurrent attacks of iritis in the right eye. Two weeks ago her right eye became uncomfortable and red, and she was found to have an intraocular pressure of 64 mm. Hg (Schiøtz). In 2 days acetazolamide, mydriatics, and topical administration of corticosteroids produced a prompt decrease of her tension to normal levels.

Findings. The vision in the right eye is 20/40 and in the left 20/25. In the right eye a few keratic precipitates can be seen, and the anterior chamber contains a few cells and a minimal flare. The pupil is dilated and fixed (due to mydriatics), and at the 2 o'clock position there is an area of brown pigmentation in contrast to the otherwise uniform blue iris (Fig. 134, A). On transillu- FIG. 134 mination there is total transmission of the red reflex in this area, and the remainder of the iris transmits no light (Fig. 134, B). The media are clear, and the fundus is normal. The left eye is normal.

Course. Topical administration of corticosteroids and mydriatics was continued for another week, at which time there were no signs of active uveitis. Two weeks after the medication was discontinued, the vision had returned to 20/20 in the right eye, and there were no further signs of anterior chamber activity. The patient was then lost to follow-up.

Postiritic focal iris atrophy

History. About 6 months ago this 26-year-old woman developed a low-grade iritis with many keratic precipitates and a mild secondary glaucoma in the left

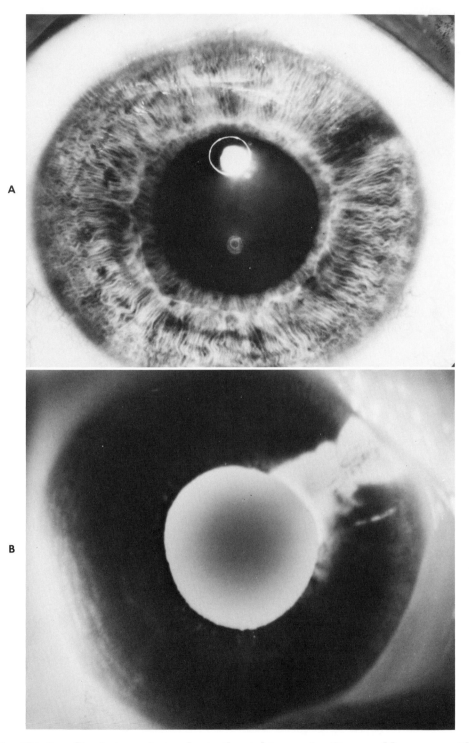

Fig. 134. *Localized stromal atrophy in the right eye of a 53-year-old woman with focal iris atrophy secondary to recurrent iritis.* **A,** At the 2 o'clock position is an area of brown pigmentation of the iris not involving the sphincter. **B,** On transillumination there is total transmission of the fundus red reflex from the pupillary margin to the periphery of the iris, indicating a focal loss of iris pigment epithelium.

236

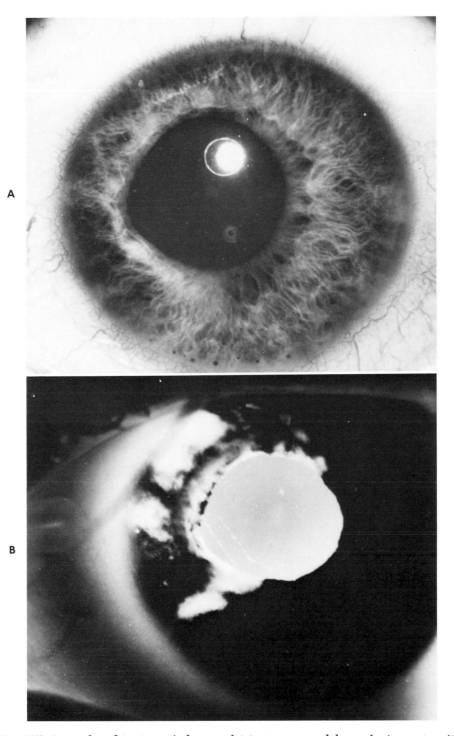

Fig. 135. *Irregular thinning of the nasal iris stroma and loss of pigment epithelium in the left eye of a 26-year-old woman with postiritic focal iris atrophy.* **A,** The pupil is irregular and retracted nasally, with thinning of the nasal iris stroma. **B,** With transillumination of the iris, visualization of the red reflex indicates total loss of pigment epithelium in an irregular pattern.

237

eye, which gradually responded to topical and systemic administration of steroids and mydriatics. In 5 months the vision had returned to normal, and there were no signs of iritis.

Findings. The vision in both eyes is 20/20 with correction. The right eye, including findings from the gonioscopic examination, is normal. In the left eye the cornea is clear except for numerous rounded nonpigmented keratic precipitates. Located inferiorly are a number of large darkly pigmented keratic precipitates.The anterior chamber is clear. The pupil is irregular, somewhat dilated, FIG. 135 and retracted nasally (Fig. 135, *A*). At the 9 o'clock position is a posterior synechia. Most of the nasal portion of the iris is thinned, and the pigment epithelium is absent in some areas, as shown by transillumination of the iris (Fig. 135, *B*). Tension is revealed by applanation tonometry is 13 mm. Hg in the right eye and 20 mm. Hg in the left. Tonography shows a normal facility of outflow in the right eye but borderline in the left. Fundus examination with dilated pupils reveals no abnormalities.

Course. Six months later there still had been no recurrence of the iritis, but gonioscopy revealed at the 8 o'clock position a peripheral anterior synechia that previously had not been present. There was only a slight increase in the degree of iris atrophy.

Optic nerve glioma and iris atrophy

History. About 1½ years ago this 16-year-old girl developed progressive loss of vision leading to blindness in her left eye. About a year ago papilledema of the left nerve head was noted. Skull x-ray films were negative. At this time she was entirely asymptomatic, but 2 months later she developed acute ocular pain. Extensive synechia formations were found, along with iris neovascularization, ectropion uveae, and corneal edema. The intraocular tension was elevated to 53 mm. Hg by applanation tonometry. For the next 5 months the tension was fairly well controlled with acetazolamide and mydriatics. Three months ago the tension again became markedly elevated, and there was practically no iris remaining. Fresh hemorrhage was visible in the fundus.

Findings. Vision in the right eye is 20/25, and the left eye is blind. The right eye is entirely normal. In the left eye there is moderate conjunctival injection, and the cornea is clear except for some diffuse pigment on the peripheral endothelium. The anterior chamber is clear but shallow, the iris is absent, and REEL XII-2 the entire equator of the lens is visible (Reel XII-2). Behind the clear lens is a vascularized yellow mass containing large irregularly dilated vessels. The tension is about 60 mm. Hg (Schiøtz).

Course. Enucleation of the left eye was performed, and the pathologic specimen showed glioma incompletely removed. Repeat x-ray films showed the left optic foramen to be 1 mm. larger than it had been a year previously. An intracranial resection of the optic nerve was performed, including unroofing of the optic foramen and removal of the remaining intraorbital optic nerve. Postoperatively, there was a marked ptosis. Two years later there were no signs of recurrence of the tumor, but the patient still had a complete ptosis. Therefore, a levator resection was performed. She was asymptomatic 1 year later, and the cosmetic result was good.

Iris atrophy with congenital glaucoma

History. At birth this 11-year-old boy was noticed to have a "white film" over his eyes; the film eventually "went away." Later he was found to have congenital glaucoma. Seven years ago an "internal clyclodialysis" was performed on both eyes because intraocular pressures had been uncontrolled medically. Postoperatively, a massive intraocular hemorrhage occurred in the right eye, and irrigation of the anterior chamber was unsuccessful, resulting in corneal hematogenous pigmentation. Gradually this eye developed band keratopathy and became blind and painful. In the past few months the left eye has required more intensive medical therapy to keep the intraocular tension normal. A month ago an enucleation was performed on the painful right eye. The recovery was uneventful.

Findings. The right eye is anophthalmic; vision in the left eye is 20/50 with correction. The left cornea is enlarged to a diameter of 15 mm. The anterior chamber is deep and the peripheral iris so markedly atrophic in many areas as to permit visualization of the iris pigment epithelium (Fig. 136). Gonioscopy FIG. 136 shows the temporal half of the angle to be closed by anterior synechias and nasally the angle structures to be poorly differentiated. The optic nerve head appears normal. The intraocular tension is 17 mm. Hg (Schiøtz).

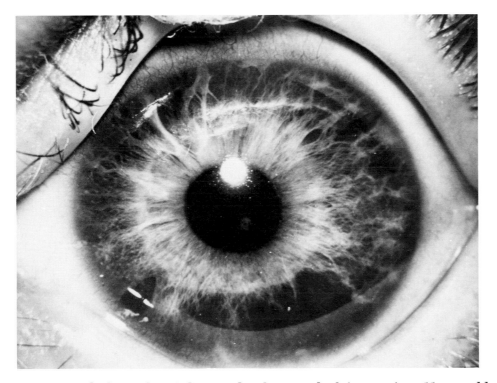

Fig. 136. *Marked atrophy of the peripheral iris in the left eye of an 11-year-old boy with congenital glaucoma.* The cornea is 15 mm. in diameter and the anterior chamber deep. The peripheral iris stroma is so thin that pigment epithelium can be visualized in many areas.

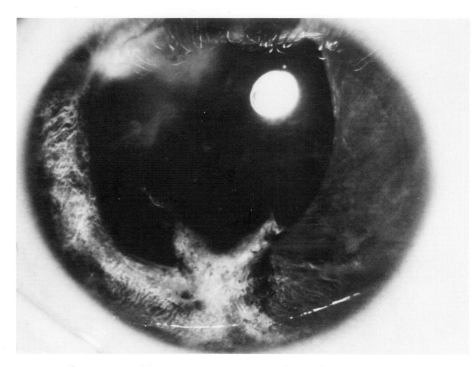

Fig. 137. *Thinning and loss of iris stroma in the right eye of a 13-year-old boy with traumatic iris atrophy.* Nasally the iris stroma is markedly thinned in contrast to the normal texture of the temporal iris. The patient had been struck in the eye resulting in a total hyphema and secondary glaucoma.

Course. The patient had a plastic prosthesis successfully fitted to the right socket. Six months later he was lost to follow-up.

Traumatic iris atrophy

History. Five years ago this 13-year-old boy was struck in the right eye by an apple; the injury resulted in a total hyphema and a markedly elevated intraocular pressure. An irrigation of the anterior chamber was performed and most of the blood removed. No hematogenous pigmentation resulted, and the corneal edema gradually cleared. The patient was found to have commotio retinae, and over the years he gradually developed a posterior subcapsular cataract.

Findings. The vision in the right eye is 20/70 with correction and in the left 20/20. In the right eye the cornea has several scars, but the apical region is clear. Superiorly there is a scar at the limbus due to the surgical procedure. The anterior chamber is deep. There is a complete iris surgical coloboma superiorly. The temporal iris is brown and of normal texture. The iris nasally is thinned and

FIG. 137   atrophic in appearance, having lost most of its pigmentation (Fig. 137). There is a dense posterior synechia inferiorly, and there are fine opacities in the anterior subcapsular region of the lens. In the posterior subcapsular region is a sheet of granular opacity. Fundus examination reveals pigmented macular changes, but the remaining fundus is normal.

Course. Five years later the vision had remained approximately the same, with no appreciable change in the lens opacities (glaucoma flecken).

Chapter 9

Tumors of the iris

FRECKLES AND NEVI OF THE IRIS

Pigment cell clusters on the surface of the iris, referred to as iris freckles, represent normal uveal cells of the iris with hyperpigmentation and increased cellularity. Clinically, they appear to lie on the surface of the iris. They are commonly found in the pupillary zone. Freckles are congenital; but like other melanocytic cells, they may become more heavily pigmented at puberty or during pregnancy.

Masses of pigmented cells somewhat elevated from the surface of the iris are referred to as nevi of the iris. Such nevi are a type of uveal melanocytosis comparable to dermal melanocytosis (blue nevi). Histopathologically, they are composed of spindle-shaped melanocytes with poorly developed dendritic processes and are often less pigmented than normal uveal melanocytes. The distinction between iris freckles and nevi is not sharp, and the two merge into each other. Sometimes iris nevi are referred to as benign melanomas, but this term is unnecessary. Nevi are also congenital and may become more pigmented during puberty and pregnancy. One histophathologic study showed that freckles and nevi are present in uveal tissue in approximately 50% of normal eyes and tend to be more frequent and larger in eyes containing a malignant melanoma of the uveal tract. The distinction between a low-grade malignant melanoma of the iris (spindle cell A type) and a nevus is difficult to make both clinically and histopathologically. It is presumed that nevi do not grow and that pigmented iris lesions that enlarge, however slowly, are probably spindle cell A type melanomas. Some spindle cell B type melanomas also have a very slow growth rate and are only locally invasive. Eyes containing multiple iris nevi are often found to have excessive pigmentation on the trabecular meshwork, presumably from degenerating cells from the nevi. Occasionally, the pigment occludes the trabecular meshwork, resulting in glaucoma. Nevi near the pupillary margin are often associated with an ectropion uveae; the pupillary border may be irregular and the reaction sluggish in the region of the nevus. Most authorities believe that all malignant melanomas of the iris arise from a preexistent nevus.

Segmental iris nevus

History. Since childhood this 25-year-old man had a "double pupil." He had no ocular symptoms except for a corneal foreign body, which caused him to go to the ophthalmologist.

Findings. The vision in both eyes is 20/20. The right eye is slightly injected, and there is an embedded corneal foreign body near the limbus. On the surface of the iris inferiorly is a fan-shaped area of heavy pigmentation extending from the 6 o'clock to the 7 o'clock position. In the left eye there is a similar area of

FIG. 138   heavy pigmentation extending from the 4 o'clock to the 6:30 position (Fig. 138). The pupils are round and respond to light normally. The posterior segment is normal.

Course. The patient did not return.

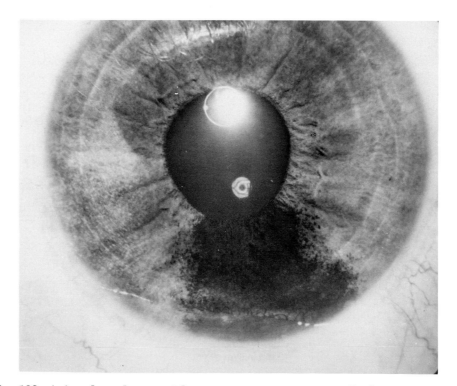

Fig. 138. *A fan-shaped area of heavy iris pigmentation in the left eye of a 25-year-old man with a segmental iris nevus.* Uniformly dark brown pigmentation extends from the 4 o'clock to the 6:30 position on the surface of the iris. In the right eye a similar area of pigmentation extends from the 6 o'clock to the 7 o'clock position.

Segmental iris nevus

History. Since birth this 47-year-old woman had a dark spot on her left iris without any change in size. She now has presbyopic symptoms.

Findings. The vision in the right eye is 20/30 and in the left 20/20. Both eyes are entirely normal except for a dark brown area of pigmentation of the left iris extending from the 2 o'clock to the 6 o'clock position (Fig. 139). This area involves the entire width of the iris, and by gonioscopy it is seen to extend up to the scleral spur. The intraocular pressure in both eyes is 18 mm. Hg (Schiøtz). FIG. 139

Course. There was no change in the iris lesions over the next 5 years.

Iris nevi and secondary glaucoma

History. Recently this 58-year-old man happened to notice that the vision in his right eye was poor. When seen by an ophthalmologist, he was found to have an elevated tension in the right eye. Reaction to a water-drinking test was positive. Pilocarpine drops were used, but they only partially controlled the glaucoma.

Findings. Vision in the right eye is hand movements at 2 feet and in the left 20/40. In the right eye there is no abnormality of the cornea, and the anterior chamber is of normal depth. A striking finding is the presence of a number of large dark brown iris nevi, particularly in the inferior half of the iris (Fig. 140). FIG. 140 The lens is clear, and the vitreous contains a number of stringy translucent opaci-

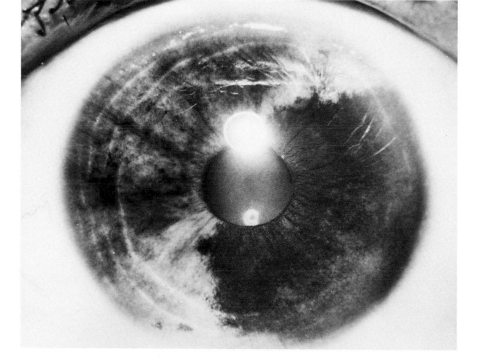

Fig. 139. *Dark pigmentation of the nasal iris of the left eye in a 47-year-old woman with a segmental iris nevus.* The dark brown pigmentation on the surface of the iris extends from the 2 o'clock to the 6 o'clock position, involving the pupillary margin and extending peripherally to the scleral spur.

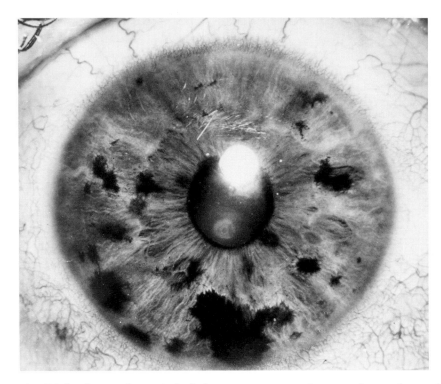

Fig. 140. *Multiple patches of dark brown pigmentation on the surface of the right eye in a 58-year-old man with iris nevi and secondary glaucoma.* Recently the patient was found to have glaucoma, with a positive reaction to a water drinking test. Gonioscopy (see Reel XII-3) shows that the angle structures of the right eye are covered with a velvety dark brown layer of pigmentation, while in the left there is only the normal tan color of the angle structures.

ties. By fundus examination the disc exhibits marked glaucomatous cupping, and in the macular region is a crescent-shaped white area, surrounded by scattered black pigment, deep to the retina. This lesion has all the appearances of a macular disciform degeneration. In the left eye the anterior segments are normal, the iris having only a few small nevi. The posterior segment is also normal except for numerous small drusen in the macular region. Gonioscopy reveals a marked difference between the two eyes. Except for the superior nasal quadrant, the angle structures in the right eye are covered with a velvety dark brown layer of pigmentation over the entire trabecular meshwork and the ciliary body band REEL XII-3 (Reel XII-3). In the left eye the trabecular meshwork is a normal tan color except for a fine light brown network of uveal meshwork overlying it. Tension by applanation tonometry is 29 mm. Hg in the right eye and 18 mm. Hg in the left. Tonography shows a decreased facility of outflow (C = 0.11) in the right eye and a normal outflow (C = 0.17) in the left eye.

Course. Intraocular pressures ranged from 22 to 40 mm. Hg in the right eye with the patient receiving pilocarpine and epinephrine drops. The vision in the left eye remained good for about 2 years, when there was sudden loss of vision to 20/100. Definite macular changes were observed, and in another year the vision

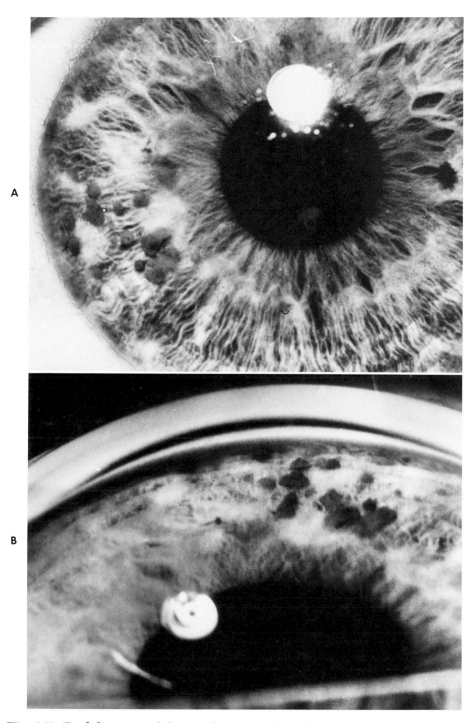

Fig. 141. *Dark brown nodules on the iris in the right eye in a 28-year-old woman with iris nevi.* **A,** Clustered together from the 8 o'clock to the 9 o'clock position on the surface of the iris are about 15 nodular nevi. **B,** By gonioscopy several more nevi are visible lying in the anterior chamber angle.

245

was reduced to 20/200. Two years later there had been no appreciable change in the appearance of the eyes, and the angle of the right eye exhibited the same extensive brown pigmentation covering the angle structures. The patient was then lost to follow-up.

Iris nevi

History. As an incidental finding this 28-year-old woman was discovered to have a number of nodules on her iris. From an ocular standpoint she is completely asymptomatic.

Findings. The vision in both eyes is 20/20. The right eye is normal, as is the left, except for about 15 dark brown nodules on the surface of the iris clustered together between the 8 and 9 o'clock positions (Fig. 141, *A*). By gonioscopy several more of these can be visualized lying in the angle of the anterior chamber (Fig. 141, *B*). Except for these nodules, the angle appears to be entirely normal. The intraocular pressures are normal and equal in both eyes.

FIG. 141

Course. When the patient was reexamined 3 years later, the findings were identical to those seen earlier.

Iris nevi

History. Since she was a young girl this 40-year-old woman had brown spots on her left iris. The patient was not sure whether there was any increase in the size of the spots.

Findings. The vision in both eyes is 20/20. The right eye is normal, and the iris contains a few nevi. The left eye is also normal except for numerous darkly pigmented nevi of the iris and one somewhat elevated lesion in the iris periphery extending from the 7 o'clock to the 8 o'clock position (Fig. 142, *A*). By gonioscopy this lesion can be seen to extend to the iris root and patchy dark pigmentation of the angle structures can be seen elsewhere (Fig. 142, *B*). Even the superior angle has an irregular dark pigmentation of all the angle structures (Fig. 142, *C*). The intraocular pressure shown by applanation tonometry is 19 mm. Hg in both eyes.

FIG. 142

Course. The patient's nevi were photographed at yearly intervals, and 4 years later they had not changed. Her vision and intraocular pressures were normal.

Iris nevus

History. Six months ago a small gray mass was noted on the iris of this 33-year-old woman. Since then it appears to have enlarged.

Fig. 142. *Numerous darkly pigmented areas on the iris in the left eye of a 40-year-old woman with iris nevi.* **A,** Most of the nevi are small and have little mass, but one is elevated at the periphery of the iris from the 7 o'clock to the 8 o'clock position. **B,** The mass as seen gonioscopically extends to the iris root but does not involve the angle structures. **C,** Elsewhere in the angle there is an irregular deposition of dark pigment on all the angle structures. The intraocular pressure is normal; 4 years later the appearance of the iris and angle was identical.

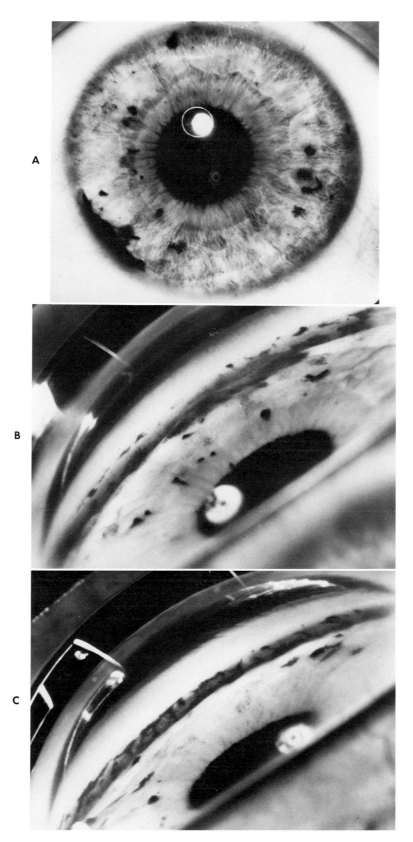

Fig. 142. For legend see opposite page.

Findings. The vision in both eyes is normal. The right eye is normal in all respects except for an elevated tan-colored mass on the mid–iris stroma at the

FIG. 143   4 o'clock position (Fig. 143, *A*). The lesion is well circumscribed and regular in contour. On the surface there is a speckling of fine dark brown pigment. Gonioscopy shows that there is no involvement of the angle structures and that the

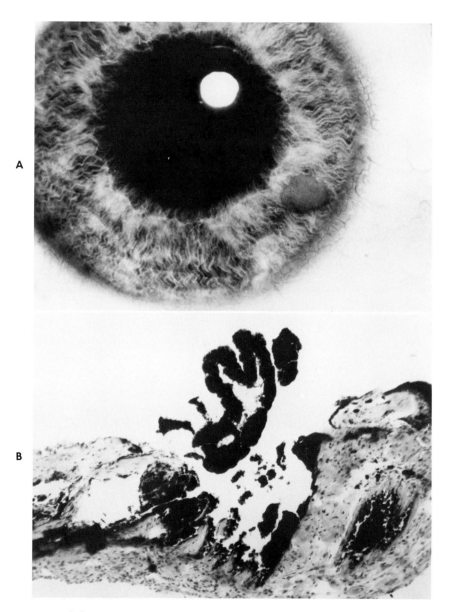

Fig. 143. *Nodular tan-colored mass on the iris stroma in the right eye of a 33-year-old woman with an iris nevus.* **A,** At the 4 o'clock position an elevated, well-circumscribed mass is covered with fine dark brown pigment. Gonioscopy (see Reel XII-4) reveals no involvement of the angle structures. **B,** Photomicrographs of lesion (following excisional iridectomy) show the tumor to be a heavily pigmented iris nevus. (H & E stain; ×400.)

angle is wide open, with visibility of the ciliary body band in most places (Reel XII-4). The left eye is normal.

REEL XII-4

Course. Local excision of the iris lesion was performed, and the recovery was uneventful. Histopathologically, the tumor was a heavily pigmented iris nevus (Fig 143, B).

Iris nevus

History. When this 31-year-old woman was seen by her ophthalmologist for a routine eye examination, a slightly raised black pigmented spot was noted in the inferior temporal quadrant of her left eye. After being questioned further, the patient said she was aware that this spot had been present since she was 9 years old. To her knowledge, it had not increased in size.

Findings. The visual acuity in the right eye is 20/12 and in the left 20/15 without correction. The intraocular tensions shown by applanation tonometry are 14 mm. Hg in both eyes. The irides are light brown in color, with multiple areas of tiny dark brown freckles scattered over the surface of each iris. In the lower temporal quadrant of the left iris is a slightly raised, darkly pigmented mass 3 mm. in diameter (Fig. 144, A). By gonioscopy it can be seen that the angle structures are uninvolved by this lesion and that except for an increase in the pigmentation of the inferior temporal trabecular meshwork the angles are normal (Fig. 144, B). The pupils are equal and react briskly to light and accommodation. Results of examination of the posterior segment are normal in both eyes.

FIG. 144

Course. The patient was followed over the next 5 years at approximately 6-month intervals. There was no change in the size of the lesion or the pupillary mobility. Vision remained at 20/12 in both eyes with correction, and intraocular tensions revealed by applanation tonometry were 17 mm. Hg bilaterally.

Iris nevus with ectropion uveae

History. Eight years ago as an incidental finding this 48-year-old woman was found to have a lesion of the iris. The patient was examined yearly during the next 8 years, and no appreciable change was found in the iris lesion.

Findings. The vision in both eyes is 20/20 with correction. In the right eye there is no abnormality except for an elevated rounded pigmented lesion involving the pupil at the 6 o'clock position (Fig. 145, A). Extending onto the tumor about 1 mm. is a layer of iris pigment epithelium that extends around from the pupillary border (ectropion uveae). The pupil is oval in shape and has a poor reaction to light inferiorly, in the region of the tumor. The remainder of the eye is normal. Intraocular pressure is 17 mm. Hg (Schiøtz).

FIG. 145

Course. For the next 13 years the patient was examined at about yearly intervals. Photographs were also repeated. There was extremely slow progression of the ectropion uveae so that the extension of the pigment epithelium increased by about 50% over this 13-year period (Fig. 145, B). The tumor mass itself increased by less than 25%. The patient's vision remained normal and the intraocular pressure the same.

Congenital nevus and angle anomaly

History. For 15 years this 41-year-old man was noted to have a brown spot on his right eye. Recently it is said to have increased. He was asymptomatic.

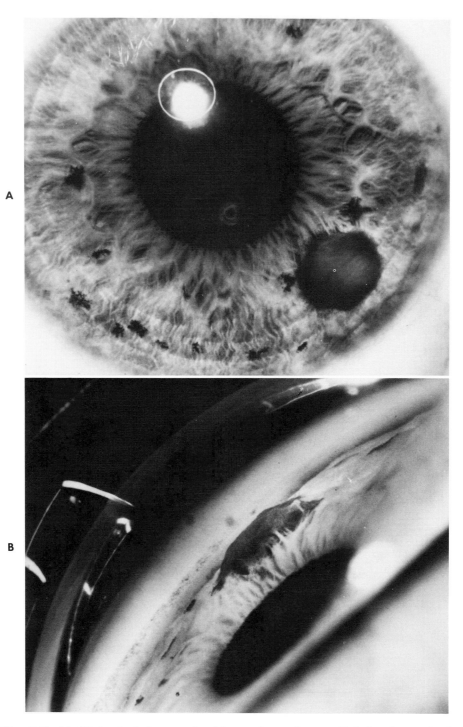

Fig. 144. *Multiple dark brown freckles and one large, slightly elevated, darkly pigmented mass in the left iris of a 31-year-old woman with an iris nevus.* **A,** In the left iris at the 4 o'clock position is a well-circumscribed elevated mass known to be present for 22 years without any change. **B,** Gonioscopy shows no involvement of the angle structures except for an increase in the pigmentation inferiorly.

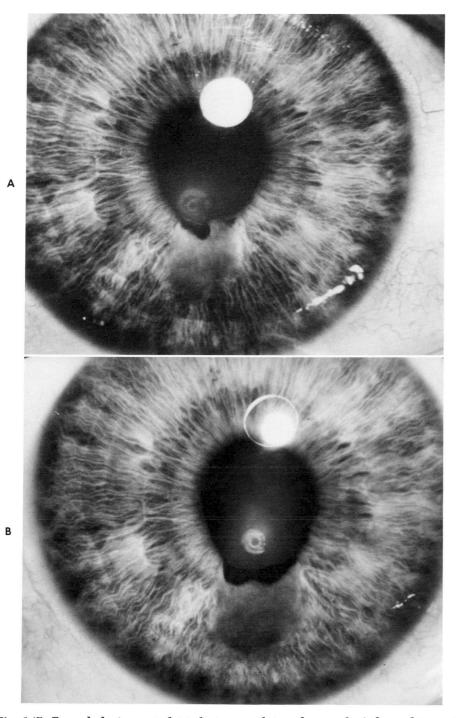

Fig. 145. *Rounded pigmented iris lesion involving the pupil of the right eye in a 48-year-old woman with an iris nevus and ectropion uveae.* **A,** At the 6 o'clock position the lesion is elevated, and iris pigment epithelium extends onto it from around the pupillary border. **B,** Thirteen years later extremely slow progression is evident by some increase in the ectropion uveae and a small increase in the size of the tumor.

251

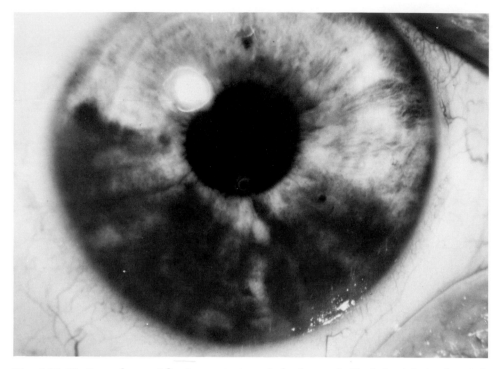

Fig. 146. *Uniform brownish pigmentation of the lower half of the iris in the right eye of a 41-year-old man with a congenital nevus and angle anomaly.* In the area of the iris pigmentation the anterior chamber is unusually deep due to posterior displacement of the iris. Gonioscopy (see Reel XII-5) shows that the angle is exceptionally wide and that the angle structures are covered by darkly pigmented fibrillar tissue.

Findings. Vision in both eyes is 20/20 with correction. The right eye has an unusually deep chamber inferiorly and uniform brownish pigmentation involving the lower half of the iris (Fig. 146). Gonioscopy shows this pigmentation to be extending into the angle (Reel XII-5). The angle is exceptionally wide, and the structures are covered by darkly pigmented fibrillar tissue that in most places extends up to Schwalbe's line. At the 5 o'clock position there is an appearance of extensive iris processes covering the ciliary body band and bridging the trabecular meshwork. Superiorly the angle is normal. In the fundus there are several nevi posterior to the equator. The anterior chamber in the left eye is of average depth; on the surface of the iris are eight or ten iris nevi having a color similar to the pigmentation of the iris in the right eye. The media and fundus are normal.

FIG. 146
REEL XII-5

Course. X-ray films showed no foreign bodies. The patient was then lost to follow-up.

MALIGNANT MELANOMAS OF THE IRIS

Melanotic masses in the iris that are observed to be enlarging are usually malignant melanomas of the iris. Melanomas are the most common intraocular

252

tumors, but those arising in the uveal tract posteriorly are more common than those of the iris. Apparently, those of the iris arise almost exclusively from pre-existing nevi; de novo instances are either very rare or nonexistent. The tumor is rarely seen in black persons. It may be solitary, multiple, or diffuse. Malignant melanomas of the iris are relatively benign as compared with the melanomas of the ciliary body and choroid. Metastasis from an iris melanoma is extremely rare, possibly in part due to earlier diagnosis because of easy visibility. Occasionally, no evidence of a tumor is visible, the only sign being a change in the color of the iris from blue to brown. This is the so-called flat melanoma of the iris in which glaucoma is frequent, due to involvement of the trabecular meshwork. Malignant melanomas of the iris tend to invade the stroma and may extend through the entire iris. A tumor may become attached to the cornea but rarely invades it. Involvement of the anterior chamber angle occurs either by pigment from the tumor, by direct invasion of the angle by the tumor, or by seeding. When enough of the angle has been involved, glaucoma results. Even Schlemm's canal may be invaded, and extension along the intrascleral plexus of vessels can carry the tumor to the outside surface of the eye, usually subconjunctivally. Occasionally, a malignant melanoma will produce an inflammatory reaction and be misdiagnosed as iritis. Rarely, the tumor bleeds, producing a hyphema that obscures the diagnosis, and may be complicated by secondary glaucoma as well.

Histopathologically, iris melanomas can usually be classified as spindle cell A, spindle cell B, or epithelioid tumors, with some mixing of the cell types as a rule. Fascicular tumors are usually spindle cell B type, while necrotic tumors are usually epithelioid. Spindle cell A type and even some spindle cell B types are of relatively low malignancy, and the majority of melanomas of the iris fall into this category. Even the epithelioid type rarely metastasizes but may be more locally invasive, with involvement of the anterior segment structures and extension into the ciliary body and even the choroid. Pigmentation of the tumor may vary from complete amelanosis, in which the tumor is whitish or pinkish and the vessels easily visible, to heavily pigmented dark brown or black masses with no vascularity visible. The most common melanotic tumor is the spindle cell A type with slender spindle-shaped cells and small flat nuclei. Nuclear chromatin may extend as a line through the center of the nucleus along its long axis. In the spindle cell B type the nuclei are larger and contain a more prominent nucleolus, and the entire cell is larger. Epithelioid cell types are composed of large irregular polygonal cells with large hyperchromatic and nucleolated nuclei. Multinucleated cells are common, and the cell walls are well defined. Mitotic figures are more commonly seen. In the spindle cell type of tumors argyrophilic reticulum fibers in relatively heavy amounts also indicate a more benign tumor.

With the knowledge that metastasis is rare, treatment of iris melanomas can now be far more conservative than in the past. Tumor masses thought not to be growing can be watched and followed photographically on the assumption that they are either nevi or spindle cell A type melanomas. In a growing tumor iridectomy will frequently remove the tumor, and in melanomas involving the angle iridocyclectomy is accepted and safe. Eyes with secondary glaucoma from

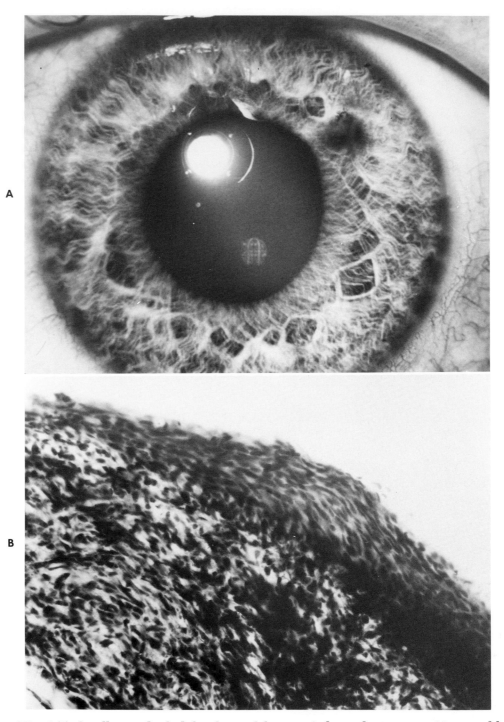

Fig. 147. *Small round, slightly elevated lesion of the right iris in a 39-year-old woman with a malignant melanoma of the iris.* **A,** The pigmented lesion is near the pupillary margin at the 2 o'clock position and produces a slight distortion of the pupil. It is covered with a grayish tissue and invades the iris stroma. **B,** Photomicrograph of the tumor shows dense pleomorphic cells overlying the anterior border layer of the iris.

invasion of the trabeculum require enucleation. Exenteration is required if extrascleral extension has occurred and even then may not be necessary in the older age group. Acquired heterochromia (indicating a diffuse or flat melanoma of the iris) associated with unilateral glaucoma requires prompt enucleation because of the more malignant tendencies of these tumors.

Malignant melanoma of the iris

History. During a routine examination this 39-year-old woman was noted to have a small pigmented spot on her right iris.

Findings. In both eyes the vision is normal. The right eye is normal except for a small brown lesion near the pupillary margin at the 2 o'clock position (Fig. 147, A). This lesion appears to invade the iris stroma and is covered with a grayish tissue. There is a slight ectropion uveae adjacent to the lesion, and there is slight distortion of the pupil. Gonioscopy shows no angle abnormalities.

FIG. 147

Course. An iridectomy was performed, with excision of the iris lesion. The histopathologic finding was dense pleomorphic cells covering the anterior border layer of the iris (Fig. 147, B).

Malignant melanoma of the iris

History. For the past several years this 11-year-old boy had a spot on his iris that has not been observed to change during the past 6 months.

Findings. Vision in both eyes is 20/20. The right eye is normal as is the left,

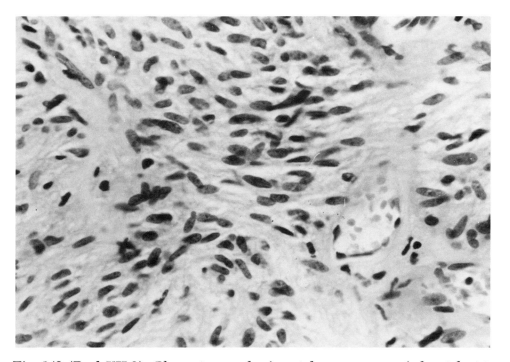

Fig. 148 (Reel XII-6). *Photomicrograph of a pink tumor mass of the right iris in an 11-year old boy with melanoma of the iris.* Histopathologically, the cell type is predominantly spindle cell A. (H & E stain; ×1600.)

REEL XII-6   except for a pink mass arising from the inferior iris in the right eye (Reel XII-6). The mass extends almost to the pupillary margin and within a few millimeters of the angle. One portion touches the cornea and is fed by two large vessels arising from the angle; the mass contains a number of small tufted vessels.

Course. Reaction to a ^{32}P test was positive. Excision of the tumor was carried out by means of the cryoprobe placed on the surface of the tumor to facilitate its complete removal. Histopathologically, the cell type was predominantly spin-

FIG. 148   dle cell A (Fig. 148). A year later there were no signs of recurrence, and the vision was 20/100 without correction but 20/20 with a high astigmatic correction.

Malignant melanoma in anterior chamber angle

History. For the past 20 years this 58-year-old man had a brown spot on his left iris. During the past 4 months it definitely became larger, without pain or redness.

Findings. Vision in the right eye is 20/20 and in the left 20/30 with correction. The right eye is normal. In the left eye there is no abnormality, except for a brown mass that appears to be arising from the peripheral iris between the 12 o'clock and the 2 o'clock position and to be in contact with the cornea for almost

FIG. 149   the same distance (Fig. 149). The mass is rounded and extends about two thirds

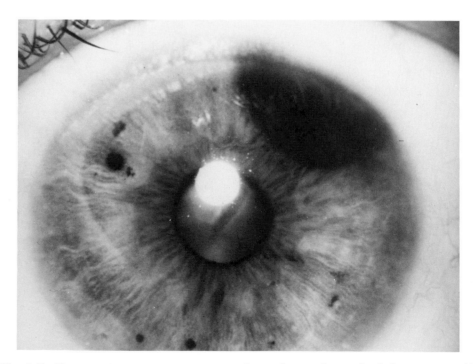

Fig. 149. *Brown iris tumor mass arising from the angle in the left eye of a 58-year-old man with a malignant melanoma.* The tumor mass is rounded, and by gonioscopy no seeding or excessive pigmentation of the adjacent angle structures can be seen. Total excision of the tumor was done by iridocyclectomy; histopathologically, it was a malignant melanoma of the spindle cell A type with extension into the ciliary body.

of the way to the pupillary margin. About five similarly colored nevi are on the surface of the iris elsewhere. Gonioscopy reveals no seeding or excessive pigmentation of the angle adjacent to the tumor mass.

Course. An iridocyclectomy was performed without vitreous loss and practically no hemorrhage. The tumor was peeled off the cornea by use of a spatula. Histopatholic diagnosis was malignant melanoma, spindle cell A type, with extension to the ciliary body. The postoperative course was uneventful, and 5 years later there was no sign of recurrence of the tumor.

Juvenile malignant melanoma of the iris

History. Since birth this 13-year-old boy has had a brown spot on his right iris. Recently there was a gradual increase in its size so it was now about twice as large. The eye became painful.

Findings. The vision in the right eye is 20/40 and in the left 20/30. The right eye is normal except for a vascularized mass of yellowish material that arises from the iris at the 4 o'clock to the 6 o'clock position. The surface of the mass is mulberry in appearance, and the pupil is distorted (Reel XII-7). About REEL XII-7 five iris freckles appear elsewhere on the iris surface. There are a few pigment clumps on the anterior capsule of the lens. The left eye is normal, with no iris freckles. The intraocular pressure is 43 mm. Hg (Schiøtz) in the right eye and 18 mm. Hg (Schiøtz) in the left.

Course. The right eye was enucleated, and the postoperative course was uneventful. Histopathologically, the tumor had invaded the entire thickness of the iris, with extension into the angle and ciliary body. In addition, nevi of the iris were undergoing malignant change (Fig. 150, A). The cell type was predomi- FIG. 150 nantly spindle cell B (Fig. 150, B). Seven years later the socket was normal, and vision was 20/20 in the left eye.

Malignant melanoma of the iris

History. For as long as he can remember, this 49-year-old man had a spot on his left eye. He was not aware of any change in the size of the spot.

Findings. The vision is 20/25 in both eyes without correction. The right eye is normal. In the left eye there are some pigment granules on the endothelium. The anterior chamber is clear, and inferiorly it is filled with a tumor mass attached to the iris and extending to the pupillary border where there is a small amount of ectropion uveae (Fig. 151, A). The central portion of the tumor almost FIG. 151 touches the cornea, and the mass extends under the external limbus. There is no reaction of the pupil in the area of the tumor. The media and fundus are normal. By gonioscopy the tumor can be seen extending onto the trabecular meshwork at the 6 o'clock position, but there is no sign of seeding or excessive pigmentation in the remainder of the angle.

Course. The patient was again seen 2½ years later, and the size of the tumor was compared photographically to its appearance on his first visit. It was apparent that there had been some increase in size, but there was no evidence of extension into other portions of the eye. Tension shown by applanation tonometry was 18 mm. Hg in the right eye and 20 mm. Hg in the left. Five years later the patient again returned; he had had pain and photophobia in the left eye

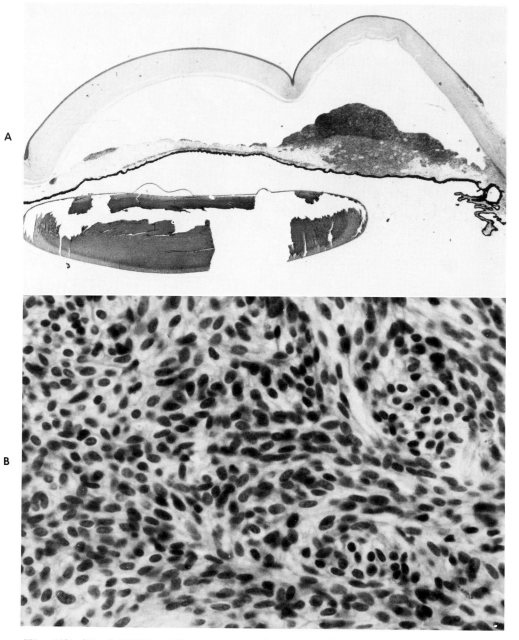

Fig. 150 (Reel XII-7). *Photomicrographs of a mulberrylike mass on the right iris in a 13-year-old boy with a juvenile malignant melanoma.* **A,** Low-power photomicrograph shows the elevated tumor mass with invasion of the entire thickness of the iris. (H & E stain; ×160.) **B,** High-power photomicrograph shows the predominantly spindle cell B type. (H & E stain; ×1600.)

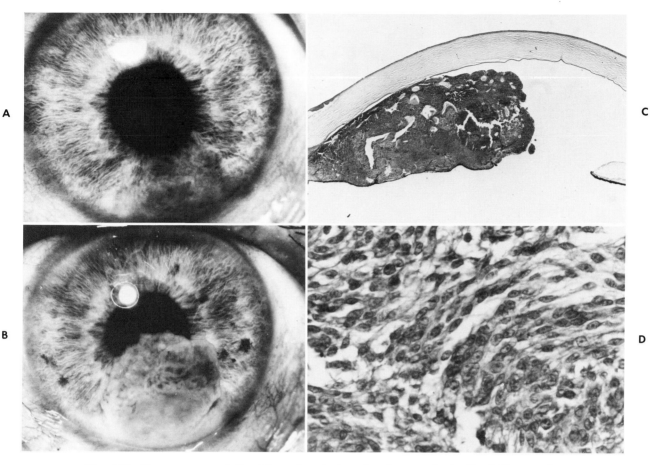

Fig. 151. *Tumor mass of the iris and anterior chamber angle in the left eye of a 49-year-old man with a malignant melanoma of the iris.* **A,** Lobulated tumor mass extends from the pupillary border into the angle from the 5 o'clock to the 7 o'clock position. By gonioscopy no seeding or excessive pigmentation can be seen. **B,** Seven and a half years later the tumor had doubled in size, occluding half of the pupil. The intraocular pressure is moderately elevated. **C,** Photomicrograph shows complete infiltration of the iris and ciliary body, with obliteration of the angle. (H & E stain; ×160.) **D,** Photomicrograph shows predominantly spindle cell B type. (H & E stain; ×1600.)

for 1 week. The tumor had more than doubled in size and now occluded half of the pupil (Fig. 151, *B*). The cornea was edematous, and there was a small hyphema. The intraocular pressure was 17 mm. Hg (Schiøtz) in the right eye and 43 mm. Hg (Schiøtz) in the left. The left eye was enucleated, and postoperative recovery was normal. Histopathologically, the tumor was found to have completely infiltrated the iris and ciliary body on the involved side, with obliteration of the chamber angle (Fig. 151, *C*). The predominant cell type was spindle cell B (Fig. 151, *D*).

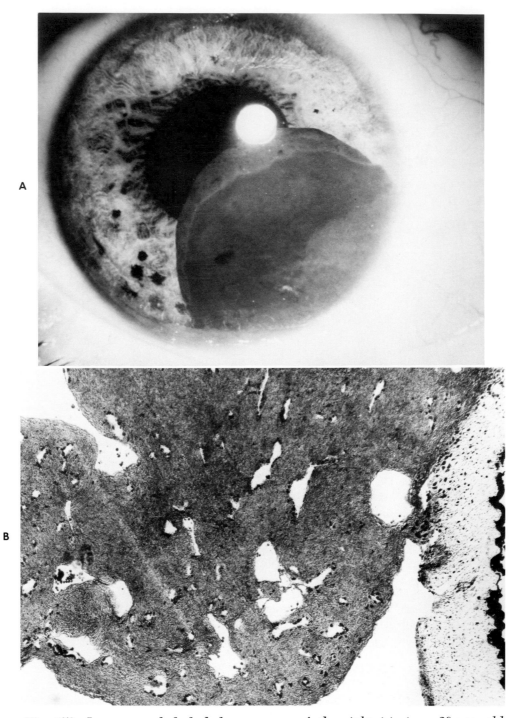

Fig. 152. *Large rounded dark brown mass of the right iris in a 30-year-old woman with a malignant melanoma of the iris.* **A,** The tumor mass partially occludes the pupil and is in contact with the cornea almost to its apex. By gonioscopy the remaining angle can be seen covered with pigment granules, and the intraocular pressure is moderately elevated. **B,** Photomicrograph shows the malignant melanoma that invades the iris, trabecular meshwork, and Schlemm's canal. (H & E stain; ×40.) The cell type is predominantly spindle cell B.

Malignant melanoma of the iris

History. Six years ago this 30-year-old woman first noticed a brown spot on her right iris. Three years ago it had grown sufficiently to be quite noticeable, and there has been a gradual increase in growth since then, with a decrease in the vision.

Findings. In the right eye there is a large rounded dark brown mass involving the angle from the 3 o'clock to the 7 o'clock position and extending halfway over the pupil (Fig. 152, *A*). The corneal epithelium is edematous FIG. 152 where the tumor is in contact with the cornea. Gonioscopy shows that most of the remaining angle is covered with fine pigment granules. The media and fundus appear normal, and the disc is normal. No abnormalities of the left eye are found. Applanation tonometry shows a tension of 32 mm. Hg in the right eye and 16 mm. Hg in the left.

Course. Reaction to a ^{32}P test was strongly positive both at 24 and 48 hours. The right eye was enucleated, and the postoperative course was uneventful. The histopathologic finding was a malignant melanoma of the iris, predominantly of the spindle cell B type, invading the trabecular meshwork and Schlemm's canal (Fig. 152, *B*).

Malignant melanoma of the iris

History. For as long as she can remember, this 30-year-old woman had a pigmented mark on her right eye. Over the past 2 months it appeared to increase in size.

Findings. The vision in both eyes is 20/20. In the right eye the anterior segment is normal except for the iris inferiorly, where there is an elevated irregular dark brown mass (Fig. 153, *A*). This mass does not extend quite to the pupil- FIG. 153 lary margin and disappears under the external limbus. There are several dark brown iris nevi, but there is no other abnormality. The posterior segment is normal. Gonioscopy shows that the tumor reaches almost to the angle structures and that there are some clumped pigment deposits on the trabecular meshwork (Fig. 153, *B*). The left eye, which is normal, contains several large iris freckles.

Course. The iris mass was totally excised, and histopathologic examination showed that it was a malignant melanoma of a mixed cell type containing considerable melanin (Fig. 153, *C*). A piece of the fresh tumor was inserted onto the iris of a living rabbit. Five months later the tissue had completely atrophied, leaving only a small area of pigment granules on the iris surface.

Malignant melanoma of the iris

History. About 1½ years ago this 54-year-old man noted blurring of vision in his right eye. He was found to have slightly reduced visual acuity, with a yellow mass on the right iris inferiorly and an intraocular pressure of 38 mm. Hg (Schiøtz). A month later an iridocyclectomy was performed inferiorly, and the histopathologic diagnosis was malignant melanoma of the iris, spindle cell B type. Vision improved to 20/70, but 2 months later a retinal detachment occurred, for which a scleral buckling procedure was performed. During the next few months the inferior portion of the lens came forward, touched the cornea, and formed a corneolenticular adhesion. The lens then became cataractous, and

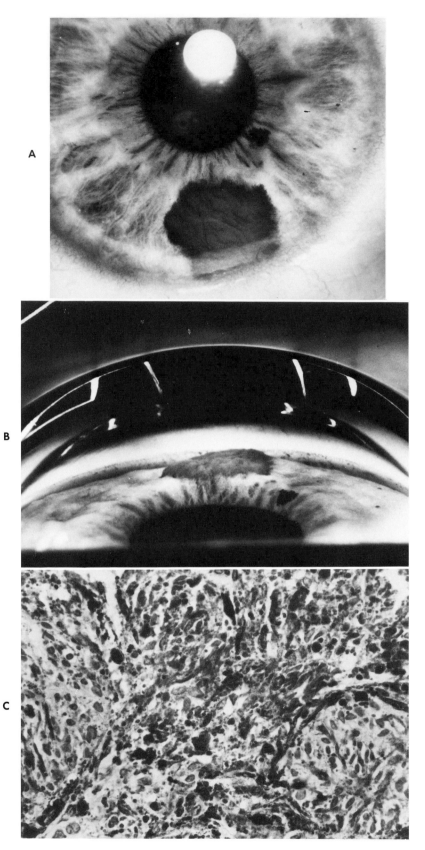

Fig. 153. For legend see opposite page.

the eye was constantly inflamed. In another 6 months there was evidence that the tumor had recurred.

Findings. The right eye is blind, and the vision in the left eye is 20/20. In the right eye there is marked conjunctival injection, with necrotic cellular debris and red blood cells located on the posterior surface of the cornea inferiorly (Reel XIII-1). There is a complete iridectomy inferiorly, and the iris is studded with small nodules, with no normal iris pattern remaining. The inferior portion of the lens appears to come into contact with the peripheral cornea, and the entire lens is cataractous. The left eye is normal.   REEL XIII-1

Course. The right eye was enucleated, and the histopathologic finding was the lens in contact with the peripheral cornea, with malignant melanoma tumor cells situated between each structure (Fig. 154, A). The cell type was predomi-   FIG. 154
nantly spindle cell B (Fig. 154, B).

Malignant melanoma of the iris

History. About 20 years ago this 40-year-old man noticed a black spot on his right eye. Two years ago there was some decrease in his vision, and about 2 months ago he found that the side vision was poor in the right eye.

Findings. The vision in the right eye is 20/30 and in the left 20/20. In the right eye there is a mass of dark pigmented material on the inferior portion of the iris extending to within about 3 mm. of the pupillary margin. The entire surface of the iris is covered with many fine pigmented spots, and there are a few iris nevi. By gonioscopy the tumor mass can be seen to extend about 3 mm. onto the cornea at the 6 o'clock position and to invade the angle over an area of several hours of the clock (Fig. 155, A). Elsewhere the angle is heavily pigmented, the   FIG. 155
lens is clear, and there is glaucomatous cupping of the disc. Confrontation field indicates an almost total loss of the nasal field. The left eye is normal, and the surface of the iris is not covered with pigmented material. Intraocular pressure in the right eye is 34 mm. Hg (Schiøtz) and in the left 20 mm. Hg (Schiøtz).

Course. The result of a ^{32}P test was equivocal, and an enucleation was carried out. Histopathologic findings were marked invasion of the angle and melanoma (Fig. 155, B) with even extension into Schlemm's canal on the opposite side of the tumor mass (Fig. 155, C). The bleached specimen showed a mixed cell type, with many epithelioid cells particularly in the aqueous (Fig. 155, D). Fifteen years later the patient was asymptomatic, and vision in his remaining eye was 20/20.

Fig. 153. *Elevated irregular dark brown iris mass on the right eye of a 30-year-old woman with a malignant melanoma.* **A,** Tumor mass extends under the external limbus at the 6 o'clock position and reaches almost to the pupillary margin. **B,** By gonioscopy the tumor can be seen reaching almost to the angle structures, and there is clumped pigment deposition on the trabecular meshwork. **C,** Photomicrograph shows a mixed cell type of malignant melanoma containing much melanin. (H & E stain; ×1600.)

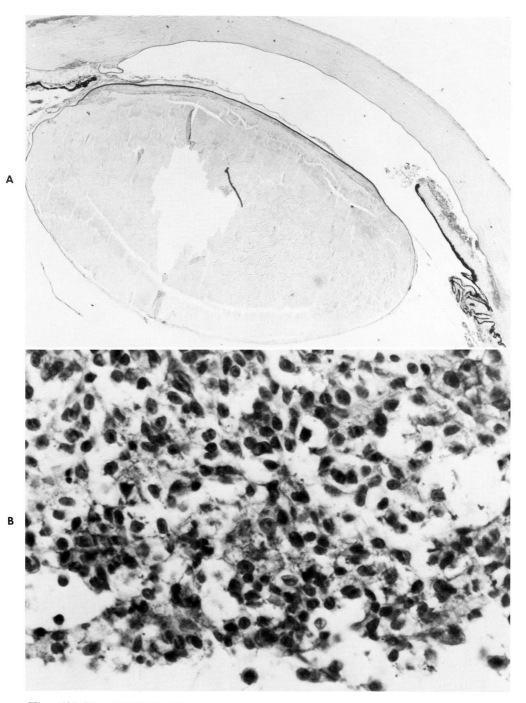

Fig. 154 (Reel XIII-1). *Photomicrographs of a recurrent malignant melanoma of the iris in a 54-year-old man.* **A,** Photomicrograph shows a complete iridectomy inferiorly and the iris superiorly studded with small nodules of the recurrent tumor. The cataractous lens is tilted forward inferiorly almost in contact with the cornea. (H & E stain; ×160.) **B,** Photomicrograph shows the cell type to be predominantly spindle cell B. (H & E stain; ×1600.)

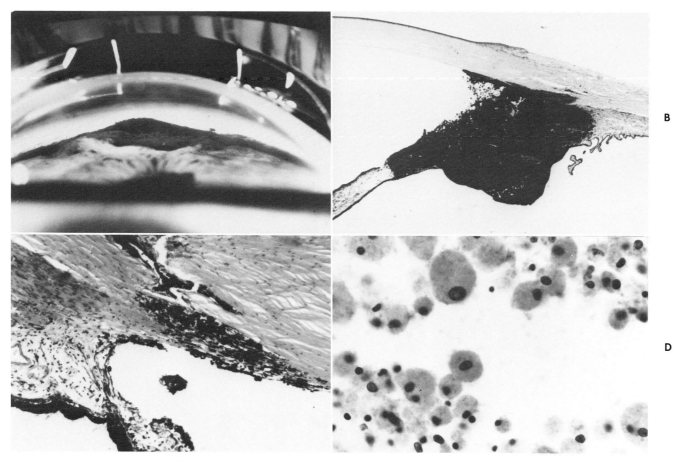

Fig. 155. *Darkly pigmented mass involving the inferior right iris in a 40-year-old man with a malignant melanoma.* **A,** By gonioscopy the tumor invades the angle, extends almost to the pupillary margin, and is in contact with the peripheral cornea. Intraocular pressure is elevated, and there is glaucomatous cupping and field defects. **B,** Photomicrograph shows marked invasion of the angle by a heavily pigmented melanoma. (H & E stain; ×40.) **C,** Photomicrograph of angle opposite the tumor shows extension of tumor cells into trabecular meshwork and Schlemm's canal. (H & E stain; ×400.) **D,** Photomicrograph shows mixed cell type with many epithelioid cells in the aqueous. (Bleached H & E stain; ×1600.)

Malignant melanoma of the iris

History. At least 14 years ago a dark spot was noticed on the right eye of this 41-year-old man. There seemed to be little change in its appearance until about a year ago, when it was thought to have enlarged slightly. Except for slight blurring, the patient had no symptoms.

Findings. Vision in the right eye is 20/40 and in the left 20/20. In the right eye the cornea exhibits some dusting of pigment on the posterior surface in the form of a Krukenberg spindle. Extending into the anterior chamber at least a

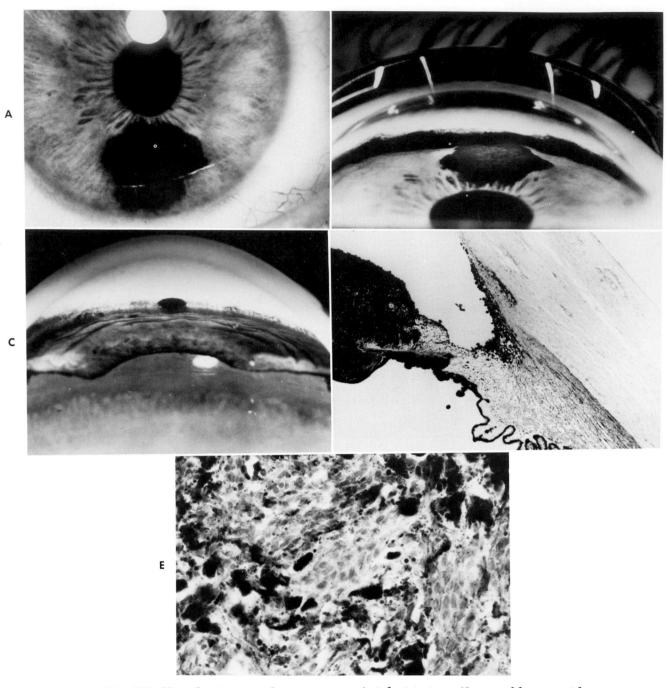

Fig. 156. *Heavily pigmented tumor mass of right iris in a 41-year-old man with a malignant melanoma.* **A,** Arising from the iris inferiorly is a dark brownish black tumor that does not quite reach the pupillary margin or external limbus. **B,** By gonioscopy the angle is filled with dark pigmented material that is not continuous with the iris mass. **C,** Gross pathologic specimen shows a satellite tumor in the superior angle. **D,** Photomicrograph shows extensive involvement of the angle, sclera, and ciliary body, adjacent to the tumor. (H & E stain; ×160.) **E,** Photomicrograph shows extensive melanin pigmentation and predominantly spindle cell B type. (H & E stain; ×1600.)

millimeter is a dark brownish black mass arising from the iris inferiorly (Fig. 156, *A*). This mass extends almost to the pupillary margin and ends about a millimeter from the external limbus. The mass does not seem to invade the iris, and the pupil reacts normally but does not fully dilate in the region of the mass. Two small nevi that have the same coloring and texture as the large mass are also visible elsewhere on the iris. Gonioscopy shows that the tumor does not extend into the angle but that the inferior angle is filled with dark pigmented material, some of which appears to have mass (Fig. 156, *B*). The superior angle also has isolated areas of excessive pigmentation. The media and fundus are normal. The left eye is normal. The intraocular pressure is 14 mm. Hg (Schiøtz) in both eyes.

Course. Enucleation was performed, and the gross pathologic specimen showed a prominent satellite tumor in the superior angle along with some increased pigmentation on the trabecular meshwork (Fig. 156, *C*). Histopathologically, there was extensive involvement of the angle adjacent to the tumor with tumor cells, and extension into the sclera and ciliary body (Fig. 156, *D*). The cell type was predominantly spindle cell B, with large amounts of melanin pigmentation throughout the tumor (Fig. 156, *E*).

FIG. 156

Malignant melanoma of the iris

History. For 35 years this 65-year-old woman had a brownish spot on her left iris. Five years ago she was found to have mild diabetes.

Findings. The vision in the right eye is 20/20 and in the left 20/200 with correction. In the right eye the anterior segment is normal, and there are early cortical lens opacities. Fundus examination reveals a number of round hemorrhages and some hard, waxy exudates. In the left eye there is a large brown vascularized mass arising from the iris and filling about one third of the temporal portion of the anterior chamber (Fig. 157, *A*). Part of the mass is in contact with the cornea, and there is a marked ectropion uveae of more than half the pupillary border. The tumor fills almost the entire temporal portion of the angle. Early cortical changes are seen in the lens, and the fundus findings are similar to those in the right eye. Intraocular tension is 21 mm. Hg (Schiøtz) in both eyes.

FIG. 157

Course. The left eye was enucleated, and a movable implant was used. Histopathologically, a large malignant melanoma was found invading the cornea and ciliary body and occluding the temporal angle (Fig. 157, *B*). The tumor was of a mixed cell type, predominantly spindle cell B and epithelioid cell (Fig. 157, *C*). Two years later the implant extruded, and it was replaced with a glass ball. Three years later at which time she was apparently having no problem with the eye, the patient died of a coronary thrombosis.

Diffuse melanoma of the iris with glaucoma

History. For about a year this 23-year-old man had decreasing vision in the left eye. One week ago this eye became red; and when seen by an ophthalmologist, he was found to have elevated intraocular pressure and only light perception in the eye. Miotics did not affect intraocular tension.

Findings. Vision in the right eye is 20/15 and in the left light perception only. The right eye is normal in all respects. In the left eye there is moderate diffuse conjunctival injection. The cornea is slightly edematous and thickened, and on

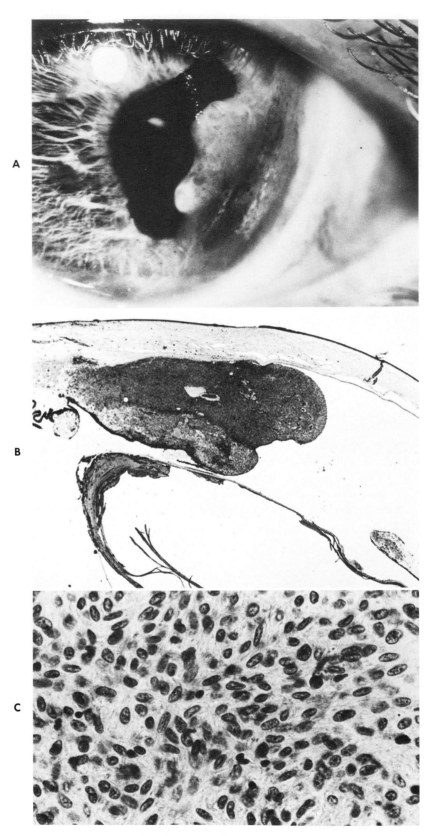

Fig. 157. For legend see opposite page.

the endothelium are a number of fine pigment granules. The anterior chamber is clear. In contrast to the right eye, the iris surface in the left eye is covered with multiple iris nevi and pigment granules (Fig. 158, A). The pupil is semidilated   FIG. 158 and reacts sluggishly. The lens is clear; the fundus shows deep glaucomatous cupping; and there are a few superficial hemorrhages near the ora. Gonioscopy of the right eye reveals no abnormalities, but in the left the entire angle is covered with a heavy deposit of dark brown granular pigment (Reel XIII-2).   REEL XIII-2 Intraocular pressure in the right eye is 18 mm. Hg (Schiøtz) and in the left 55 mm. Hg (Schiøtz).

Course. Acetazolamide, ephinephrine (1%) drops, and topical administration of corticosteroids were initiated; but even with intensive use they produced no appreciable change in the intraocular pressure. Because of the possibility of a malignant melanoma, enucleation was performed. The histopathologic findings were a diffuse malignant melanoma of the iris, with cells blocking the trabecular meshwork. The cell type was predominantly epithelioid, with some cells containing much melanin and others almost amelanotic (Fig. 158, B).

Flat melanoma of the iris

History. For over a year this 38-year-old man noted a change in the color of his left eye from blue to chocolate brown. Four years ago he was seen by an ophthalmologist, who noted excessive pigmentation along the inferior border of the pupil of the left eye and considered it to be a congenital ectropion uveae. During the past week the patient noted decreased vision in the left eye. He stated that the vision in his right eye had been poor all his life due to a "lazy eye."

Findings. The vision in the right eye is 20/200 and in the left 20/30. No abnormalities of the right eye can be found; the iris is light blue with a prominent grayish blue sphincter (Fig. 159, A). In the left eye there is mild con-   FIG. 159 junctival injection and some bedewing of the corneal epithelium centrally. There are also several leukomas due to old corneal injuries; the largest leukoma involves the temporal portion of the pupillary area (Fig. 159, B). The anterior chamber is clear and of normal depth. The entire iris is a dark brown, and a sheetlike broad, flat mass of pigmented tissue completely replaces all the iris crypts. In the more peripheral portion of the iris, strands of iris stroma are visible through the dense brown pigment. There is a marked ectropion uveae most prominent inferiorly, and this is composed of darker brown, smoother pigmented tissue. The pupil reacts poorly to light. The media and fundus appear normal.

Fig. 157. *Large brown vascularized mass of the left iris in a 65-year-old woman with a malignant melanoma.* **A,** The mass is in contact with the cornea, and there is a marked ectropion uveae, with a distorted pupil. **B,** Low-power photomicrograph shows the large tumor mass filling the angle of the anterior chamber and invading the peripheral cornea and ciliary body. (H & E stain; ×40.) **C,** Photomicrograph of tumor shows a mixed cell type, predominantly spindle cell B and epithelioid. (H & E stain; ×1600.)

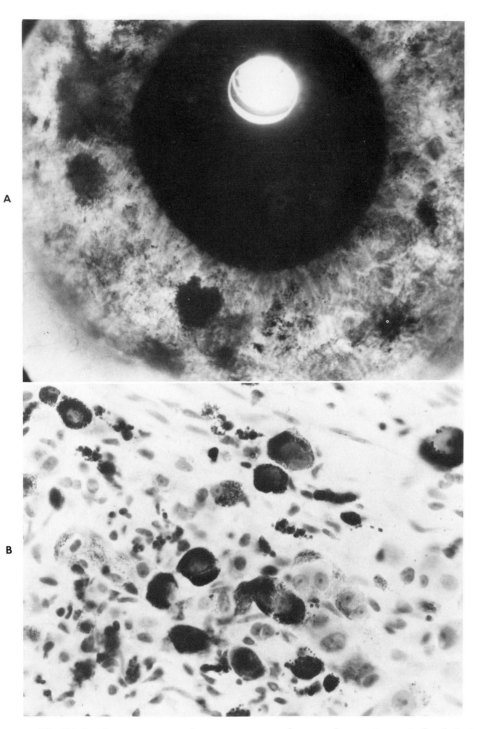

Fig. 158. *Multiple iris nevi and pigment granules on the surface of the left iris in a 23-year-old man with diffuse melanoma of the iris and secondary glaucoma.* A, Almost the entire surface of the iris is covered with irregular pigmentation, and the pupil is semidilated and reacts sluggishly. By gonioscopy (see Reel XIII-2) the entire angle has a heavy deposit of dark brown pigment. Intraocular pressure is markedly elevated. B, Photomicrograph shows both heavily pigmented and almost amelanotic cells of predominantly epithelioid type. (H & E stain; ×1600.) Histopathologically, the tumor was diffusely spread throughout the iris, and tumor cells blocked the trabecular meshwork.

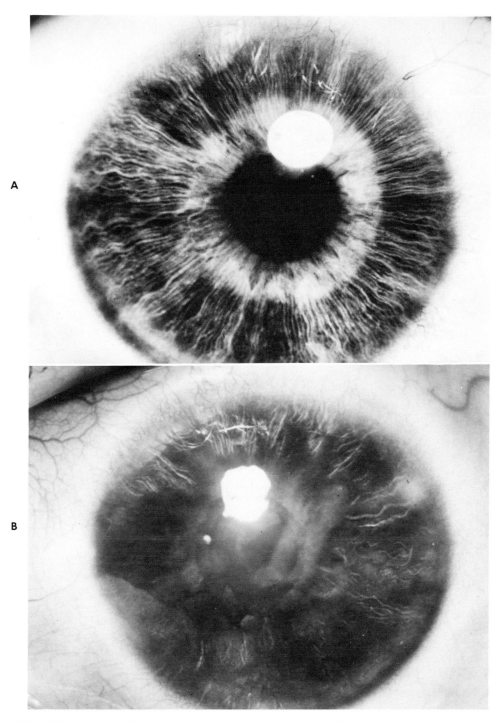

Fig. 159. *Recent change in color of the left iris from blue to chocolate brown in a 38-year-old man with a flat melanoma of the iris.* **A,** In the right eye the iris is light blue and has a prominent sphincter. **B,** In the left eye most of the iris is chocolate brown, with some peripheral iris strands still visible. There is a marked ectropion uveae, and the intraocular pressure is markedly elevated. Histopathologically, the tumor involves the anterior chamber angle, ciliary body, and sclera. The cell type is spindle cell B.

Gonioscopy reveals no angle abnormalities. The intraocular tension in the right eye is normal but in the left is 55 mm. Hg (Schiøtz).

Course. A trephine procedure was performed; but there was recurrent pain, and the intraocular tension again became uncontrollable. It became obvious that a tumor was present, so enucleation was performed 1 year later. The histopathologic finding was a flat melanoma of the iris that had extensively involved the angle of the anterior chamber, ciliary body, and sclera. The cell type was spindle cell B, and the secondary glaucoma appeared to be due to pigment cells within the trabecular meshwork. The patient was then lost to follow-up.

Malignant melanoma of the choroid with iris and episcleral extension

History. Two years ago this 67-year-old woman noted a black spot on her left eye. She did not know whether it had increased in size, but she had no symptoms related to it. The eye had always been "weak."

Findings. Vision in the right eye is 20/30 and in the left 20/200 with correction. No abnormality can be found in the right eye, but in the left there is a black mass under the conjunctiva extending from the 5 o'clock to the 6 o'clock position adjacent to the limbus. From the 4 o'clock to the 6 o'clock position in the peripheral iris is a similar dark brown tumor that appears to extend into the angle (Fig. 160, *A*). The pupil dilates well with mydriatics. There is an immature cataract, and the fundus is normal. No abnormalities of the left eye are found.

FIG. 160

Course. The eye was enucleated, and the postoperative recovery was uneventful. Histopathologically, the choroidal melanoma had completely invaded the ciliary body, extended into the anterior chamber, and spread into the episcleral region (Fig. 160, *B*). The cell type was spindle cell B and epitheloid (Fig. 160, *C*). Nine months later the patient was apparently in good health and had no ocular symptoms.

Melanoma of the iris with iritis and glaucoma

History. Recently this 63-year-old man was found to have an iritis and elevated intraocular pressure in his left eye.

Findings. The vision in the right eye is 20/20 and in the left 20/30. The right eye is normal. In the left eye there is moderate conjunctival injection. The cornea is clear, but the anterior chamber contains many cells and some flare. A pigment ring remains on the anterior capsule of the lens following posterior synechial formation. There are numerous small areas of pigmentation on the surface of the iris, and inferiorly is a mass that extends from the angle to the pupillary

---

Fig. 160. *Black mass under the conjunctiva and in the peripheral iris in the left eye of a 67-year-old woman with a malignant melanoma. A,* The tumor at the 6 o'clock position in the peripheral iris and under the conjunctiva is a dark brown mass. **B,** Photomicrograph shows a choroidal melanoma that had invaded the ciliary body, with extension into the anterior chamber and the episcleral region. (H & E stain; ×160.) **C,** The cell type is spindle cell B and epithelioid. (H & E stain; ×1600.)

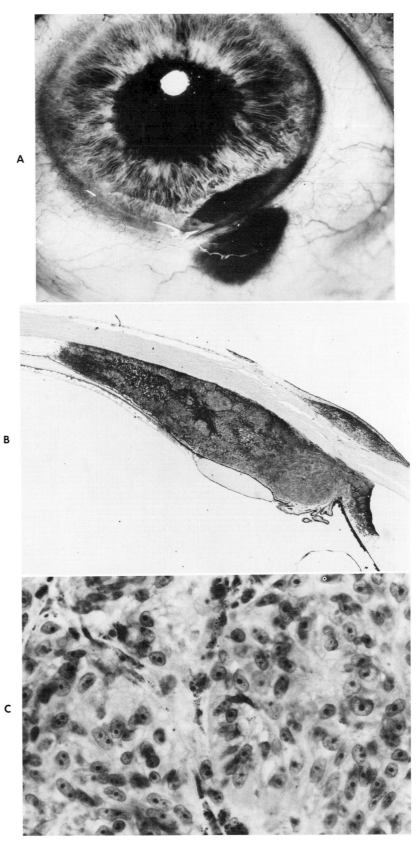

Fig. 160. For legend see opposite page.

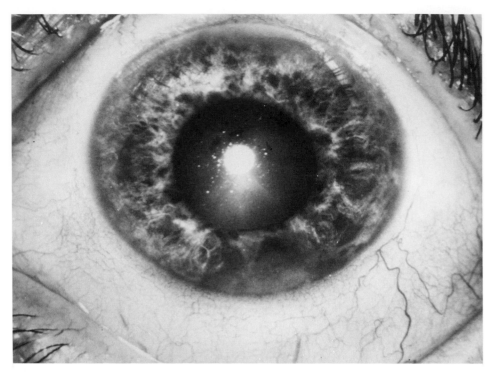

Fig. 161. *Pigmented mass of the left iris in a 63-year-old man with a malignant melanoma and secondary iritis and glaucoma.* The tumor mass extends from the inferior angle to the pupillary margin, and gonioscopy reveals that the inferior angle is filled with tumor mass. On the anterior lens capsule is a pigment ring due to posterior synechia formation. The patient had iritis and an elevated intraocular pressure. Histopathologically, the mass was a malignant melanoma of spindle cell B type that had invaded the trabecular meshwork.

FIG. 161 margin (Fig. 161). Gonioscopy reveals that the angle is completely filled inferiorly with the tumor mass. The intraocular pressure is 45 mm. Hg (Schiøtz).

Course. Reaction to a ^{32}P test was negative. Treatment was instituted with mydriatics, systemic administration of corticosteroid, and acetazolamide. Over the next month there was no appreciable improvement in the iritis and glaucoma, and the iris lesion appeared to be enlarging. Enucleation was performed, and the postoperative recovery was uneventful. The histopathologic diagnosis was malignant melanoma of the iris, with invasion of the angle and trabecular meshwork. There was no necrosis, and the cell type was spindle cell B. Six years later the left eye had a vision of 20/25 with correction, and the patient appeared to be in good health.

NONPIGMENTED IRIS TUMORS

Iris tumors without pigment are rare, and the most common of these are the muscle tumors (leiomyomas). These are very slow growing and are derived from the dilator or sphincter muscle of the iris. Although of neuroectodermal origin, they are histopathologically indistinguishable from leiomyomas elsewhere

274

in the body and have a slowly progressive benign course. Iris leiomyomas arising from the sphincter are salmon-colored, while those from the dilator are usually pigmented.

Most neuroectodermal tumors involving the iris are neurofibromas and are frequently associated with neurofibromatosis (von Recklinghausen's disease). They are congenital benign tumors, with very slow growth, and are seen as multiple small, elevated nodules anywhere on the iris (p. 168). Neurolemmomas arise from sheaths of nerves in the ciliary body. Vascular tumors, or hemangiomas, are occasionally seen in the stroma of the iris and usually remain stationary over a long period of time. Various reticuloses giving rise to the lymphomas can produce iris tumors that are difficult to differentiate from other types.

Metastatic tumors constitute one of the more common nonpigmented iris neoplasms, although they are much less frequent in the iris than in the choroid. Of the primary sources of such metastatic tumors, the breast is most common, followed by the lung. Retinoblastoma may seed into the anterior chamber and thus can be considered a metastatic tumor. As these lesions grow, they frequently become necrotic and produce a secondary iritis.

Leiomyoma of the iris

History. For some time this 22-year-old man was aware of a pinkish mass on his right eye. Since early life he had poor vision in both eyes, and 8 years ago surgery for strabismus was performed on the muscles of the right eye.

Findings. The vision in both eyes is 20/70. There is a pendular nystagmus in all directions of gaze; other findings of the skin and eyes are consistent with partial albinism. In the right eye the entire iris is light blue except for a small elevated pink mass involving the periphery of the iris at the 7 o'clock to the 9 o'clock position (Reel XIII-3). The moderately elevated mass appears to invade REEL XIII-3 the iris stroma, and on its surface are a number of fine blood vessels. The media and fundus are normal. No abnormalities are found in the left eye.

Course. Reaction to a ^{32}P test was negative, and a local excision of the lesion was performed. Histopathologic findings were those of typical cellular structure of a leiomyoma with a Masson trichrome stain (Fig. 162) and myofibrils visible FIG. 162 in the phosphotungstic acid–hematoxylin stain.

Retinoblastoma

History. One month ago a peculiar white reflex was noted in the right pupil of this 3-year-old girl.

Findings. External examination of both eyes reveals no abnormalities. With the right pupil dilated, a retrolenticular mass that is yellowish and that has on its surface a number of prominent blood vessels can be seen (Fig. 163, A). It occupies FIG. 163 almost the entire pupillary area, and there is a hemorrhage at the 2 o'clock position. Examination of the fundus of the left eye shows no abnormality.

Course. The right eye was enucleated. At the time of enucleation the left eye was thoroughly examined, and no abnormality was found. Histopathologic diagnosis was retinoblastoma with involvement of the choroid, nerve head, sclera, and episclera. Postoperative convalescence was uneventful until 6 months later, when a spontaneous hyphema developed in the left eye. As the blood absorbed, a pinkish tumor could be seen extending around the periphery of the iris from the 2 o'clock to the 7 o'clock position (Fig. 163, *B*). Examination of the patient while she was under anesthesia showed no fundus lesion to be present. Examination of the right socket showed no signs of tumor, but aspiration of the anterior chamber of the left eye showed tumor cells typical of retinoblastoma. Metastatic series showed no signs of metastasis, but a bone marrow aspirate showed clumps of tumor cells typical of retinoblastoma. Three weeks later the tumor in the anterior chamber had doubled in size, and the entire iris was nodular (Reel

REEL XIII-4

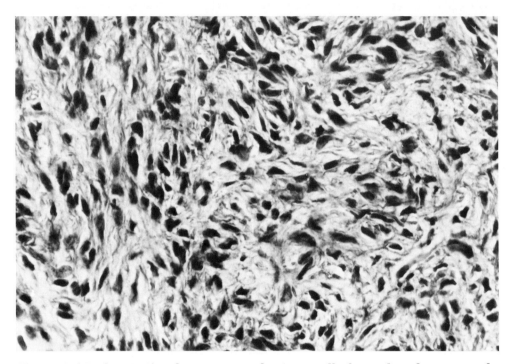

Fig. 162 (Reel XIII-3). *Photomicrograph of a small elevated pink mass in the peripheral iris of a 22-year-old man with a leiomyoma.* Histopathologically, the cellular structure is typical of a leiomyoma. (Masson stain; ×1600.)

Fig. 163. *Retrolenticular mass in the right eye and iris tumor in the left in a 3-year-old girl with retinoblastoma.* **A,** In the right eye a yellowish mass is immediately behind the lens and contains prominent blood vessels and hemorrhage. The eye was enucleated, and extensive retinoblastoma was found. **B,** Six months later a pinkish tumor of the left iris was found, but there was no fundus lesion. An anterior chamber tap showed typical retinoblastoma tumor cells. Three weeks later the tumor had doubled in size (see Reel XIII-4). **C,** In another 3 weeks the entire iris was nodular and the anterior chamber half filled with tumor. **D,** In 3 more weeks there was proptosis, corneal ulceration, and further filling of the anterior chamber with tumor. **E,** Photomicrograph shows the iris to be minimally involved but the anterior chamber to be filled with necrotic tumor cells. (H & E stain; ×40.)

276

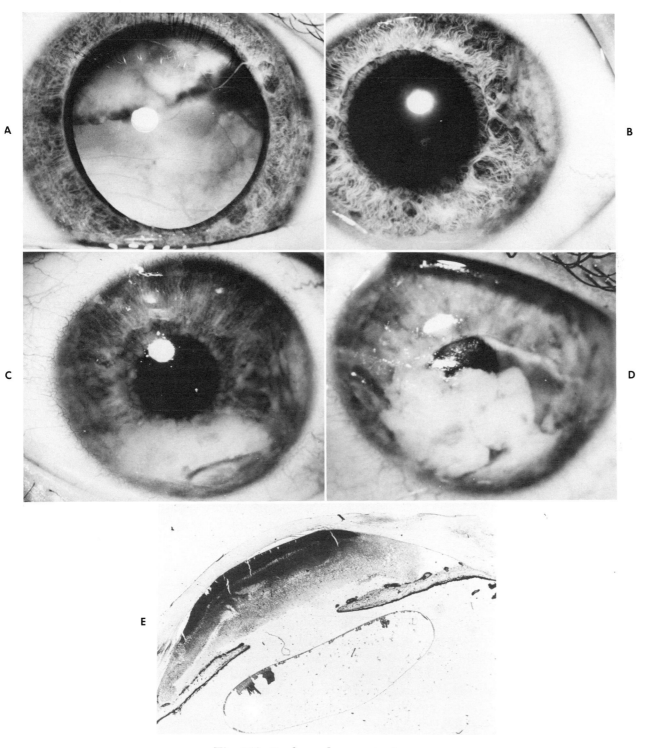

Fig. 163. For legend see opposite page.

XIII-4). Plans were made to treat the left eye with x-radiation and nitrogen mustard, but she was found to have a hemoglobin level of 7.2. Several weeks later a mass was noted in her left mandible, and x-ray films confirmed diffuse infiltration by tumor. In another week a metastatic lesion of the left femur was identified, and the anterior chamber was about half filled with tumor tissue and most of the iris infiltrated with tumor nodules (Fig. 163, C). There was also evidence of recurrence of the tumor in the right orbit and metastasis to the skull. With the patient receiving biweekly injections of thio-TEPA her condition improved remarkably. Proptosis of the left eye then became apparent and progressed markedly over a period of the next 2 weeks, at which time the cornea became ulcerated and the anterior chamber further filled with tumor cells (Fig. 163, D). Histopathologic examination showed the iris to be minimally involved but the anterior chamber to be full of necrotic tumor cells (Fig. 163, E). Two weeks later she died.

Seeding of retinoblastoma in anterior chamber

History. Two weeks ago this 3-year-old girl was noted to have "white spots" on her right eye. Since then, they have increased in number. She had no pain or redness. Three other siblings are entirely well.

Findings. In the right eye there is minimal conjunctival injection. The cornea is clear except for a number of white avascular masses attached to the posterior surface near the limbus (Fig. 164, A). Similar masses, also avascular, are attached to the iris. By gonioscopy it can be seen that tumor masses involve the angle structures as well (Fig. 164, B). Examination of the fundus with the patient's pupil dilated reveals a massive tumor filling the vitreous cavity and obscuring any view of the fundus. Examination of the left eye, including the fundus with the patient's pupil dilated, shows no abnormalities.

FIG. 164

Course. An aspiration of the anterior chamber was performed, and the aqueous was studied on smears. The cells found were compatible with retinoblastoma or neuroblastoma. An enucleation was performed, and the postoperative course was uneventful. Histopathologic examination showed the entire eye to be massively involved with retinoblastoma invading the anterior chamber, iris, ciliary body, and optic nerve head. Microscopically, typical retinoblastoma cells were evident, with many pseudorosettes throughout the tumor (Fig. 164, C). Nine months later the patient died of generalized metastasis.

Fig. 164. *White avascular masses on the cornea and iris and in the chamber angle in the right eye of a 3-year-old girl with seeding of a retinoblastoma.* **A,** White nodules on the posterior surface of the cornea and iris in an otherwise normal anterior segment. **B,** Gonioscopy shows that similar tumor masses involve the angle structures. Examination of the fundus showed a massive tumor filling the vitreous cavity, and an anterior chamber tap showed retinoblastoma cells. **C,** Photomicrograph shows typical retinoblastoma cells with pseudorosettes. The tumor had invaded the anterior chamber, iris, ciliary body, and optic nerve head. (H & E stain; ×1600.)

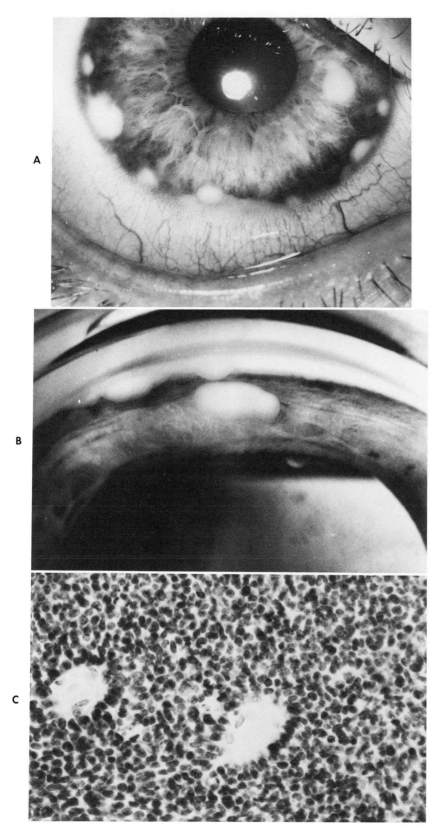

Fig. 164. For legend see opposite page.

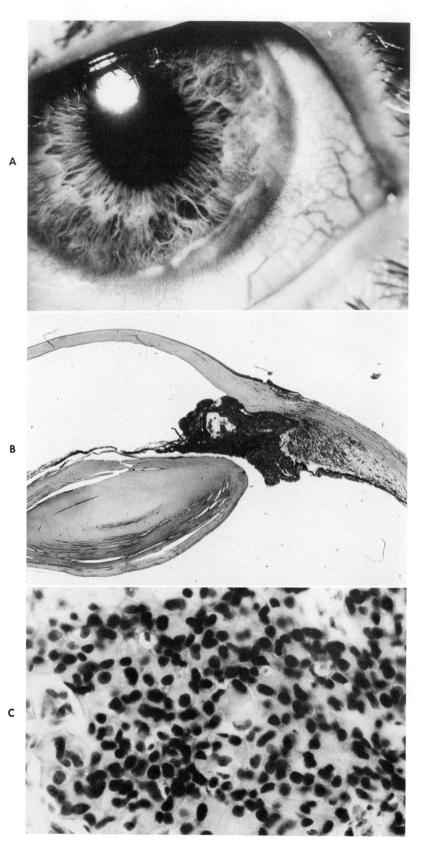

Fig. 165. For legend see opposite page.

Metastatic carcinoma of the iris

History. Nine years ago this 50-year-old woman had a right radical mastectomy for carcinoma with metastatic involvement of the regional lymph nodes. This was followed by x-ray therapy applied to the right axilla and supraclavicular area. Four years ago she developed pleurisy in the right chest, and a pleural tap yielded fluid that contained malignant cells. X-ray findings of the chest were also consistent with pulmonary metastases. Testosterone propionate was given over a period of 6 months, but her condition did not improve. Moreover, she was also discovered to have a choroidal metastasis with a secondary separation of the retina in the left eye. Treatment was then changed to stilbestrol, and there was a marked regression of the lung and choroidal metastases. Stilbestrol was continued, and there were no further signs of metastatic disease for 2 years. The patient then developed ascites; the fluid was positive for tumor cells. An x-ray castration was then carried out. Six months ago there was an increase in the field defect of the right eye and also a tumor in the angle of the anterior chamber. Further studies showed a recurrence of the metastasis in the lungs, liver, and bone. Within the next 6 months there was gradual increase in the size of the tumor of the angle.

Findings. The vision in the right eye is 20/30 and in the left 20/200. The right eye is normal. In the left eye the conjunctiva is moderately injected, and there is a nonpigmented mass that fills the angle from the 2 o'clock to the 6 o'clock position (Fig. 165, A). In some places there are small nodules on the mass and FIG. 165 fine blood vessels covering its surface. There are a number of posterior synechias adjacent to the iris tumor. The fundus shows an extensive pigmentary change superiorly, with retinal atrophy, but no obvious tumor mass. Intraocular pressure in the right eye is 21 mm. Hg and in the left 11 mm. Hg (Schiøtz).

Course. Stilbestrol therapy was continued, and mydriatic drops were administered to the left eye, but there was gradual progression of the tumor. The patient was asymptomatic except for the visual loss. Three months later the tumor had increased in size, and there were a number of prominent nodules over its surface (Reel XIII-5). The vision was reduced to hand movements, and REEL XIII-5 the vitreous was so hazy that the retina could not be visualized. The left eye was enucleated, and the postoperative course was uneventful. Histopathologic diagnosis was extensive adenocarcinoma involving most of the anterior chamber and infiltrating the ciliary body and choroid (Fig. 165, B). Microscopically, there were many nests of tumor cells interspersed with fibrous proliferation (Fig. 165,

---

Fig. 165. *Nonpigmented peripheral tumor mass of the left iris in a 50-year-old woman with metastatic carcinoma.* **A,** The tumor mass extends from the 2 o'clock to the 6 o'clock position and is composed in some places of small nodules. Three months later nodules covered almost the entire surface of the tumor (see Reel XIII-5). The patient had a radical mastectomy 9 years previously and is known to have metastasis. **B,** Photomicrograph shows iris tumor with infiltration of the ciliary body and choroid. (H & E stain; ×16.) **C,** Photomicrograph shows nests of tumor cells interspersed with fibrous proliferation. (H & E stain; ×1600.)

281

C). A year later the patient had a gallbladder attack, and a cholecystectomy was performed, at which time "tumors" were found in her liver. A month later she died, presumably of her metastatic disease.

Lymphoblastic lymphoma

History. Two weeks ago this 15-year-old girl developed blurred vision in the right eye, followed by photophobia, redness, and tearing. Topical and systemic administration of corticosteroids, mydriatics, and acetazolamide were used for the treatment of her "uveitis." Antibiotics (chloramphenicol and erythromycin) were also given systemically. The right eye became progressively worse.

Findings. Vision in the right eye is accurate light projection and in the left 20/30. The conjunctiva of the right eye is markedly injected, and there is bedewing of the corneal epithelium. The lower half of the anterior chamber is filled with blood (hyphema), and through the cloudy aqueous in the upper half of the anterior chamber the iris, which has a markedly irregular surface, can be

REEL XIII-6   seen (Reel XIII-6). From the 10 o'clock to the 11 o'clock position there is a prominent elevation of the iris, and the entire surface is covered with various-sized hemorrhages and some dilated vessels. The media cannot be visualized, and there is no red fundus reflex. The left eye is normal. Intraocular pressures are 40 mm. Hg (Schiøtz) in the right eye and 18 mm. Hg (Schiøtz) in the left. General physical examination shows a hepatosplenomegaly, with the liver edge palpable 9 cm. below the costal margin.

Course. Reactions to multiple skin tests, including tests for histoplasmosis, blastomycosis, coccidiomycosis, and tuberculosis, were negative. Reactions to the various blood studies and urinalyses were also negative. The sedimentation rate was 30 mm./hr., and the cerebrospinal fluid was normal. Bone marrow aspiration revealed only hypocellular marrow. Since various liver and spleen studies were not diagnostic, an open liver biopsy was performed. The findings were consistent with lymphoblastic lymphoma, although reticulum cell sarcoma was also considered a possibility. Corticosteroids administered systemically and cyclophosphamide (Cytoxan) were initiated, but there was a marked downhill course with the development of ascites. The patient died 3 weeks later.

Chapter 10

Traumatic conditions of the iris

TRAUMATIC IRIDODIALYSIS AND SYNECHIA FORMATION

Separation of the iris from the ciliary body is referred to as an iridodialysis. The most common cause is a direct blow to the eye with a relatively small object, such as a ball, bb shot, or stone. Iridodialyses also occur during surgical procedures either by intention or by inadvertence. The iris sphincter produces a constant pull on the attachment at the ciliary body. The iris is thinnest at its periphery, which is the most common location of tears. Generally, only one segment of the iris is involved, although multiple or even complete iridodialyses have occurred. A crescent-shaped black opening is always seen, due to the pull of the sphincter. The pupil is distorted and displaced away from the iridodialysis. Zonules and even the lens may be visible through the opening. Almost invariably a hemorrhage is associated with the trauma and may obscure the iris defect. Because of their anterior chamber involvement, the complications and treatment of hyphemas have already been discussed (Chapter 3, p. 72).

Treatment of small iridodialyses is usually not required; and even the larger ones, particularly those located superiorly, cause no symptoms. Some visual loss will occur if an iridodialysis is in the interpalpebral region, and particularly if the pupil is displaced so that iris covers the axial portion of the eye. Diplopia may result, as well as impairment of visual acuity. Probably the most satisfactory treatment is the surgical replacement of the iris root to the scleral lip of a limbal incision by attachment with fine synthetic suture material (10-0 Nylon). A simpler operative procedure is conversion of the iridodialysis into a complete coloboma by iridotomy or iridectomy.

Another condition closely related to iridodialysis is the traumatic recession of the anterior chamber angle, which is also commonly associated with blunt trauma to the anterior segment. This recession is actually a tear into the ciliary body (Chapter 14, p. 353). Another result of blunt trauma is traumatic cyclodialysis, in which there is an opening into the suprachoroidal space.

283

Anterior synechias attached to a scar are a common complication of perforating wounds of the cornea or limbal region. As aqueous is lost from the eye, the iris comes into contact with the perforation. Frequently, because of the pressure of aqueous still remaining in the anterior chamber, the iris is pushed through the wound. The incarcerated iris may plug the wound, resulting in spontaneous re-formation of the anterior chamber. However, organization and fibrosis occur in the incarcerated iris, and a permanent anterior synechia (adherent leukoma) is produced. Surgical intervention can correct this condition, especially if an iridectomy is performed to avoid further iris incarceration. With a fresh wound, a small prolapse may be reposited; and with careful suturing of the wound and finally air injection, synechias may be prevented. In longstanding adherent leukomas the possible adverse consequences of freeing the synechia may outweigh the advantages. If such an attempt is made, filling the anterior chamber with air may avoid recurrence of the synechia formation.

When the perforating wound is at the limbus, pigment proliferation of the prolapsed pigment epithelium may occur under the conjunctiva and thus simulate a malignant melanoma of the peripheral iris or ciliary body. Gonioscopic examination easily determines that the cause is trauma.

Traumatic iris hemorrhage and iridodialysis

History. Yesterday this 15-year-old boy was struck in the right eye by a branch of a tree. The eye was painful and the vision reduced.

Findings. Vision in the right eye is 20/100 and in the left 20/20. In the right eye there is moderate conjunctival injection, and there is a corneal abrasion near the limbus at the 7 o'clock position. In the inferior anterior chamber is a mass of vitreous protruding through a large iridodialysis extending from the 5 o'clock to the 7 o'clock position. On the surface of the vitreous mass is a layer of red blood cells that extend just above the upper edge of the pupil and that outline REEL XIII-7 the extent of the vitreous mass (Reel XIII-7). The edge of the iridodialysis has a ragged appearance due to the eversion of the pigment epithelium of the iris. From the 9 o'clock to the 12 o'clock position at the base of the iris is a blood clot. Considerable blood is also lying on the iris just basal to the iridodialysis. The lens and fundus are difficult to view, but the lens appears to be in place, and there is no evidence of retinal detachment. The left eye is normal.

Course. Three days later much of the hemorrhage had cleared, and the patient was asymptomatic. He was then lost to follow-up.

Traumatic iridodialysis

History. Three weeks ago this 31-year-old man was struck in the right eye by the nozzle of a fire hose. A massive hyphema occurred, which gradually absorbed, but was followed by a secondary glaucoma, which was controlled by acetazolamide and miotics.

Findings. The vision in the right eye is 20/40 with correction and in the left 20/20. The right eye is white, and the cornea is clear. The iris is totally detached from its root from the 8 o'clock to the 1 o'clock position superiorly. It is displaced nasally and inferiorly, being rolled upon itself and producing an oval FIG. 166 pupillary opening (Fig. 166). The lens is clear, and the posterior segment is

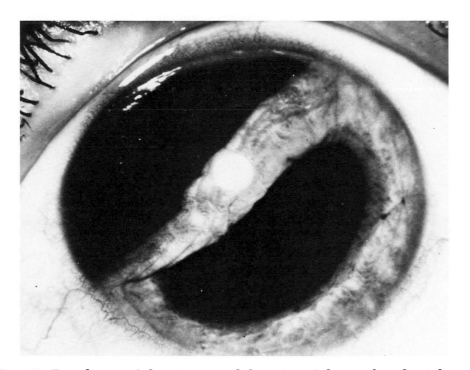

Fig. 166. *Detachment of the iris root and distortion of the pupil in the right eye of a 31-year-old man with a traumatic iridodialysis.* The detached iris is rolled up on itself, and gonioscopy shows the iris to be cleanly torn from the root from the 8 o'clock to the 1 o'clock position. The patient was struck by the nozzle of a fire hose.

normal. By gonioscopy the iris can be seen to have been cleanly torn from the root, leaving intact the ciliary processes and a normal trabecular meshwork. In a few places the zonules are broken, and a small amount of vitreous is prolapsed anteriorly. The left eye is normal. The intraocular pressure is 17 mm. Hg (Schiøtz) in both eyes.

Course. Three months later a repair of the iridodialysis was performed in which the peripheral edge of the iris was sutured to the scleral lip. The patient was then lost to follow-up.

Pillar synechia (traumatic)

History. This 40-year-old man had a spot on his right eye for as long as he can remember. As a child he had a red, sore right eye for several weeks but has been asymptomatic ever since.

Findings. Vision in the right eye is 20/40 and in the left 20/20 with correction. The right eye requires a large astigmatic correction. In the cornea there is a dark bluish black structure at the 6 o'clock position near the limbus (Fig. 167). FIG. 167 Attached to this area on the cornea are strands of iris stroma that extend almost to the pupillary margin, but the pupil is round. Gonioscopy reveals a large pillar synechia attaching to the posterior surface of the cornea; inside the cornea is dark pigmented material that has the appearance of pigment epithelium

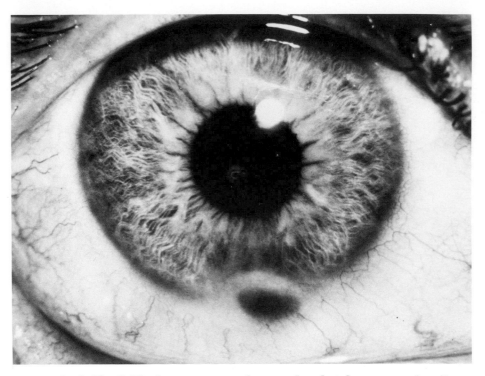

Fig. 167. *Dark bluish black structure in the peripheral right cornea of a 40-year-old man with a traumatic pillar synechia. By gonioscopy (see Reel XIV-1) a large pillar synechia is attached to the posterior surface of the cornea, with no involvement of the chamber angle. As a child, the patient apparently had a corneal perforation.*

REEL XIV-1　　(Reel XIV-1). Except for several clumps of pigment, the angle is open and normal. The posterior segment of the eye is normal, and there are no abnormalities in the left eye.

　　Course. Seven years later there had been a slight increase in the limbal opacity of the right cornea. Eleven years after that there was no appreciable change in the cornea or the angle of the anterior chamber.

TRAUMATIC IRITIS

　　Acute or chronic iritis may follow an injury to the anterior segment. If trauma, including surgery, is sufficiently severe, the entire uveal tract may be inflamed. Minor contusions of the iris will produce an inflammatory reaction, with cells and aqueous flare in the anterior chamber. More severe injuries may result in fibrinous iritis, which in turn may be obscured if hyphema is also present. Even in the absence of bacterial infections, severe generalized uveitis can follow a perforation of the globe, particularly when there is a retained intraocular foreign body. The acute reaction is probably associated with some tissue necrosis, but in the more chronic type a hypersensitivity to uveal pigment or lens cortex (p. 207) may be involved.

286

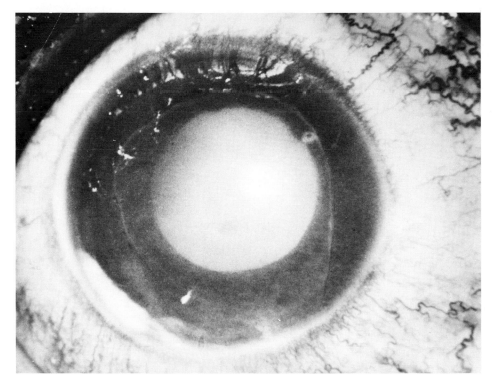

Fig. 168. *A rounded fibrin mass and a small hypopyon in the right eye of an 11-year-old boy with traumatic iritis.* The pupil is semidilated and the lens diffusely cloudy. Recently the patient was struck in the eye with a paper clip shot from a rubber band.

Regardless of the cause, topical and systemic administration of corticosteroids is usually of benefit if a bacterial infection is not involved. In addition, removal of an intraocular foreign body or irrigation of cortex from the anterior chamber may be an essential therapeutic procedure. Occasionally, secondary glaucoma may require appropriate treatment, but more commonly the eye is hypotensive; and when the injury is sufficiently severe, phthisis bulbi may ensue.

Traumatic iritis

History. Three days ago this 11-year-old boy was struck in the right eye with a paper clip shot from a rubber band. When he was examined the same day, the intraocular pressures and the vision in both eyes were equal and normal. Fundus examination revealed a peripheral detachment in the right eye and some retinal hemorrhages. Yesterday his vision dropped to light perception only, and the eye became painful.

Findings. The vision in the right eye is light perception and in the left 20/25. In the right eye there is marked conjunctival injection, and the cornea is clear. The anterior chamber is filled with a rounded fibrin mass, and there is 1-mm. hypopyon inferiorly (Fig. 168). The pupil is semidilated (mydriatics), and the FIG. 168

287

lens appears to be diffusely cloudy. No visualization of the vitreous or retina can be obtained. The left eye is normal. The intraocular pressure in both eyes is 15 mm. Hg (Schiøtz).

Course. Systemic administration of corticosteroids and antibiotics was instituted, along with local administration of antibiotics and mydriatics. The next day there was some increase in the anterior chamber reaction, and an elevated area of the conjunctiva was noted near the inner canthus. Since a conjunctival and possibly scleral laceration was suspected, an exploration was performed. During this procedure a conjunctival and scleral perforation was found and sutured. In addition, a small abscess of the medial rectus muscle was excised. Cultures were taken, which subsequently showed no growth. Postoperatively, the eye was mushy soft; despite intensive antibiotic and corticosteroid therapy, the anterior chamber continued to show signs of moderate activity. A month later the vision was only light perception. The anterior chamber was clear, but the anterior vitreous appeared to be organized in a yellowish mass containing new blood vessels typical of an organizing vitreous abscess. Eight months later there was a mature cataract, and the eye was blind. In another 6 months the eye had become phthisical and had developed a gross hyphema, which caused severe pain. An enucleation was performed, and the histopathologic diagnosis was angle recession, cyclitic membrane, old perforating injury, hyphema, retinal detachment, optic atrophy, and gliosis. Six months later the boy sustained a lid and corneal laceration with a piece of glass in his remaining eye, which required corneal suturing. Healing was uneventful, and he was then lost to follow-up.

TRAUMATIC RUPTURES OF THE IRIS SPHINCTER

Blunt trauma to the anterior segment of the eye results in lacerations or tears of the pupillary border and sphincter. The degree of involvement may be so slight that only by transillumination of the iris can the defect be visualized. Sometimes only a small area of the anterior stroma over the sphincter is involved, whereas in other instances multiple minute ruptures of the pupillary border occur. More extensive changes involve tears, usually multiple, into and sometimes through the iris sphincter. In severe injuries, the pupillary border and sphincter may be so extensively traumatized that no normal architecture of the sphincter remains. Complications of such injuries are hyphema, which almost always occurs with tears into the sphincter, and traumatic mydriasis. Later, the sphincter region may gradually become atrophic and fibrotic, and the pupil remains permanently dilated. In most cases there is no treatment.

Traumatic mydriasis and tear of the iris sphincter

History. Two months ago this 41-year-old man was struck in the left eye by an elbow. Immediately following the injury the patient was found to have a marked subconjunctival hemorrhage, cells and flare in the anterior chamber, and minimal macular edema, with decrease of vision to 20/30. Subsequently, a subretinal hemorrhage developed nasally.

Findings. Vision in the right eye is 20/20 and in the left 20/30. The right eye is normal; but in the left the pupil is dilated, fixed, and irregular, particularly inferiorly (Fig. 169). At the 6:30 position there is a prominent tear of the stroma

FIG. 169

288

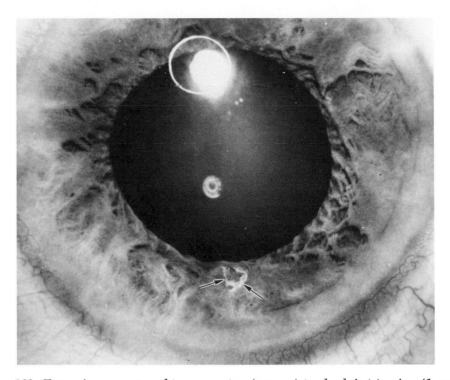

Fig. 169. *Tear of stroma in sphincter region (arrows) in the left iris of a 41-year-old man with a traumatic tear in the iris sphincter.* The pupil is dilated, fixed, and irregular (traumatic mydriasis), and by gonioscopy a recession of the angle temporally can be seen. The patient's eye was struck by an elbow.

overlying the sphincter of the iris. Subcapsular lens opacities consisting of spokes are seen within the pupil. Gonioscopy shows a recession of the angle temporally. Nasal to the disc there is some residual subretinal hemorrhage. Intraocular tension is 14 mm. Hg (Schiøtz) in both eyes.

Course. Six weeks later the pupil still was dilated and reacted poorly to light. There had been little change in the subcapsular lens opacities. The retinal hemorrhage had disappeared, but the macular region exhibited an irregular appearance, presumably due to the preexisting macular edema. The vision was still reduced to 20/25. The patient was then lost to follow-up.

Traumatic tears in the iris sphincter

History. About a year ago this 53-year-old woman was severely injured during a robbery. A few months later she developed blurred vision; and about 5 months ago she was given glasses, which restored her vision to normal.

Findings. The vision is 20/20 in both eyes with a +15.50 sphere on each eye. Both eyes are essentially the same, with normal corneas, vitreous prolapse in the anterior chambers, and pupils that are irregular due to multiple tears into the sphincter (Fig. 170). The lenses, which can be seen in the inferior fundus, change their location with change in the position of the patient's head. The remainder of the fundus is normal. The intraocular tension is 20 mm. Hg. (Schiøtz) in both eyes.

FIG. 170

289

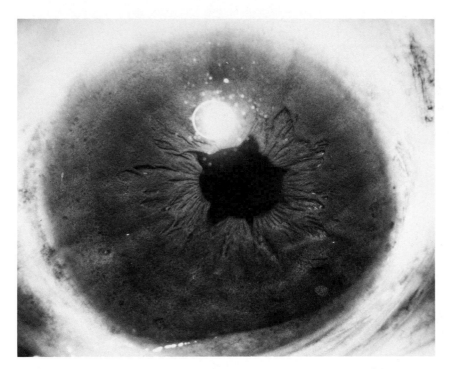

Fig. 170. *Multiple tears in the pupillary margin of a 53-year-old woman with traumatic tears in the iris sphincter.* Six tears into the iris sphincter, vitreous prolapse into the anterior chamber, and subluxation of the lenses occurred when the patient was severely beaten.

Course. A year later the ocular findings were essentially the same, and the patient was then lost to follow-up.

Traumatic tears in the iris sphincter

History. Five days ago this 14-year-old boy was struck in the right eye by a model airplane. The next day he was found to have a microscopic hyphema, corneal abrasions, traumatic mydriasis, and retinal edema and hemorrhage. There was no recurrence of the hyphema, and his vision improved slightly during his hospitalization.

Findings. Vision in the right eye is 20/70 and in the left 20/30. The right cornea is clear and lustrous, and the anterior chamber is deep, without cells or flare. The

FIG. 171 pupil is dilated and fixed, with multiple tears of the sphincter muscle (Fig. 171). The lens is clear except for a few pigment granules on the anterior capsule. Fundus examination reveals that the disc is normal but that superotemporally to the disc is an area of edema and hemorrhage; and there is some edema of the macula, typical of commotio retinae. The left eye is normal except for the pupil, which although of normal size (3.5 mm.) is slightly irregular and reacts very poorly to light.

Course. Over the next 4 months there was gradual improvement of the vision in the right eye to 20/30 with correction. Field examination showed a binasal

290

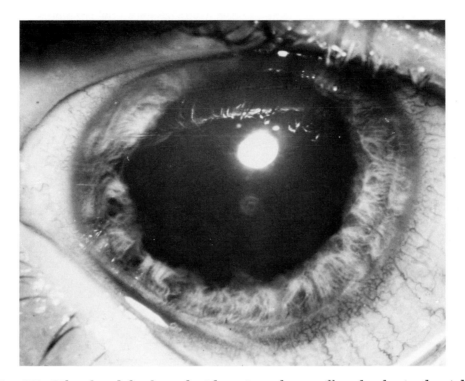

Fig. 171. *Dilated and fixed pupil with an irregular pupillary border in the right eye of a 14-year-old boy with traumatic tears in the iris sphincter.* Multiple irregular tears involve most of the sphincter muscle due to blunt trauma to the eye. The patient also has a commotio retinae.

constriction, which could not be explained. When the patient was seen 3 years later, the same field defect was present, but not as large in the left eye as previously. The patient was then lost to follow-up.

FOREIGN BODIES INVOLVING THE IRIS

Corneal perforation by a low-velocity foreign body may result in the foreign body's becoming enmeshed in the iris stroma or falling into the inferior anterior chamber angle. The reaction of the iris to most foreign bodies is minimal and sometimes nil when the eye is free of infection. The reaction depends largely on the type of foreign body and is similar to that from foreign bodies elsewhere in the eye (p. 60). Iron and steel foreign bodies, the most common, may cause recurrent episodes of iritis over a period of many years, usually with siderosis, but not if a high-grade steel is involved or if the foreign body becomes encapsulated. Siderosis involves not only the iris but also all other tissues of the eye and particularly the lens, vitreous, and retina. It is due to the gradual breakdown into ferrous ions and the deposition of iron in the tissues immediately in contact with the foreign body (direct siderosis) or by diffusion of ferrous ions throughout the eye (indirect siderosis). The latter is the most common and serious, producing in the iris a rusty yellowish brown discoloration, in striking contrast to the other eye, especially if the iris is blue (heterochromia iridis). Another effect of long-standing siderosis is mydriasis, which results from damage to the sphincter muscle of the iris. Siderosis lentis with cataract formation is more serious. Disseminated retinal degeneration is the most serious complication. If of sufficiently long duration, a secondary glaucoma develops. Less commonly, copper, when embedded in the iris, may produce a greenish discoloration of the iris. The typical sunflower cataract is frequently seen. Chalcosis of the retina and secondary glaucoma are rare. Inert foreign bodies, such as particles of sand, glass, and methylmethacrylate (Plexiglas), can remain in the iris for years without untoward effects.

Steel foreign body on the iris

History. Four years ago this 46-year-old man developed redness and soreness in his left eye and was found to have a rusty-appearing foreign body on his iris. This foreign body apparently was causing an iritis, and topical administration of corticosteroids produced a prompt remission of his symptoms and a clearing of the iritis. He had a history of a foreign body hitting his eye at age 6. Further examination showed the patient to have some lens opacities, but there was no evidence of siderosis iridis. Removal of the foreign body was suggested, but the patient did not return until today because of a recurrence of his iritis during the past week.

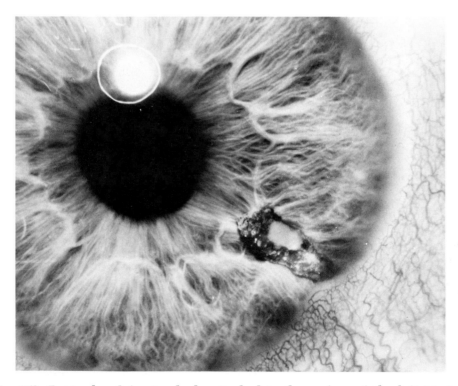

Fig. 172. *Rust-colored foreign body attached to the surface of the left iris in a 46-year-old man with a steel foreign body.* There is an old corneal scar near the limbus and moderate anterior chamber reaction. The patient has had recurrent attacks of iritis from a foreign body that apparently entered his eye 40 years ago.

Findings. Vision in the right eye is 20/20 and in the left 20/400 without correction. The right eye is normal, but in the left there is a ciliary flush and moderate diffuse conjunctival injection. There is an old scar of the cornea at the 4 o'clock position near the limbus, and immediately below this is a rust-colored foreign body attached to the surface of the iris (Fig. 172). The anterior chamber   FIG. 172 contains moderate cells and flare; the pupil reacts normally; and there is a minimal cortical cataract. The fundus is normal.

Course. Topical treatment with corticosteroids and mydriatics was initiated, and in 1 week the iritis had completely subsided. X-ray films again showed a foreign body in the region of the iris. Refraction showed that the vision in the left eye had increased to 20/40. The foreign body was removed 4 months later. During the procedure a peripheral iridectomy was necessary because of the firm adhesion of the foreign body to the iris. The postoperative course was uneventful, and the patient's corrected vision was 20/40.

Siderosis iridis and lentis

History. A year ago a chip flew from a grinder into the left eye of this 40-year-old man. He was treated for corneal abrasions. No x-ray film was taken. About 7 months later vision in his left eye became blurred, and he noticed that his iris had changed color. The loss of vision was due to a cataract. X-ray films taken a month ago showed a foreign body that appeared to be localized in the upper eyelid rather than in the globe.

Findings. Vision in the right eye is 20/20 and in the left 20/200. The right eye is normal, and the iris is blue. In the left eye the iris is yellowish brown, and the pupil reacts only slightly to light (Fig. 173). The lens is cataractous, containing   FIG. 173 brown spots of pigment (Reel XIV-2). Gonioscopy shows scattered pigment of   REEL XIV-2

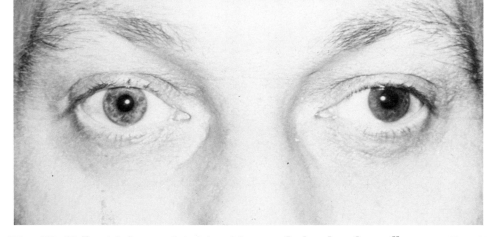

Fig. 173. *Yellowish brown left iris with a marked reduced pupillary reaction to light in a 40-year-old man with siderosis iridis and lentis.* The lens (see Reel XIV-2) is cataractous and contains brown spots of pigment. A year ago a steel chip flew into the patient's eye.

the angle but no foreign body. With a dilated pupil there is also no foreign body visible. The Berman-Moorhead locator fails to show any evidence of a foreign body. X-ray films, however, indicate a minute foreign body 5 mm. behind the vertex of the cornea and 8 mm. below the axis.

Course. By the use of a giant magnet the iris bulged at the 5 o'clock position, and the foreign body was moved into the anterior chamber. Through a keratome incision the foreign body was drawn from the anterior chamber with a magnet. Postoperatively the patient did well. One and a half years later a mature cataract and a secondary glaucoma had developed, and a lens extraction was performed. Subsequently, the glaucoma was not controlled, and bullous keratopathy developed. Seven years later his vision was reduced to 20/200, and the intraocular tension was in the 40's and 50's. A scleral filtering procedure was performed, and a good bleb formed initially. This subsequently needed revision and again failed. An additional filtering procedure was performed inferiorly and was unsuccessful. Finally, cauterization of the cornea was performed, resulting in relief of the bullous keratopathy.

Siderosis iridis and lentis

History. More than a year ago this 40-year-old man was struck in the left eye with a piece of steel. Recently his vision deteriorated.

Findings. Vision in the right eye is 20/20 and in the left light perception. The

FIG. 174 right eye is normal in all respects, and the iris is blue (Fig. 174, *A*). In the left eye there is a small corneal scar of the upper temporal quadrant and a hole in the iris just below the scar (Fig. 174, *B*). The anterior chamber is clear, and the iris is yellow-brown, with a decrease in clarity of the stromal pattern. There is a mature cataract, with many brown subcapsular deposits.

Course. X-ray films showed no foreign body, and attempts to locate a foreign body with a giant magnet were unsuccessful. It was felt that the retina was also damaged by the siderosis, and no further treatment was undertaken. Three months later the patient returned because of pain in the eye, and his intraocular tension was found to be 63 mm. Hg (Schiøtz). Treatment with pilocarpine (4%) and epinephrine (1%) promptly reduced the intraocular pressure to normal. In 3 months the eye again became painful; there were cells in the anterior chamber, and the intraocular pressure was markedly elevated. Enucleation was performed, and the histopathologic diagnosis was siderosis bulbi, with iron staining of the corneal lamellae, iris stroma, ciliary epithelium, sclera, retina, and optic disc. No foreign body was found.

Sand on the iris

History. About 12 years ago this soldier stepped on a land mine, which embedded numerous pieces of sand and stone in the lids and globe of the right eye. The left eye was involved to a much lesser extent.

Findings. Vision in the right eye is 20/20 and in the left 20/25. The lids of the right eye contain multiple small foreign bodies. The cornea is clear except for a few foreign bodies in the lower half and several scars near the limbus inferiorly

FIG. 175 (Fig. 175). To two of these scars are attached pillar synechias, which apparently represent areas of limbal perforation. On the surface of the iris are at least

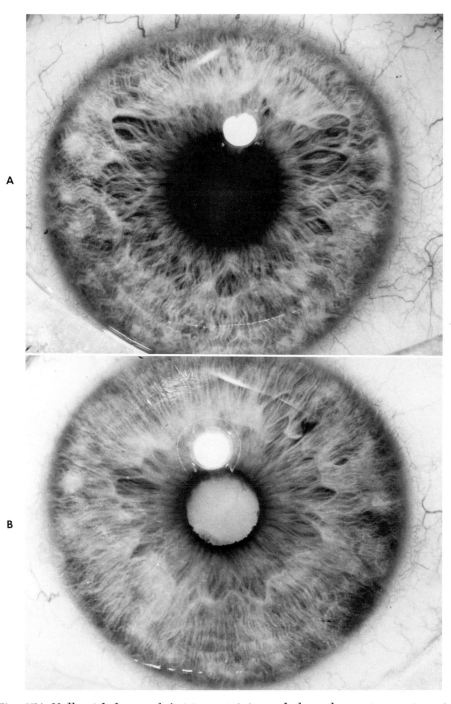

Fig. 174. *Yellowish brown left iris containing a hole and a mature cataract in a 40-year-old man with siderosis iridis and lentis.* **A,** The right iris is light blue, with a distinct iris pattern. **B,** The left iris is yellowish brown, with a decrease in clarity of the stromal pattern. A mature cataract contains many brown subcapsular deposits. A piece of steel penetrated the eye more than a year ago.

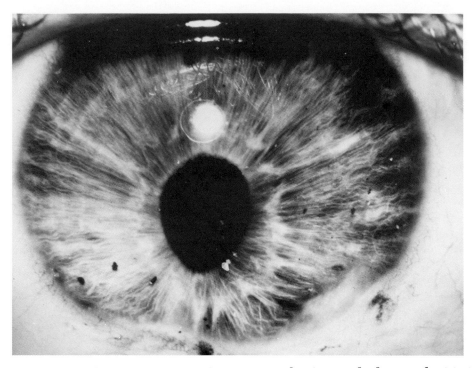

Fig. 175. *Multiple corneal scars and many irregular foreign bodies on the iris in a man who stepped on a land mine 12 years ago.* The foreign bodies are apparently pieces of sand and stone that penetrated the cornea.

30 foreign bodies of various types, colors, and size. At the 12 o'clock position there is a hole in the iris. The pupil is ovoid and displaced inferiorly due to the peripheral anterior synechias. In the left eye no foreign bodies are visible, but there is considerable epithelial edema in the lower half of the cornea, without apparent cause, although undetected foreign bodies settled in the inferior portion of the angle are a possibility. The remainder of the eye is normal.

Course. The patient was lost to follow-up.

Glass embedded in the iris

History. About 6 months ago this 22-year-old man was struck with a beer bottle, and a piece perforated the right cornea and lodged in the iris. There was vitreous loss and lens material in the anterior chamber. The cornea was repaired; and postoperatively there was a flat chamber due to a choroidal detachment, which was drained. Within a few months the eye no longer showed signs of irritation, and the glass migrated to a location just under the iris. A cataract formed, but the upper portion of the pupil remained clear. Recently there has been some atrophy of the iris overlying the piece of glass and slow progression of the lens opacity.

Findings. Vision in the right eye is counting fingers at 10 feet and in the left 20/20. The cornea of the right eye has a dense linear scar inferiorly, which has a large blood vessel leading to it from the limbus. The scar is attached on its

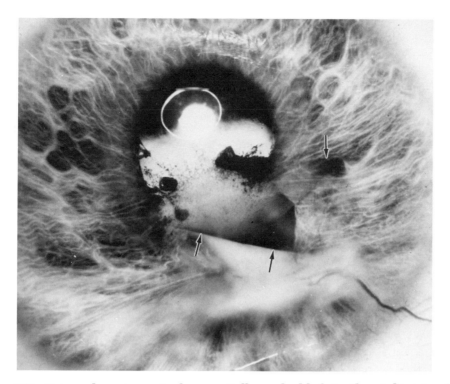

Fig. 176. *Triangular piece of glass partially embedded in the right iris of a 22-year-old man who was struck with a beer bottle.* The glass (arrows) is partially covered with iris stroma and extends to the lower portion of the pupil into a cataract. By transillumination (see Reel XIV-3) the entire piece of glass can be visualized.

posterior surface to a membrane that extends down to the lower portion of a piece of glass partially embedded in the iris (Fig. 176). About half the glass is FIG. 176 covered with intact iris stroma, and the portion immediately below the pupil extends into cataractous lens tissue. Above this in the upper third of the pupil is an area that appears to be clear lens. By transillumination it is possible to visualize the entire piece of glass (Reel XIV-3). The fundus cannot be visualized. REEL XIV-3

Course. No appreciable change occurred during the next 5 years.

Intraocular Plexiglas particles and hole in the iris

History. About 3 years ago this 25-year-old pilot was flying his plane when an antiaircraft shell exploded over the cockpit and shattered the Plexiglas dome. There was immediate marked loss of vision in his right eye and some blurring in his left.

Findings. Vision in the right eye is hand movements and in the left 20/20. In the right cornea are numerous shiny white foreign bodies at various levels. The anterior chamber is formed and the pupil round. A few similar foreign bodies are also embedded in the iris stroma, and at the 5 o'clock position there is a hole through the iris. The lens is densely opacified, and no view of the fundus can be obtained. By gonioscopy a number of white foreign bodies can be visu-

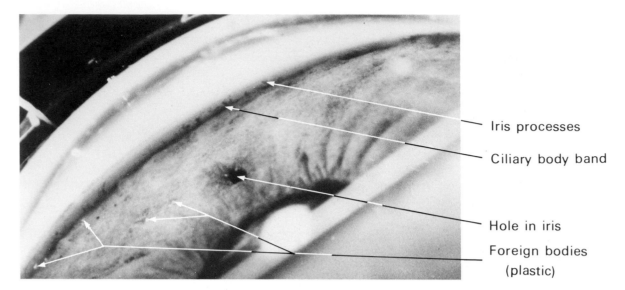

Iris processes

Ciliary body band

Hole in iris

Foreign bodies (plastic)

Fig. 177 (Reel XIV-4). *Numerous shiny white foreign bodies in the cornea, iris, and chamber angle in a 25-year-old man with intraocular Plexiglas particles. One foreign body perforated the iris, leaving a hole and producing a cataract. The patient was a military pilot, and an antiaircraft shell exploded, shattering his Plexiglas dome.*

REEL XIV-4 alized in the angle and on the surface of the iris (Reel XIV-4 and Fig. 177).
FIG. 177   The hole in the iris is easily visible. The angle is wide open and contains a number of pigmented iris processes. The left eye is normal except for a few white foreign bodies in the superficial cornea.

Course. Fifteen years later the patient was asymptomatic, and a mature cataract still remained in the right eye.

TRAUMATIC CYSTS OF THE IRIS

The introduction of conjunctival or corneal epithelial cells into the iris by a perforating injury may result in an inclusion cyst of the iris either shortly after the injury or after a delay of years. Such cysts are epithelial-lined cysts that continue to enlarge slowly and thus require treatment. The most common cause of inclusion cysts is surgery involving the iris; the progression and treatment of these inclusion cysts are discussed in Chapter 11 (p. 302).

The so-called pearl cyst typically develops around the follicle of a retained lash in the anterior chamber. This cyst differs from the implantation type in that it has a solid appearance and is composed of densely packed cellular material with a glistening surface, enmeshed in the iris. Only occasionally does a true serous cyst occur in association with a cilium in the iris. As the pearl cyst gradually enlarges, iridocyclitis and glaucoma may develop.

Traumatic cyst of the iris

History. About a year ago this 15-year-old boy was struck in the right eye with a piece of broken glass. This resulted in a corneal perforation, with an iris

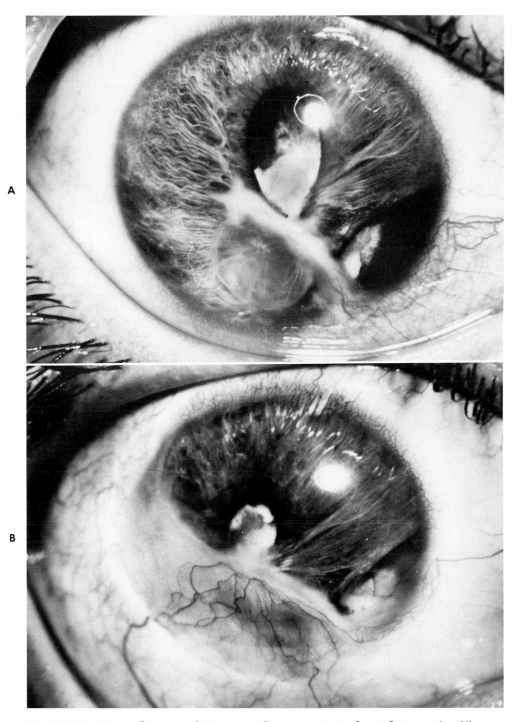

Fig. 178. A, *Corneal scar and iris cyst adjacent to it in the right eye of a 15-year-old boy with a traumatic cyst of the iris.* An iridodialysis is present nasally, and there is a dense cataract. A year ago the patient was struck with a piece of glass. **B,** Because the cyst continued to enlarge, cryotherapeutic applications were made, and a large iridectomy was performed. Subsequently, the cyst recurred but remained stationary.

299

prolapse and a secondary hyphema. Following surgical repair, an adherent leukoma and a cataract developed. Four months ago an iris cyst developed in the area of the leukoma, and it gradually enlarged.

Findings. Vision in the right eye is counting fingers at 1 foot and in the left 20/15 with correction. In the right eye there is a diagonal scar involving the inferior half of the cornea and ending at the limbus at the 5 o'clock position (Fig. 178, *A*). Just beneath the scar is a cyst that arises from the iris and touches the cornea. Nasally there is an iridodialysis through which opacified cortex is visible. The pupil is oval and displaced upward, and through it can be seen more opacified lens material. No fundus view can be obtained. The left eye is normal.

FIG. 178

Course. Over the next year the cyst in the anterior chamber continued to enlarge until it filled almost the entire temporal half. The chamber was opened, and the cyst was excised. Cryotherapeutic applications were made to the involved posterior surface of the cornea, and a large iridectomy was performed. Four months postoperatively the cornea was hazy and vascularized in the area of the excision of the cyst (Fig. 178, *B*). There was further progression of the cataract, and a pupillary membrane developed. Five months later excision of the pupillary membrane was performed, along with a large iridectomy superiorly. The postoperative course was uneventful. A few months later the cyst recurred, but over

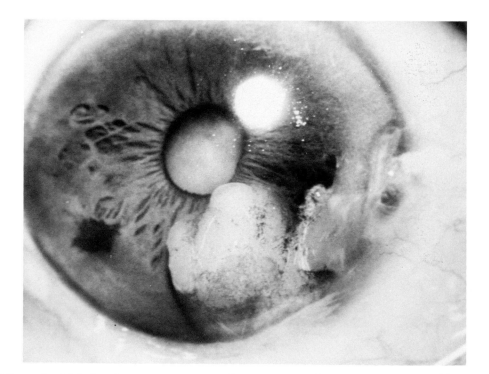

Fig. 179. *Multilocular cystic mass of the inferior right iris in a 72-year-old man with a traumatic cyst of the iris.* The cyst is sufficiently elevated to almost touch the cornea, and nasally at the limbus is the old scar where the injury occurred 54 years ago.

the next year it remained stationary. The patient was comfortable; his vision was counting fingers.

Traumatic cyst of the iris

History. At 18 years of age this 72-year-old man's right eye was cut by a wire. Six years ago he was found to have a cyst of the iris, and since then he developed a mature cataract.

Findings. The vision in the right eye is accurate light projection and in the left 20/20. In the right eye there is a multilocular cyst of the nasal and inferior iris (Fig. 179). At the 3 o'clock position near the limbus is a scar from an old FIG. 179 perforating injury of the cornea. The cyst inferiorly is elevated so that it almost touches the cornea. By gonioscopy the angle is open, but the cyst appears to be extending posteriorly into the ciliary body. There is a mature cataract that obscures any view of the posterior segment. The left eye is normal. The intraocular pressure in both eyes is 17 mm. Hg (Schiøtz).

Course. It was recommended that a cataract extraction be performed, but the patient was then lost to follow-up.

Chapter 11

Medical and surgical iatrogenic conditions of the iris

IRIS CYSTS

Cysts of the pupillary border of the iris commonly occur in patients using echothiophate (Phospholine) iodide or demecarium bromide (Humorsol) over a prolonged period of time. It is more likely to occur in younger patients. Even the weak concentrations of echothiophate used in children for the correction of esotropia may lead to multiple black cysts that frequently involve the entire pupillary margin and occasionally completely fill the pupillary aperture. The use of phenylephrine drops along with the miotic drops usually prevents the development of the cysts; and with discontinuance of the miotic, the cysts gradually disappear. Complications from such cysts are minimal. If the miotic is required to control glaucoma, phenylephrine should be added to the medication.

The most common cyst involving the iris stroma is the iris implantation cyst (iris inclusion cyst, traumatic serous cyst of the iris). This type of cyst most commonly occurs following a surgical procedure but may also be associated with trauma. Generally, it is thought that a surgical error in technique somehow allows conjunctival epithelium to be embedded in the iris stroma. Cysts that are similar in appearance are thought to be congenital, parasitic, or degenerative; these may still be traumatic despite the absence of history or evidence of an injury (Chapter 10, p. 298). The cyst may develop within weeks, but more typically it appears years after the surgery or injury. The typical serous cyst of the iris has a thin transparent anterior wall that is sufficiently clear to allow observation of the cloudy contents with a slit-lamp biomicroscope. This cellular debris can be seen floating freely within the cyst. Although most cysts are rounded and unilocular, they may be multilocular and have an irregular surface. The posterior wall of the cyst is made up of compressed iris stroma, and the pigment epithelium of the iris cannot usually be visualized. It can be anywhere on the iris, but it is not uncommon to find it near the periphery, where it can involve the iridocorneal angle and become attached to the cornea itself. With enlargement, a low-grade iritis may ensue, and later an increase in intraocular pressure may occur. Cysts are known to rupture spontaneously, resulting in a severe inflammatory reaction and secondary glaucoma. Following such a rupture the cyst wall may again close off, and the cyst may re-form. Even with corneal involvement there is usually no corneal edema. With gradual increase in size of the cyst over a period of time, the entire anterior chamber may be filled.

It is important that treatment be instituted early to avoid involvement of additional portions of the eye. Excision has the best chance of success, especially if the cyst does not rupture during the procedure. However, many cysts are not amenable to such treatment because of their size and their involvement of the iridocorneal angle and the cornea. Good results have been reported with electrolysis, in which an electrode is placed inside the cyst, resulting in destruction of its epithelial lining. In other hands the results of this procedure have been poor, with an extensive inflammatory reaction; in addition, recurrences are common. Injection of various irritant chemicals such as phenol, iodine, 50% dextrose solution, and radioactive materials have been attempted after aspiration of the contents of the cyst. Leakage of such solutions into the anterior chamber, however, may be followed by a marked inflammatory reaction and permanent damage or even loss of the eye. Ionizing radiation is apparently of limited value. Probably the most satisfactory treatment is the use of both photocoagulation and cryocoagulation, procedures that can be used with a fair degree of safety and repeated a number of times if necessary.

Pupillary margin cyst

History. Two years ago the right eye of this 5-year-old girl was noted to turn in when she was tired. Cycloplegic refraction showed no significant hyperopia, and she was treated with echothiophate ($\frac{1}{16}$%) daily. This was increased to twice a day; but since the esotropia continued, a recession of the right medial rectus and resection of the right lateral rectus were performed a year ago. Her condition was greatly improved; but since there was still some turning in when she was tired, echothiophate ($\frac{1}{16}$%) once a day was continued. A month ago the esotropia increased, even though the girl was given echothophiate ($\frac{1}{8}$%) daily. Cysts of the pupillary margin were visible but did not interfere with her vision.

Findings. Vision in each eye is 20/30. There is intermittent esotropia, occurring more when the patient focuses on near objects than on those more distant, and the eyes are normal except for numerous small, dark brown cysts that protrude from the pupillary margin in both eyes (Reel XIV-5).

REEL XIV-5

Course. A recession of the left medial rectus was performed and was followed by residual esophoria of about 5 prism diopters. In about a year the eyes were again noted to turn in when the patient was tired, so the use of echothiophate ($\frac{1}{16}$%) at bedtime was resumed, and the cysts that had practically disappeared reappeared but not to as great an extent. With this treatment she had no esophoria or esotropia even when she was tired.

Miotic-induced iris cysts

History. Almost a year ago this 39-year-old man was discovered to have open angle glaucoma in the right eye. After 2 months of treatment with pilocarpine and epinephrine drops in both eyes, control was not adequate in the right eye, and echothiophate (⅛%), administered twice a day only to the right eye, was added to the regimen. The intraocular pressure was well controlled, but 7 months later the patient was found to have a large cyst of the iris in the pupillary opening of the right eye that did not resolve with the use of phenylephrine (10%) drops daily for 1 week.

Findings. Vision in the right eye is 20/30 and in the left 20/15. The cornea of the right eye is normal and the anterior chamber of moderate depth. The pupil is markedly constricted, and the iris is normal; but there are small dark brown FIG. 180 cysts occluding most of the pupil (Fig. 180). These can be seen to arise from the pigment epithelium of the iris at the pupillary margin. The fundus cannot be visualized. In the left eye the pupil is about 2 mm., and there are no cysts of the pupillary margin. Examination of the fundus is normal except for questionable glaucomatous cupping of the disc.

Course. The use of echothiophate iodide was discontinued; in 1 month the cysts had markedly regressed, and in 3 months they were completely gone. Five

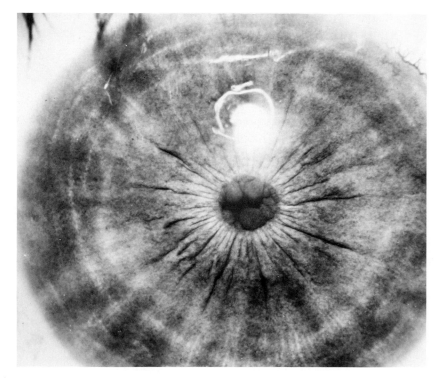

Fig. 180. *Multiple dark brown cysts in the right pupil of a 39-year-old man with miotic-induced iris cysts.* The cysts occlude most of the pupil and arise from iris pigment epithelium. Echothiophate iodide was required to control his open angle glaucoma.

years later the patient's condition was still well controlled by pilocarpine (4%) and epinephrine (1%) drops. At this time the discs were found to be unchanged, and medications were discontinued. Repeated tonography showed the outflow to be considerably improved, and for the past year without the patient receiving any medications whatever the intraocular pressures in either eye have never been above 22 mm. Hg as shown by applanation tonometry.

Iris inclusion cyst

History. Ten years ago this 78-year-old man had a cataract extraction in the left eye and 5 years ago in the right eye. Except for borderline pressures, he had no difficulty, and his vision was satisfactory. A week ago a transparent cyst was seen on the surface of the iris in the left eye.

Findings. Vision in the right eye is 20/30 and in the left 20/50 with aphakic correction. The right eye is aphakic but otherwise normal. In the left eye there is a translucent cyst involving the anterior chamber angle adjacent to the temporal iris pillar (Reel XIV-6). The cyst wall is incorporated in the corneal scar and REEL XIV-6 produces a backward bulge of the pigment epithelium of the iris. There is a complete surgical coloboma superiorly, and the vitreous face is behind the iris plane. Both eyes and discs are normal. Intraocular pressure is 30 mm. Hg (Schiøtz) in both eyes, and tonography shows a facility of outflow in the glaucomatous range.

Course. Periodic checks on the size of the cyst showed it to remain stationary over the next 4 years. The intraocular pressures remained in the upper 20's, and for several years there was no field defect or change in the discs. However, finally a nasal step and saucerization of the disc were found, so miotics were instituted, resulting in good control of intraocular tensions. Two years later the patient was doing well; he was then lost to follow-up.

Iris inclusion cyst

History. One and a half years ago this 57-year-old man noticed intermittent halos in the left eye. When he was first seen by an ophthalmologist 6 months ago, the tension was slightly elevated in the right eye and was 56 mm. Hg (Schiøtz) in the left. Both discs were "cupped," and there was "exfoliation of the lens capsule" in the left eye. Despite intensive medical therapy, the intraocular pressure in the left eye was uncontrolled; therefore, a trephine filtering procedure was performed. A month postoperatively a small iris cyst was noted near the iridectomy superiorly. Over the next 4 months this gradually enlarged.

Findings. Vision in the right eye is 20/30 and in the left 20/40. The right eye, including the optic nerve head, is normal. The left eye shows slightly conjunctival injection, with a flat filtering bleb superiorly. The anterior chamber is clear, and the iris has a peripheral iridectomy at the 12 o'clock position. Below the iridectomy and nasal to it is a cyst involving the sphincter and two thirds of the width of the iris (Fig. 181, *A*). The anterior wall of the cyst is thin, and its contents FIG. 181 appear to be clear. Fundus examination reveals glaucomatous cupping of the disc. The intraocular tension is 16 mm. Hg (Schiøtz) in both eyes. Visual fields are normal.

Course. Because the iris cyst appeared to be enlarging, it was incised with

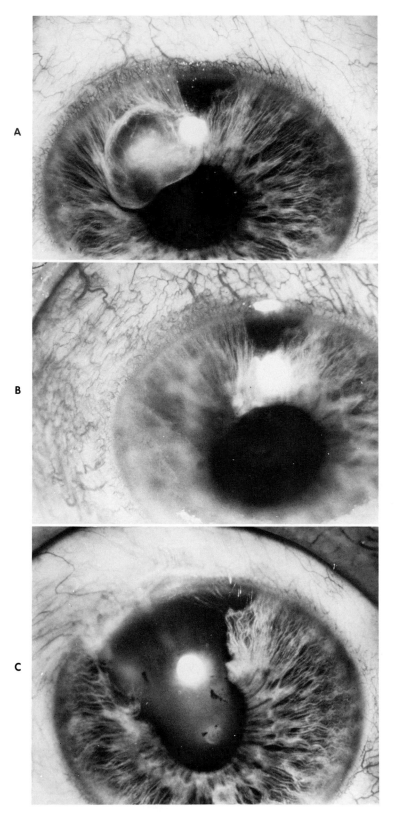

Fig. 181. For legend see opposite page.

a Wheeler knife. Two days postoperatively, examination showed marked flare and cells, corneal edema, and moderate elevation of intraocular pressure. Treatment with mydriatics, corticosteroid and epinephrine drops, and hot compresses produced some improvement in 5 days; but a moderate flare and cells and considerable corneal edema remained (Fig. 181, B). The vision was reduced to counting fingers at 1 foot. There was gradual resolution of the iritis and corneal edema, but a month later the iris cyst recurred. Because of its progressive enlargement, the cyst was totally excised. The postoperative recovery was uneventful. The intraocular tension was well controlled with the patient receiving no medication. Eight months later there were no signs of recurrence of the cyst, and a large sector iridectomy was visible from the 10 o'clock to the 1 o'clock position (Fig. 181, C). Ten years later the patient had bilateral cataract extractions. A postoperative hemorrhage in the left eye produced a dense pupillary membrane, resulting in reduction of vision to 20/200 in this eye, while the right eye was correctable to 20/25.

Iris inclusion cyst

History. Seven years ago this 67-year-old man had a cataract extraction performed on the right eye and 4 years ago on the left. Two years ago a retinal detachment in the left eye was unsuccessfully reattached. A year ago he developed a detachment in the right eye, which was successfully reattached. Six months ago he had another scleral buckling operation on his left eye, which was successful. During the past few months he developed a cyst of the iris in the left eye, which has gradually enlarged.

Findings. Vision in the right eye is 20/20 and in the left 20/200. The right eye is aphakic, and the fundus examination shows a successful scleral buckling procedure. In the left eye there is a cyst of the nasal iris, extending into the pupil. The cyst involves the angle structures from the 9 o'clock to the 11 o'clock position (Fig. 182, A). The eye is aphakic; there is evidence of extensive retinal surgery;   FIG. 182
and the posterior retina is in place.

Course. During the next 4 months there was gradual enlargement of the cyst until it extended almost across the entire pupil (Fig. 182, B). Total excision of the cyst was performed, requiring a basal iridectomy. The patient was then lost to follow-up.

Fig. 181. *Cystic mass involving the pupillary margin in the left eye of a 57-year-old man with an iris inclusion cyst. A,* The anterior wall of the cyst is thin, and its contents are clear. There is a peripheral iridectomy superiorly where a trephine filtering procedure was performed. B, Following incision of the cyst with a knife, there was a marked inflammatory reaction in the anterior chamber, with corneal edema and increased intraocular pressure. C, A large sector iridectomy followed the excision of the cyst, which had recurred and had become larger than ever.

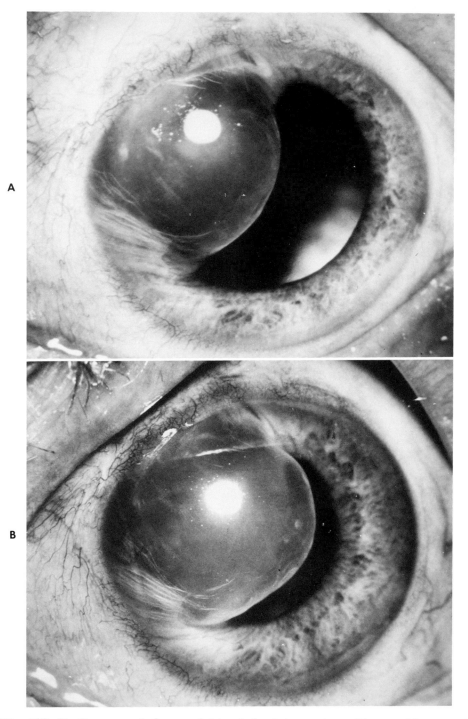

Fig. 182. *Cystic mass of the nasal iris of the left eye in a 67-year-old man with an iris inclusion cyst.* **A,** About half of the pupil is occluded, and a portion of the chamber angle is involved. Four years ago the patient had a cataract extraction. **B,** Enlargement of the cyst in 4 months occluded almost the entire pupil. An excisional iridectomy was performed.

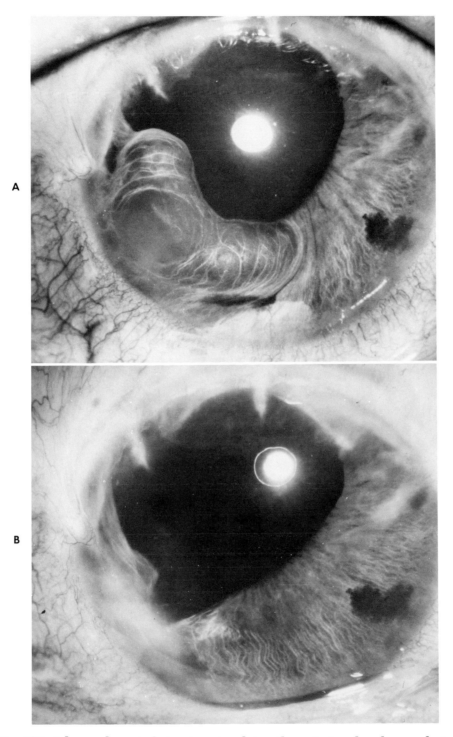

Fig. 183. *A large elongated structure involving the anterior chamber angle in the right eye of a 45-year-old man with an iris implantation cyst.* **A,** The cyst involves almost the entire inferior and temporal iris with a large area of corneal contact. The surgical coloboma superiorly was done when the cataract extraction was performed 2 years ago. **B,** Following the application of an insulated electrocautery needle inside the cyst, the cyst was apparently obliterated.

Medical and surgical iatrogenic conditions of the iris

Iris implantation cyst

History. Two years ago this 45-year-old man had an intracapsular cataract extraction performed on the right eye. Recovery was uneventful, and vision was normal with aphakic correction. Several months ago he was noted to have a cyst on the iris in the right eye, which rapidly enlarged.

Findings. Vision in the right eye with correction is 20/40 and in the left 20/25. The cornea of the right eye is clear. The anterior chamber is of average depth except where there is a large cyst that extends from the 6 o'clock to the 11 o'clock position, involving the entire width of the iris (Fig. 183, A). The cyst extends into the angle of the anterior chamber from the 7 o'clock to the 9 o'clock position and comes into contact with the peripheral cornea. The iris has a full iridectomy, and the vitreous face is at the iris plane except where it sweeps upward to come into contact with the wound superiorly. The left eye is normal in all respects. Intraocular tension is 14 mm. Hg (Schiøtz) in the right eye and 16 mm. Hg (Schiøtz) in the left.

FIG. 183

Course. Because of the angle involvement, excision of the cyst was not attempted. Instead, following evacuation of the cyst contents, an insulated electrocautery needle was placed into the cyst in several areas, and a low-voltage current was used to coagulate the cyst wall. This produced an opacity of the adjacent cornea, with almost the entire temporal half of the cornea becoming edematous postoperatively. A month later the cornea was almost completely clear, and the cyst was invisible (Fig. 183, B). Two years later there was only a small area of cystic-appearing iris at the 9 o'clock position. At this time an intracapsular cataract extraction was performed on the left eye, and the patient obtained a vision of 20/20 with correction. Six years later he developed an inferior retinal detachment in the left eye, and a scleral buckling procedure was performed, which resulted in a vision of 20/40.

Iris implantation cyst

History. Two years ago this 39-year-old man had an unplanned extracapsular cataract extraction in the right eye. The cataract, as well as an iridodialysis, was caused by an old BB gun injury at age 16. Following the extraction the patient obtained a vision of 20/20 and was asymptomatic. Two months ago he was found to have a large cyst of the iris involving the temporal angle. A month ago this cyst was evacuated, but within a week it had reformed.

Findings. The vision in the right eye is 20/40 with aphakic correction and in the left 20/25. There is some conjunctival injection in the right eye, and the cornea is clear. The anterior chamber is deep except temporally, where a large iris cyst extends from the 7 o'clock to the 11 o'clock position, touching the cornea peripherally and extending almost to the pupillary margin (Fig. 184, A). The anterior wall of the cyst is thin, and cellular debris can be seen within the cyst cavity. The posterior wall extends well back into the vitreous and can be seen projecting into the pupil. The eye is aphakic, and the vitreous face is behind the pupil, which has a sector iridectomy superiorly. The fundus is normal. The left eye is normal. The intraocular pressure is 18 mm. Hg (Schiøtz) in both eyes.

FIG. 184

Course. Following another aspiration the cyst promptly reformed. Again the cyst was evacuated; but this time, in addition photocoagulation was applied to

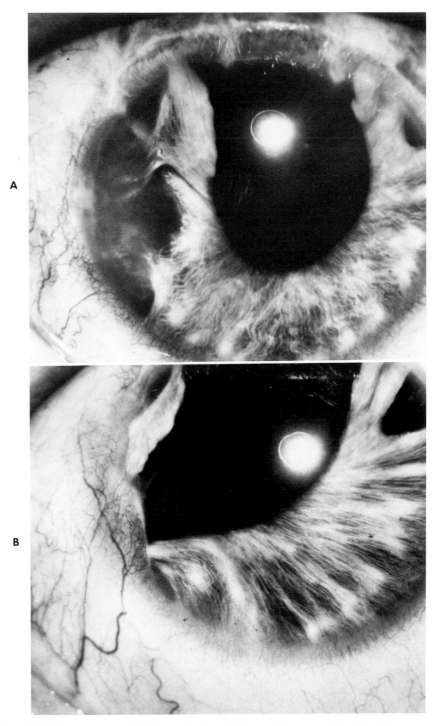

Fig. 184. *Large cyst of the peripheral iris, with extensive involvement of the cornea and chamber angle in the right eye of a 39-year-old man with an iris implantation cyst.* **A,** The cyst has a thin anterior wall and contains cellular debris. A surgical coloboma is present superiorly associated with the cataract extraction performed 2 years ago. **B,** Following several aspirations and photocoagulation of the cyst walls, a year later a small cyst developed inferiorly. Photocoagulation and finally cryocoagulation were used; 18 months later the cyst had not recurred.

the collapsed cyst walls. In another 3 months there was a slight recurrence, and the cyst was again aspirated and photocoagulated. One year later the cyst re-appeared between the 7 and 8 o'clock positions (Fig. 184, *B*). Gonioscopy showed that at the 10 o'clock position there was a questionable small cyst that appeared to extend into the ciliary body. Photocoagulation was again performed. Six months later the cyst definitely was growing behind the ciliary body; it was therefore evacuated and extensively frozen with a cryoprobe. Eighteen months later there was no sign of recurrence.

POSTOPERATIVE COMPLICATIONS

Iris prolapse occurring within a few days of cataract extraction should be repaired surgically as soon as possible. An exception might be where the pro-lapse is very small and completely covered with conjunctiva. Excision of the pro-lapsed iris is usually preferable to repositing it. After resuturing, a bubble of air in the anterior chamber may avoid adherence of the iris to the repaired wound. In a late iris prolapse, conjunctiva tissue usually covers the prolapsed iris; it may be allowed to remain unless a filtering cicatrix with hypotony occurs. In this event, a procedure similar to that with early iris prolapse is carried out, but the wound edges must be carefully cleaned before resuturing.

Adherence of the iris to the wound is a common complication of cataract sur-gery. If only iris tissue is involved, there is usually no untoward effect except for irregularity of the pupil. Hyaloid membrane incarcerated in the wound can re-sult in organization of the vitreous and possible retinal detachment. When iris or vitreous is attached to the wound and cornea, permanent corneal edema may result, necessitating surgical intervention. If the attachment is not too extensive, introduction of the cyclodialysis spatula through a limbal incision followed by injection of air in the anterior chamber is usually successful.

Infection of a filtering bleb may occur in thin-walled blebs; in actuality, there may be minute openings in the wall, which means that there is direct continuity between the outside of the eye and the anterior chamber. The fact that these eyes are usually hypotonic also may contribute to the ease with which infection enters the bleb. The earliest sign of infection is localized hyperemia and a milky appearance of the bleb. Within a matter of hours the bleb may become white and more elevated. The anterior chamber contains many cells, with a developing hypopyon. If the condition is not treated promptly, panophthalmitis may develop rapidly, resulting in loss of the eye.

A smear and culture of both the conjunctiva and aqueous obtained by means of an anterior chamber tap must be performed. Multiple topical and systemic antibiotic therapy should be initiated and modified according to the results of the smear and of the culture and sensitivity determinations. It is gen-erally agreed that systemic administration of corticosteroids is also indicated in an attempt to save the filtering bleb. Usually in milder infections, and occasionally even in the presence of a severe infection, the bleb continues to function.

All patients with thin-walled blebs should be given a prophylactic antibiotic drop at least once a day. In addition, they should be warned of the possibility of an infection and the importance of immediate treatment.

Anterior segment necrosis of the eye may occur as a complication of retinal detachment surgery and more rarely following the detachment of three or more muscles in strabismus surgery. Interference with the anterior or posterior ciliary circulation is probably the responsible mechanism. In retinal detachment surgery the most common cause is excessive diathermy over the long ciliary arteries.

Signs of anterior segment necrosis usually begin within a few days after the operation, when the cornea becomes diffusely edematous and a marked striate keratopathy develops. The tension is usually low but initially may be elevated, particularly when an encircling scleral implant has been used. Iridocyclitis, without hypopyon, is a common early sign, but without a yellow reflex from the fundus as seen in endophthalmitis. In a short time there is iris atrophy, with pigment dispersion, posterior synechia formation, and diffuse opacification of the lens. Choroidal detachment, hyphema, and finally phthisis bulbi may occur. Although the exact mechanism of anterior segment necrosis is not fully understood, it is believed that the occlusion of both long posterior ciliary arteries, with loss of blood supply to the anterior segment, is the most important factor. Interference with the circulation of the anterior ciliary artery can also produce a mild anterior segment necrosis, but the most severe type is encountered when muscles are removed in combination with diathermy, as in extensive retinal detachment surgery. The use of cryotherapy rather than diathermy apparently avoids this serious complication. Treatment of anterior segment necrosis involves the use of corticosteroids both systemically and topically and of mydriatics for the iridocyclitis. Because of the similarity between anterior segment necrosis and early endophthalmitis, antibiotics are administered systemically until the diagnosis is evident. Despite the extensive involvement of the anterior segment, the posterior segment remains normal, and good visual acuity may be salvaged.

Iris prolapse

History. Three months ago this 43-year-old man was struck in the right eye with a chip of wood. He developed a traumatic hyphema and a severe secondary glaucoma that could not be controlled by medical treatment even after the hyphema had absorbed. There was a traumatic dislocation of the lens, with cataract formation. A month after the injury, the intraocular pressure was 60 mm. Hg (Schiøtz), and a trephine procedure was performed. The postoperative course was uneventful. A month later intraocular pressure again became elevated despite intensive medical treatment. The cataract was now mature, and the anterior chamber was shallow. An intracapsular cataract extraction was performed. There were no postoperative complications until 2 weeks postoperatively, when a dehiscence was noted at the site of the cataract wound inferiorly. The dehiscence gradually increased, resulting in an iris prolapse, but the intraocular pressure remained normal.

Findings. Vision in the right eye is 20/200 and in the left 20/20. There is moderate injection of the right eye and an iris prolapse from the 6 o'clock to the 8 o'clock position, completely covered by conjunctiva (Reel XIV-7). Two partially absorbed catgut sutures can be seen along the healed incision, and a somewhat flat bleb is visible superiorly. There is a moderate striate keratopathy. The pupil is widely dilated. The eye is aphakic. The vitreous face is intact, and the fundus normal. The left eye is normal.

REEL XIV-7

313

Course. Since the prolapse continued to enlarge slightly during the next month, an excision of the staphyloma was performed, and the defect was repaired. The postoperative course was uneventful, except that a week later the intraocular tension was found to be in the 30's despite frequent use of glycerol taken orally. A cyclodialysis was performed, resulting in normalization of the intraocular pressure. Two years later the tension remained normal with the patient using pilocarpine drops, and his vision was 20/30 with an aphakic correction.

Synechial attachment to cataract wound

History. Sixteen years ago this 72-year-old man had painless loss of vision in both eyes, more pronounced in the right. Nine years ago he had a cataract extraction in the right eye and obtained 20/20 vision. About 8 months ago he was found to have a retinal detachment involving the macula in the right eye. This was successfully reattached with a scleral buckling procedure, but the visual result was poor. Therefore, an intracapsular cataract extraction was performed on the left eye, resulting in 20/25 vision with aphakic correction.

Findings. Vision in the right eye is 20/200 and in the left 20/25 with correction. The right eye is aphakic, with a surgical coloboma superiorly and a reattached retina posteriorly, with folds in the macular region. The left eye is also aphakic, with a surgical coloboma superiorly, an intact vitreous face at the pupillary plane, and a normal fundus. Gonioscopy reveals an adherence of the iris FIG. 185 to the corneal wound at the 2 o'clock position (Fig. 185). This broad, truncated

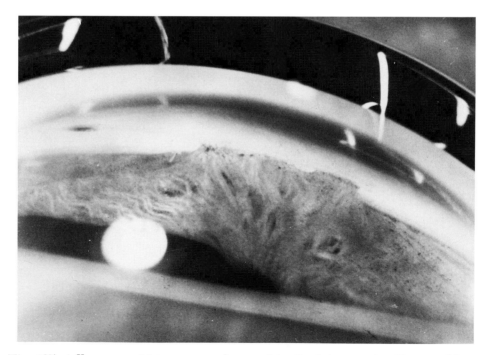

Fig. 185. *Adherence of iris to corneal wound in the left eye of a 72-year-old man with synechial attachment to a cataract wound.* As seen by gonioscopy, the peripheral iris shows a broad, truncated synechia that bridges the trabecular meshwork.

synechia appears to bridge the trabecular meshwork, and the corneoscleral wound edges are in good apposition. Elsewhere the angle is wide open and moderately pigmented. Intraocular pressure is 17 mm. Hg (Schiøtz) in the right eye and 19 mm. Hg (Schiøtz) in the left. Tonography shows a normal facility of outflow in both eyes. Fields are normal in both eyes except for a small nasal step on the right.

Course. Six months later the retina of the right eye redetached, and the patient underwent another scleral buckling procedure, with reattachment of the retina. A few months later the retina again redetached, and further surgery was attempted, but without success. The patient was then lost to follow-up.

Infected trephine bleb

History. Three years ago this 65-year-old man was found to have markedly elevated intraocular pressures in both eyes. The left eye had a marked field loss and could not be controlled with medical therapy. A trephine filtering procedure was performed, resulting in good control of the intraocular pressure. Two weeks ago the left eye became red and crusted, and 3 days ago it became painful.

Findings. Vision in the right eye is 20/40 and in the left light perception

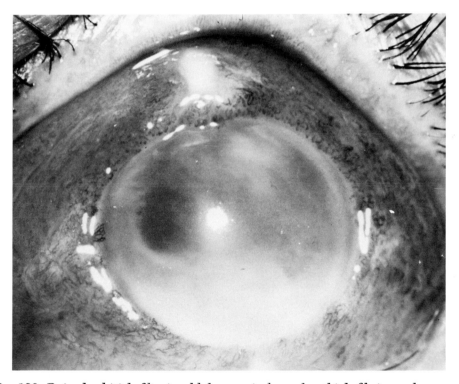

Fig. 186. *Raised whitish filtering bleb superiorly and a thick fibrinous hypopyon in the left eye of a 65-year-old man with an infected trephine bleb.* The center of the bleb appears to contain purulent material that apparently has extended into the anterior chamber through the trephine opening made 3 years ago. Cultures showed *Staphylococcus aureus;* but despite intensive antibiotic therapy, enucleation was required.

FIG. 186 only. The right eye is normal, but the left is markedly injected and chemotic. At the 12 o'clock position is a raised whitish bleb with a center that appears to contain purulent material (Fig. 186). The cornea is thickened and opacified. The anterior chamber is filled with a thick fibrinous hypopyon. The iris cannot be visualized.

Course. Cultures were taken, and intensive antibiotic therapy was initiated. There was no improvement, and the cultures revealed *Staphylococcus aureus.* Four days later the left eye was enucleated; postoperative recovery was uneventful.

Anterior segment necrosis

History. Five weeks ago this 62-year-old man experienced a sudden loss of vision in the left eye due to a vitreous hemorrhage. Over the next 3 weeks there was sufficient clearing of the hemorrhage to visualize a giant tear that involved about two thirds of the equatorial region. A scleral buckling procedure was performed that required the removal of three rectus muscles and a 360° scleral implant. Diathermy was applied to the entire bed, which in some places

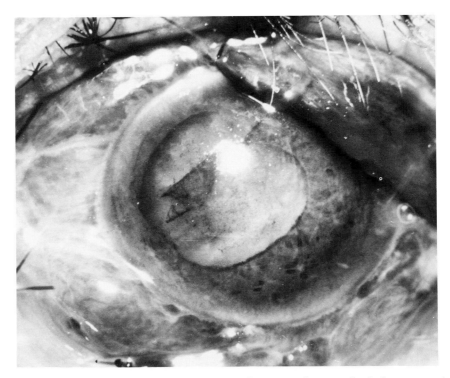

Fig. 187. *Chemosis, corneal edema, striate keratopathy, marked thinning of the iris, and cataract formation in the left eye of a 62-year-old man with anterior segment necrosis.* Following a 360° scleral implant for a detached retina 5 weeks ago, there was shallowing of the anterior chamber, followed by a persistent corneal epithelial defect, iris atrophy, and lens opacities. Six months later the eye appeared to have become blind (questionable light perception).

was more than 16 mm. wide. At the end of the procedure the retina was flat and the intraocular pressure normal. However, on the first postoperative day the tension was found to be elevated to 50 mm. Hg (Schiøtz); and marked corneal edema, conjunctival chemosis, and a shallow anterior chamber were present. Medical therapy lowered the intraocular pressure somewhat; but because of the shallow anterior chamber and the possibility of pupillary block, a peripheral iridectomy, re-formation of the anterior chamber, and a posterior sclerotomy were performed. Moderate amounts of subchoroidal fluid were released, but postoperatively the anterior chamber remained shallow. In addition to the corneal edema, there was rapid opacification of the lens cortex. The iris became atrophic, and a large, persistent corneal epithelial defect developed. The eye became very soft, with a flat anterior chamber. A week later the cornea was much clearer, but the lens opacity had become denser.

Findings. The vision in the right eye is 20/20 and in the left there is light perception only. The right eye is normal in all respects. In the left eye there is marked chemosis, moderate corneal edema, striate keratopathy, and an epithelial defect involving about half the cornea (Fig. 187). The anterior chamber FIG. 187

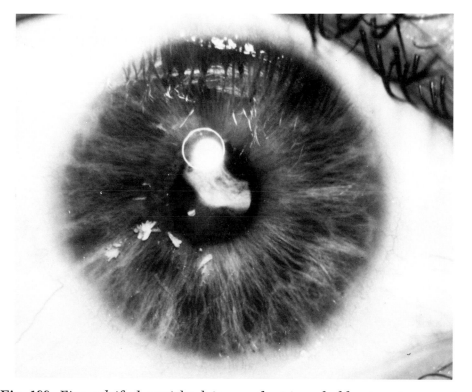

Fig. 188. *Fine calcified particles lying on the iris and old cataract remnants in the right pupil of a 24-year-old man with a rubella cataract.* At age 1 bilateral cataract extractions were performed, and subsequently glaucoma developed in both eyes.

317

is almost flat, and the iris is markedly thinned, with extensive posterior synechia formations to the intumescent lens. The tension is 12 mm. Hg by applanation tonometry.

Course. During the next week the epithelial defect became larger, the cornea more edematous, the iris more atrophic, and the lens totally opaque. Treatment consisted of systemic and topical administration of corticosteroids and mydriatics. Six months later the anterior chamber had formed, and the cornea had cleared; but the eye remained very soft, and an intumescent cataract was present. There was questionable light perception.

Calcific lens cortex on the iris

History. The mother of this 24-year-old man had rubella during the first trimester of her pregnancy. The patient was born with bilateral cataracts and partial deafness. At age 1 he had bilateral cataract operations. Six years ago he was found to have glaucoma in both eyes, from which the left eye has now become blind. Medical therapy of the right eye has controlled the intraocular tension.

Findings. The vision in the right eye is 20/50 and in the left light perception. There is a fine pendular nystagmus, and both eyes exhibit microcornea. In the right eye the cornea is clear and the anterior chamber unusually deep. The iris is atrophic, and on its surface lie a number of fine calcified-appearing particles that are similar to old cortical and capsular remnants that are within the pupil

FIG. 188 (Fig. 188). The portions of the fundus that can be visualized are normal. In the left eye the cornea is grossly edematous, and the anterior chamber is deep. Similar particles lie on the surface of the iris. The intraocular tension in the right eye is 20 mm. Hg (Schiøtz) and in the left 63 mm. Hg (Schiøtz).

Course. Over the next 6 years the glaucoma in the right eye was medically controlled. The left eye developed extensive rubeosis iridis.

COMMON OPERATIONS PRIMARILY INVOLVING THE IRIS

The peripheral iridectomy is performed for angle closure glaucoma, following the acute episode or prophylactically in the fellow eye. The procedure is curative unless the angle is closed permanently with anterior synechias due to the duration of the angle closure. Peripheral iridectomy is also important in the treatment of iris bombé. A complication of peripheral iridectomy is the appearance of a flat or shallow anterior chamber postoperatively. This may be due to a wound leak, but malignant glaucoma must always be kept in mind (p. 33). Occasionally, only stroma is removed, leaving a layer of pigment. Other complications in surgical technique involve making the incision too far posteriorly, with excision of ciliary body rather than iris tissue. Another involves incarceration of iris in the wound, which may eliminate the opening between the anterior and posterior chamber, causing the procedure to be completely ineffective. Posterior synechias may develop in the presence of a mild iritis; this can be avoided by the use of topically administered corticosteroids and phenylephrine drops.

Cyclodialysis attempts to form a cleft in the angle of the anterior chamber that will communicate with the suprachoroidal space. The effectiveness of the procedure probably depends more on separating the ciliary body and choroid from the sclera, with suppression of aqueous formation, rather than on providing drainage of aqueous from the anterior chamber into the suprachoroidal space. A complication involved in the cyclodialysis procedure is a more severe glaucoma from trauma to the angle structures if the cleft fails to remain open. Severe hemorrhage is fairly common postoperatively and may be responsible for a marked elevation in the intraocular pressure and closure of the cleft. Extreme hypotony is, unfortunately, common with cyclodialysis and may result in ciliary body and choroidal separation, which can reach the macula and reduce the visual acuity. Cataract formation is common. Because of the unpredictable results, it is generally thought that cyclodialysis should be limited to aphakic eyes.

The various types of filtering procedures involve the principle of creating an opening from the anterior chamber to the subconjunctival space in the hope of forming a filtering bleb. The most common are iridencleisis, trephination, and scleral cautery. Complications of filtering procedures are many and depend somewhat on the exact procedure used. However, some complications common to all the filtering operations are buttonholing of the conjunctiva, postoperative flat anterior chamber, hemorrhage, cataract formation, and hypotony. In general, the filtering procedure of choice is that with which the surgeon is most comfortable and familiar and with which he has had the best results.

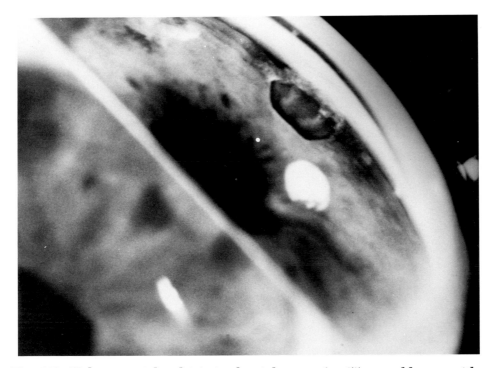

Fig. 189. *Hole in peripheral iris in the right eye of a 55-year-old man with a peripheral iridectomy for acute glaucoma.* Gonioscopy reveals that the angle is narrow but open, and through the peripheral iridectomy the ciliary processes can be visualized.

Peripheral iridectomy for acute glaucoma

History. Eighteen months ago this 55-year-old man developed blurred vision and halos in the right eye. This was followed by severe pain and marked loss of vision. After symptoms had persisted for about 12 hours, he consulted his ophthalmologist who, after administering intensive miotic therapy, performed a peripheral iridectomy. The anterior chamber angle of the left eye was narrow, and a prophylactic peripheral iridectomy was performed on that eye. Postoperatively the intraocular pressures were normal, and the patient was asymptomatic.

Findings. The vision in the right eye is 20/20 and in the left 20/30. In the right eye the anterior segment is normal except for a peripheral iridectomy. The media and fundus are also normal. In the left eye there is a peripheral iridectomy at the 2 o'clock position and some nuclear sclerosis of the lens. Gonioscopy of both eyes reveals a narrow but open angle; in the left eye the peripheral iridectomy is at the root of the iris, and through it can be visualized FIG. 189 the ciliary processes (Fig. 189). Intraocular pressures are in the normal range.

Course. For the next 5 years there was gradual decrease in vision in both eyes due to nuclear sclerosis. The intraocular pressure was found to be 26 mm. Hg (Schiøtz) in the right eye, and miotics were used at bedtime. Six years later the medications were discontinued, and subsequently the intraocular pressure was found to be only 22 mm. Hg (Schiøtz) in the right eye and 17 mm. Hg in the left. The lens changes have still not progressed to the stage requiring cataract extraction.

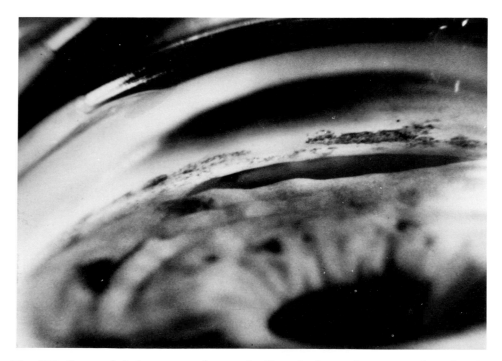

Fig. 190. *Large cleft between sclera and ciliary body in the temporal angle of a 55-year-old man with a cyclodialysis cleft.* The scleral spur has been detached, and through the cleft the inner scleral wall can be visualized. The procedure was performed about 4 years ago; since then, the pressure has remained low.

Cyclodialysis cleft

History. For a number of years this 55-year-old man had chronic open angle glaucoma. About 4 years ago he developed cataracts, and bilateral cataract extractions were performed. Two years ago the intraocular pressure in the left eye remained in the mid 30's despite intensive medical therapy, and a cyclodialysis was performed. Since then the intraocular pressure remained between 10 and 15 mm. Hg (Schiøtz).

Findings. Vision in both eyes is 20/40 with correction. Both eyes are aphakic, and in the left there is an open cyclodialysis cleft in the temporal angle as revealed by gonioscopy (Fig. 190). Moderate irregular pigmentation can be seen FIG. 190 on the trabecular meshwork and in some places extending onto the peripheral cornea. Through the cleft can be visualized the inner surface of the sclera.

Course. The patient was lost to follow-up.

Iridencleisis filtering procedure

History. Three years ago this 15-year-old girl was found to have a markedly elevated intraocular pressure in her left eye. She gave a history of seeing occasional halos around lights but had no other ocular symptoms. Her father, her paternal grandmother, and two paternal aunts had glaucoma. While she was taking miotics, she had a wide diurnal variation of pressure in both eyes, ranging from 4 to 49 mm. Hg during the same week, highest at about midday. Fields showed a Bjerrum scotoma in both eyes and decreased vision in the left. An iridencleisis was performed on the left eye, and the postoperative course was uneventful. The pressure was then well controlled, but the right eye remained in the glaucomatous range despite maximum medical therapy. Accordingly, 2 weeks later an iridencleisis was performed on the right eye. Again the postoperative course was uneventful, and intraocular tensions remained in the teens or lower.

Findings. The vision in the right eye is 20/25 and in the left 20/30. In both eyes there are large filtering blebs superiorly and visualization of the pigment epithelium deep in the bleb. The anterior chambers are deep, and there is a superior coloboma in each eye. The media are clear, and the discs show mild glaucomatous cupping. By gonioscopy an opening can be seen at the 12 o'clock position just anterior to the trabecular meshwork (Reel XV-1). The iris extends REEL XV-1 through this corneal opening and in part can be seen on the outside of the eye through the transparent cornea. The field in the right eye is normal, but in the left there is a prominent nasal step.

Course. Over the next 2 years the tensions remained low, and there was no change in the patient's vision or fields. She was then lost to follow-up.

Trephine filtering procedure

History. Four years ago this 67-year-old woman was discovered to have chronic open angle glaucoma and a large Bjerrum scotoma in the right eye. Intraocular pressure in the right eye was not controlled by medical therapy, and a year later a trephine filtering procedure was performed. Following this, the anterior chamber became flat, and a posterior sclerotomy and paracentesis resulted in the formation of the anterior chamber. Although the tension was normal and a good conjunctival bleb formed, a cataract gradually developed. Two years ago cataract extraction in the right eye was performed from below, and since then the intraocular pressures have varied between 7 and 14 mm. Hg (Schiøtz). The intraocular pressure in the left eye had remained in the low 20's with the patient receiving maximal medical therapy, but because of a maturing cataract a combined cyclodialysis and cataract extraction was performed 1 year ago. The postoperative course was uneventful.

Findings. Vision in the right eye is 20/30 and in the left 20/20 with correction. In the right eye there is a large elevated filtering bleb superiorly. The cornea is clear, and there is a deep anterior chamber except inferiorly where some peripheral anterior synechias are attached to the area of the wound for the cataract extraction. There is a peripheral iridectomy superiorly, and the eye is aphakic. The disc appears atrophic and cupped superiorly. Gonioscopy shows a round opening in the peripheral cornea at the 12 o'clock position (Reel XV-2). Inferiorly there is a broad peripheral synechia extending to the cataract wound. In the left eye the anterior chamber is deep, and the eye is aphakic. There are two peripheral iridectomies superiorly. No cyclodialysis cleft is visible. The optic nerve head shows minimal glaucomatous cupping. The intraocular pressure is 15 mm. Hg in the right eye and 8 mm. Hg in the left as shown by applanation tonometry.

REEL XV-2

Course. For the next 3 years the intraocular pressure remained within the normal range with the patient receiving no medication. When she was last seen, the intraocular pressure was 13 mm. Hg in the right eye and 19 mm. Hg in the left as shown by applanation tonometry, and the vision was normal.

Bibliography for part two

Bell, R., and Font, R. L.: Granulomatous anterior uveitis caused by *Coccidioides immitis*, Amer. **74**:93-98, July 1972.

Bertelsen, T. I., Drablös, P. A., and Flood, P. R.: The so-called senile exfoliation (pseudo-exfoliation) of the anterior lens capsule, a product of the lens epithelium, fibrillopathia epitheliocapsularis, Acta Ophthal. **42**:1096-1113, 1964.

Boyle, G. L., Gwon, A. E., Ainn, K. M., and Leopold, I. H.: Intraocular penetration of carbenicillin after subconjunctival injection in man, Amer. J. Ophthal. **37**:754-759, May. 1972.

Chandler, P. A.: Atrophy of the stroma of the iris, endothelial dystrophy, corneal edema, and glaucoma, Amer. J. Ophthal. **41**:607-615, April 1956.

Cogan, D. G., Kuwabara, T., Kinoshita, J., Sudarsky, D., and Ring, H.: Ocular manifestation of systemic cystinosis, Arch. Ophthal. **55**:36-41, Jan. 1956.

deVeer, J. A.: Pathologic findings in cases of retained nonmetallic foreign bodies, Amer. J. Ophthal. **31**:615, May 1948.

Donaldson, D. D.: The significance of spotting of the iris in mongoloids, Brushfield's spots, Arch. Ophthal. **65**:26-31, Jan. 1961.

Dugmore, W. N.: 11-year follow up of a case of iris leiomyosarcoma, Brit. J. Ophthal. **56**:366-367, April 1972.

Duguis, I. M.: Anterior segment necrosis following retinal detachment surgery, Trans. Ophthal. Soc. U. K. **87**:171-178, 1967.

Duke-Elder, S.: System of ophthalmology. Vol. 8, Diseases of the outer eye; conjunctiva, cornea, and sclera, St. Louis, 1965, The C. V. Mosby Co.

Duke-Elder, S.: Textbook of ophthalmology. Vol. 6, Injuries, London, 1954, Henry Kimpton.

Duke-Elder, S., and Perkins, E. S.: System of ophthalmology. Vol. 9, Diseases of the uveal tract, St. Louis, 1966, The C. V. Mosby Co.

Elgjo, K., and Opsahl, R.: Metastasis to the chamber angle from mucoid breast carcinoma, Acta Ophthal. **42**:881-883, 1964.

Feingold, M., Shiere, F., Fogels, H. R., and Donaldson, D.: Rieger's syndrome, Pediatrics **44**:564-569, Oct. 1969.

Find, B. S.: Free-floating pigmented cyst in the anterior chamber, a clinicohistopathologic report, Amer. J. Ophthal. **67**:493-500, April 1969.

Fitzpatrick, T. B., and Quevedo, W. C.: Albinism. In Stanbury, J. B., Wyngaarden, J. B., and Fredrickson, D. S., editors: The metabolic basis of inherited disease, New York, 1960, McGraw-Hill Book Co., pp. 326-337.

Fitzpatrick, T. B., Zeller, R., Kukita, A., and Kitamura, H.: Oculodermomelanocytosis, Arch. Ophthal. **5**; 830-832, Dec. 1956.

Fonda, G.: Characteristics and low-vision corrections in albinism, a report of 161 patients, Arch. Ophthal. **68**:754-761, Dec. 1962.

Francois, J., Hanssens, M., Coppieters, R., and Evens, L.: Cystinosis, Amer. J. Ophthal. **73**:643-650, May 1972.

Francois, P., and Corbel, M.: Le syndrome atrophie essentielle et progressive de l'iris, Bull. Soc. Ophthal. Fr. **65**:137-142, 1965.

Freeman, H. M., Hawkins, W. R., and Schepens, C. L.: Anterior segment necrosis, Arch. Ophthal. **75**:644-650, May 1966.

Gladstone, R. M.: Development and significance of heterochromia of the iris, Arch. Neurol. **21**:184-192, Aug. 1969.

Grant, W. M., and Walton, D. S.: Distinctive gonioscopic findings in glaucoma due to neurofibromatosis, Arch. Ophthal. **79**:127-134, Feb. 1968.

Henderson, J. R., and Benedict, W. L.: Essential progressive atrophy of the iris, Amer. J. Ophthal. **23**:644-650, 1940.

Hogan, M. J., and Zimmerman, L. E.: Ophthalmic pathology, Philadelphia, 1962, W. B. Saunders Co.

Horven, I.: Exfoliation syndrome, a histological and histochemical study, Acta Ophthal. **44**:790-799, 1966.

Hoskins, H. D., Jr., and Shaffer, R. N.: Rieger's syndrome; a form of iridocorneal mesodermal dysgenesis, J. Pediat. Ophthal. **9**(1):26-30, 1972.

Huerkamp, B.: Zwei Typen des progressiven durchgreifenden Irisschwundes, Klin. Monatsbl. Augenheilkd. **121**:656-662, 1952.

Iwamoto, T., Jones, I. S., and Howard, G. M.: Ultrastructural comparison of spindle A, spindle B, and epithelioid-type cells in uveal malignant melanoma, Invest. Ophthal. **11**:873-889, Nov. 1972.

Mamo, J. B., and Azzam, S. A.: Treatment of Behçet's disease with chlorambucil, Arch. Ophthal. **84**:446-450, Oct. 1970.

Mamo, J. B., and Baghlassarian, A.: Behçet's disease; a report of 28 cases, Arch. Ophthal. **71**:4-14, Jan. 1964.

Manor, R. S., and Sachs, W.: Spontaneous hypema, Amer. J. Ophthal. **74**:293-295, Aug. 1972.

Maumenee, A. E.: An approach to the study of uveitis. In Clinical methods in uveitis, Fourth Sloan Symposium, St. Louis, 1968, The C. V. Mosby Co.

Miller, D., Farley, V. H., McLaughlin, R., and Sullivan, G. E.: A light-shielded spectacle for albino patients, Ann. Ophthal. **4**:611-612, Aug. 1972.

Naumann, G., Font, R. L., and Zimmerman, L. E.: Electron microscopic verification of primary rhabdomyosarcoma of the iris, Amer. J. Ophthal. **74**:110-117, July 1972.

Reese, A. B.: Tumors of the eye, ed. 2, New York, 1963, Paul B. Hoeber, Inc.

Rosselet, E., Saudan, Y., and Zenklusen, G.: Les effets de l'azathioprine (Imuran) dans la maladie de Behçet, premiers resultats therapeutiques, Ophthalmologica **156**:218-226, 1968.

Scheie, H. G.: Gonioscopy in diagnosis of tumors of the iris and ciliary body, Arch. Ophthal. **51**:288-300, March 1954.

Schlaegel, T. F., Jr.: Recent advances in uveitis, Ann. Ophthal. **4**:525-552, July 1972.

Schwartz, D. E.: Herpes zoster ophthalmicus with nasociliary nerve involvement, Amer. J. Ophthal. **74**:142-144, July 1972.

Scialfa, A. C.: Ocular albinism in a female, Amer. J. Ophthal. **73**:943-948, June 1972.

Tarkkanen, A.: Pseudoexfoliation of the lens capsule, Acta Ophthal. Suppl. **71**:84-86, 1962.

Wilson, W.: Iris cyst treated by electrolysis, Brit. J. Ophthal. **48**:45-49, Jan. 1964.

Witmer, R.: Etiology of uveitis, Ann. Ophthal. **4**:615-625, Aug. 1972.

Wolter, J. R.: Double embolism of the central retinal artery and one long posterior ciliary artery followed by secondary hemorrhagic glaucoma, Amer. J. Ophthal. **73**:651-657, May 1972.

Zimmerman, L. E.: Ocular lesions of juvenile xanthogranuloma, nevoxanthoendothelioma, Trans. Amer. Acad. Ophthal. **69**:412-442, May-June 1965.

Part three

CILIARY BODY

The functions of the ciliary body are important. Contraction of the ciliary muscle releases the tension on the zonules attached to the lens, which in turn allows the lens to become more convex and focuses the eye for near objects. The ciliary epithelium has a vital function producing aqueous humor at a constant rate with maintenance of a proper intraocular pressure and flow through the posterior and anterior chamber.

Anatomically, the ciliary body is triangular in cross section, with its base at the iris and angle recess and the apex continuous with the anterior choroid at the ora serrata. Its external surface is separated from the sclera by the suprachoroidal space, and the internal surface is in contact with the vitreous. The anterior portion of the internal surface is made up of the corona ciliaris, from which about 80 ciliary processes arise. The posterior portion of the internal surface is the orbiculus ciliaris, or pars plana, which is continuous with the retina posteriorly. External to the corona ciliaris and orbiculus ciliaris is the major portion of the ciliary body, the ciliary muscle. The ciliary muscle may be divided into three groups of fibers: meridional, radial, and circular. The meridional fibers occupy the external portion of the ciliary body and are inserted into the scleral spur. The radial and circular muscle fibers are located more anteriorly and internally, and their fibers are arranged as their names imply. The circular fibers, which are probably most important in the function of accommodation, continue to develop after birth; they are more developed in the hyperopic eye than in the myopic. The ciliary processes have a vascular connective tissue core covered by ciliary epithelium. External to the ciliary processes is a vascular layer, which is directly continuous with the vessels of the choroid. The inner surface of the ciliary processes is covered by an internal limiting membrane to which the zonular fibers of the lens are attached. The ciliary epithelium itself is composed of two layers of cells that in adults are firmly united at the ora serrata. The outer layer of cells is pigmented, while the inner layer has no pigment except near the iris root. It is generally assumed that this inner layer has a secretory function and produces aqueous humor.

In contrast to the iris, when the ciliary body is subjected to trauma there is a definite tissue reaction. There is fibroblastic proliferation and resulting cicatrization. Pigment cell proliferation from the pigmented ciliary epithelium is common. As with the iris, the ciliary body is particularly susceptible to inflammatory reactions, with a resultant cyclitis. The iris almost always is involved; therefore, the process is an iridocyclitis, which may be due to various exogenous, endogenous or, as is commonly the case, unknown causes.

Inasmuch as the ciliary body is the source of aqueous humor, it is responsible for the increased intraocular pressure in glaucoma when the outflow channels no longer function. When both medical and surgical treatment of glaucoma has failed, it is common to resort to a direct attack on the ciliary body itself. Thus cyclodiathermy and, more recently, cyclocryotherapy have been used to reduce the aqueous secretory activity of the ciliary body by making a portion of it either temporarily or permanently nonfunctional. However, if a sufficient amount of the ciliary body becomes atrophic from any cause, phthisis bulbi and loss of the eye may follow.

Chapter 12

Congenital conditions of the ciliary body

DICTYOMA (MEDULLOEPITHELIOMA)

An embryonic neoplasm arising from the embryonic or fetal tissues of the nonpigmented ciliary epithelium is commonly referred to as a dictyoma but more properly should be called a medulloepithelioma. It is a relatively benign tumor, usually observed at birth or becoming apparent in early childhood, and must be differentiated from the more common retinoblastoma. The name dictyoma was given to indicate the netlike appearance of the tumor due to medullary epithelial bands. Verhoeff was the first to emphasize its embryonal character. In contrast to retinoblastoma, dictyoma is not familial and never multicentric in origin or bilateral. Histopathologically, the dictyoma, or medulloepithelioma, consists of cells arranged in sheets, rosettes, and amorphous masses. In contrast to retinoblastomas, in dictyomas there are more medullary sheets and more mucoid in the stroma, but there are fewer small rosettes and less necrosis and calcification. Portions of the tumor may simulate embryonic retina. The so-called pure medulloepithelioma contains elements that closely resemble medullary epithelium. However, it may also contain structures derived from the secondary optic vesicle or optic cup, such as retinal pigment epithelium, ciliary epithelium, vitreous, and neuroglia. In the teratoid medulloepithelioma, heteroplastic elements are present, the most common of which is hyaline cartilage and the next most common a tissue resembling brain. Skeletal muscle has also been described; thus the tumor may resemble a moderately well-differentiated rhabdomyosarcoma.

The tumor is slow growing and extends locally into the surrounding tissues, commonly the root of the iris, and into the angle, where it may obstruct aqueous outflow. Frequently it is light in color and therefore may be misdiagnosed as a retinoblastoma. Enucleation is required. The histopathologic diagnosis carries a far better prognosis than that in retinoblastoma.

Congenital conditions of the ciliary body

Dictyoma (medulloepithelioma) of the ciliary body

History. This 5-year-old girl was referred to an ophthalmologist by her pediatrician for examination and evaluation of a white lesion in her right eye. Further questioning revealed that her mother had noticed a whitish spot in the eye for the past 2 months.

Findings. With Allen cards the vision is 8/30 in the right eye and 20/30 in the left. The tension in both eyes is 14 mm. Hg (Schiøtz). Examination reveals that the right eye has a pearl-white lobulated mass, with prominent vessels, that extends superiorly from the angle into the anterior chamber over the iris, causing

REEL XV-3   the right pupil to be semicircular (Reel XV-3). Also extending superiorly into the anterior chamber through the pupil are several cysts, some of which are covered with iris pigment epithelium. By direct and indirect ophthalmoscopy the fundus is normal except for a slightly elevated white mound located just anterior to the ora serrata from the 11 o'clock to the 1 o'clock position. The left eye is completely normal.

Course. The patient was seen 1 month later, and the mass had definitely enlarged. The eye was enucleated, and the pathologic diagnosis was dictyoma of the ciliary body arising from the nonpigmented epithelium. Histopathologically, the ciliary body, iris, and anterior chamber were invaded with the typical net-

FIG. 191   like polycystic tissue seen in the dictyoma (Fig. 191, *A*). Microscopically, there were many true rosettes (Fig. 191, *B*). The patient's postoperative course was uneventful. Over the next 3 years the patient was seen yearly, and results of all examinations were normal. Vision in the left eye was 20/20. Cosmetically, the motility and the appearance of the prosthesis were excellent.

CYSTS OF THE CILIARY BODY

Frequently bilateral and generally considered congenital in origin, cysts of the ciliary body usually manifest themselves as localized narrowing of the chamber angle. Although this is best determined by gonioscopy, a localized smooth and rounded bulge of the extreme periphery of the iris may signal a cyst of the peripheral iris or ciliary body. Scleral transillumination usually differentiates these cysts from solid tumors, and a lack of inflammatory signs differentiates them from inflammatory masses. With a maximally dilated pupil such cysts can easily be visualized gonioscopically between the iris and the anterior surface of the lens. They are smoothly rounded. Some are darkly pigmented, while others are almost transparent, depending on the portion of the ciliary epithelium from which they are derived.

If the cysts are multiple, which is frequently the case, a subacute angle closure glaucoma or occasionally a typical picture of acute angle closure glaucoma may develop. The angle varies considerably in width, depending on the location of the cyst, being closed where the cyst is sufficiently large to push the iris against the trabecular meshwork. Such a picture is almost pathognomonic of a cyst of the ciliary body. If an iridectomy is performed, the cyst may be visible through the iridectomy. Puncture of an iris cyst in phakic patients is hazardous, and therefore a large basal iridectomy is the treatment of choice and usually avoids further angle closure. With an ordinary peripheral iridectomy the angle does not open as in acute angle closure glaucoma, although sometimes the glau-

328

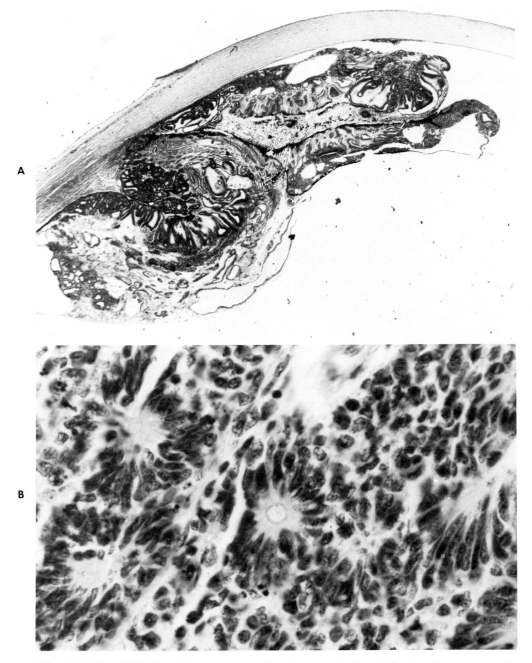

Fig. 191 (Reel XV-3). *Photomicrographs of a pearl-white lobulated mass extending from the angle over the iris in the right eye of a 5-year-old girl with a dictyoma of the ciliary body.* **A,** Low-power photomicrograph shows netlike polycystic tissue arising from the nonpigmented epithelium of the ciliary body. (P.A.S. stain; ×40.) **B,** High-power photomicrograph shows true rosettes typical of a dictyoma.

329

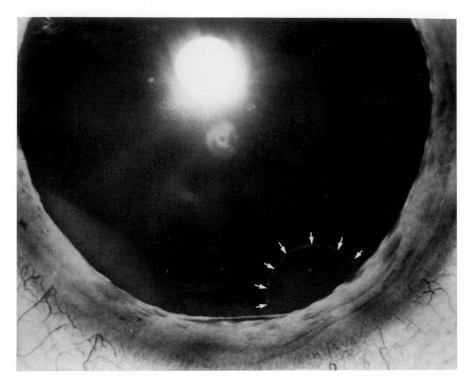

Fig. 192. *Smoothly rounded transparent cystic structure at pupillary margin in left eye of a 41-year-old man with cysts of the ciliary body.* By gonioscopy (see Reel XV-5) the cyst can be seen to arise from the ciliary processes and to push the iris forward against the trabecular meshwork.

coma can then be controlled medically. Where permanent peripheral anterior synechias have formed, a filtering operation may be necessary. In rare cases multiple cysts on the iris or ciliary body may produce excessive pigment and simulate a pigmentary glaucoma.

Cysts of the ciliary body

History. Fourteen years ago this 28-year-old man was struck in the left eye; the injury resulted in a corneal perforation and iris prolapse. A large basal iridectomy was performed, and the eye healed uneventfully. Recently the patient sustained a blow to the eye, which resulted in a subconjunctival hemorrhage. During ocular examination cysts were found.

Findings. The right eye is normal. In the left eye there is a subconjunctival hemorrhage inferiorly. Temporal to the apex of the cornea is a dense scar; attached to the scar is a large iridocorneal adhesion (adherent leukoma). Inferiorly there is a large basal iridectomy exposing the ciliary processes. Gonioscopy reveals three cysts of the ciliary body (Reel XV-4). At the 5 o'clock position there is a large cyst with a lightly pigmented wall extending well out into the anterior chamber. At the 6 o'clock position a small cyst with a translucent wall extends out to the edge of the iris, and at the 7 o'clock position another cyst with a moderately pigmented wall extends only to the edge of the partially excised iris.

REEL XV-4

330

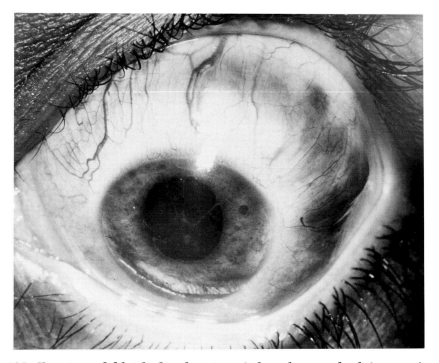

Fig. 193. *Ectasia and bluish discoloration of the sclera in the left eye of a 21-year-old girl with ciliary staphylomas and glaucoma.* Since birth, the eye was poor, and congenital iris defects were present. Because the eye was blind and the intraocular pressure markedly elevated, the eye was enucleated.

Except for irregular granular pigment deposits on the anterior capsule of the lens, there is no opacity of the lens. The posterior segment is normal.

Course. The patient was lost to follow-up.

Cysts of the ciliary body

History. As an incidental finding this 41-year-old man was noted to have a bulge in the iris of the left eye. He had no symptoms referable to this lesion.

Findings. The right eye is normal in all respects, but in the left there is a localized rounded convexity of the peripheral iris at the 5 o'clock position. With the pupil maximally dilated, a smoothly rounded translucent cyst that elevates the iris off the lens and projects into the anterior chamber can be seen (Fig. 192). By gonioscopy the cyst can be seen to arise from the ciliary processes and to close the angle by pushing the iris forward against the meshwork (Reel XV-5). One other small translucent cyst can be seen on an adjacent ciliary process. Elsewhere the angle is normal, with moderate granular pigmentation on the trabeculum. Intraocular pressure in both eyes is 20 mm. Hg (Schiøtz).

Course. The patient was lost to follow-up.

FIG. 192

REEL XV-5

CONGENITAL CILIARY STAPHYLOMAS

Eyes with congenital anomalies and secondary glaucoma are prone to develop thinning of the sclera over the region of the ciliary body. An ectasia of the sclera occurs, and a bluish discoloration appears due to visualization of the ciliary body. This results in the so-called ciliary staphyloma and is usually seen in eyes that are blind or have a markedly reduced vision. Ciliary staphylomas are also associated with chronic glaucoma, trauma, and chronic scleritis. The condition is discussed in more detail in Chapter 14 (p. 359).

Congenital anomalies, glaucoma, and ciliary staphylomas

History. The vision in the left eye of this 21-year-old girl was poor. Recently she had vague symptoms in the eye.

Findings. Vision in the right eye is 20/15 and in the left accurate light projection. The right eye is normal. In the left eye the cornea is smaller than normal. Except for the 6 o'clock to the 10 o'clock position, there is an ectasia FIG. 193 and bluish discoloration to the sclera over the ciliary body region (Fig. 193). The cornea exhibits a mild band keratopathy. The anterior chamber is of normal depth. The fibrillar pattern of the iris surface is absent, and there is no collarette. On the pupillary margin are a number of strands of iris tissue extending to the apical region, where they attach to each other. There are a few opacities centrally in the anterior capsule of the lens, where some of the persistent pupillary membrane remnants attach. The lens is otherwise clear, but there is a diffuse haziness to the vitreous, which affords only a poor view of the disc and some of the vascular pattern. Intraocular pressure is 53 mm. Hg (Schiøtz).

Course. Four years later there had been some increase in the extent of the staphyloma, but the patient was asymptomatic. In another 3 years the eye had become blind, and there had been further increase in the staphyloma. The eye had a poor appearance; therefore, the patient agreed to enucleation. Postoperatively there was no complication, and histopathologically the eye showed extensive staphylomas, with atrophy of the ciliary body, closure of the angle by extensive peripheral anterior synechia formation, and glaucomatous cupping of the disc.

Chapter 13

Tumors of the ciliary body

TUMORS OF THE CILIARY BODY

Primary tumors of the ciliary body can be divided into two general categories: epithelial and stromal. The ciliary body has an inner lining of two layers of cuboidal cells that are of neuroectodermal origin—the ciliary epithelium. The inner layer, with the basement membrane facing the vitreous, is nonpigmented; while the outer layer, which faces the stroma, is pigmented. Although rare, benign tumors of the nonpigmented epithelium, such as adenomatous hyperplasias and papillomas, do occur. Medulloepitheliomas, although also rare, are more common and more important than benign tumors of the nonpigmented epithelium; and represent embryonic neoplasms arising from embryonic or fetal tissues. Medulloepitheliomas are discussed in Chapter 12 (p. 327) because of their congenital origin. Tumors that contain one or more heteroplastic elements (the most common is hyaline cartilage) are referred to as teratoid medulloepitheliomas, in contrast to "pure" medulloepitheliomas, which closely resemble the medullary epithelium of the ciliary body; but in addition pure medulloepitheliomas may contain structures resembling tissues derived from the secondary optic vesicle or optic cup. The adult counterpart of the medulloepithelioma is usually designated as an "adenocarcinoma" due to its more glandular configuration and the more highly differentiated cells that it contains. The malignancy of these tumors varies widely. Mixed epithelial tumors composed of both the pigmented and nonpigmented epithelial layers are usually associated with a reactive hyperplasia in traumatized or otherwise diseased eyes.

Melanomas of the ciliary body arise from the stroma and may contain any of the cell types of the ciliary body stroma. They do not differ histologically from tumors of the choroid; therefore, it is frequently difficult to differentiate the two. The most benign pigmented tumor of the ciliary body is the nevus, which is identical to nevi found in the choroid. The melanocytoma (magnocellular nevus) is similar to the melanocytoma of the nerve head. Malignant melanomas of the ciliary body are less common than those of the choroid and more common than those of the iris. They frequently extend either into the iris or choroid or both. Usually the initial sign of malignant melanomas of the ciliary body is the appearance of a dark mass at the periphery of the iris, which pushes the iris aside, producing folds and an oval pupil. Sometimes there is a forward bulge of the iris, without iris disinsertion. With further growth of the tumor, the lens may become cataractous (often only adjacent to the tumor mass) or dislocated. When the tumor extends posteriorly, the choroid is invaded, and the retina may be detached. Extrabulbar extension through one of the anterior emissaries may be revealed as a scleral pigmented nodule. As in malignant melanomas of the iris, the tumor may release pigment, especially when there is necrosis, which is more common than in other uveal melanomas. The pigment is carried into the anterior chamber and may result in glaucoma due to deposition in the trabecular meshwork and a decreased facility of outflow. Occasionally, an iritis is the initial sign in a melanoma of the ciliary body, presumably secondary to necrosis, and it will usually not respond to the conventional treatment for iritis.

Classification of melanomas of the ciliary body is the same as that of the iris and choroid. Callender's classification seems to be the most useful with spindle cell A, spindle cell B, epithelioid, fascicular, necrotic, and mixed cell types. The amount of pigmentation varies considerably, and some of the epithelioid type are almost amelanotic and therefore difficult to differentiate from metastatic carcinomas.

Other rare primary tumors of the ciliary body are neurolemmomas, neurofibromas, gliomas, and hemangiomas.

Metastatic tumors in the ciliary body are rare, being more common in the choroid and even in the iris.

The treatment of tumors of the ciliary body in the past was almost universally enucleation. However, when there is no sign of spread of the tumor and its size is still relatively small, an iridocyclectomy may result in removal of the tumor, with preservation of the eye. The approach may be corneal or scleral or a combination of both. Where the tumor is firmly attached to the sclera, a lamellar scleral resection can be done and the inner lamella removed with the tumor. A number of successful operations using such procedures are reported. It must be realized that at least some malignant melanomas are low-grade spindle cell A or spindle cell B type; and even though total resection is not accomplished, the chances of metastasis are small, and recurrences, if they do occur, develop slowly.

Malignant melanoma of the ciliary body

History. This 27-year-old woman was seen this morning because of a minor injury to her left eye, which produced a subconjunctival hemorrhage. The pupil was noted to be abnormally shaped, and a tumor mass was found when the pupil was dilated. She was unaware of any ocular symptoms prior to her injury.

Findings. The vision in the right eye is 20/20 and in the left 20/40. The right eye is normal. In the left eye there is a small subconjunctival hemorrhage

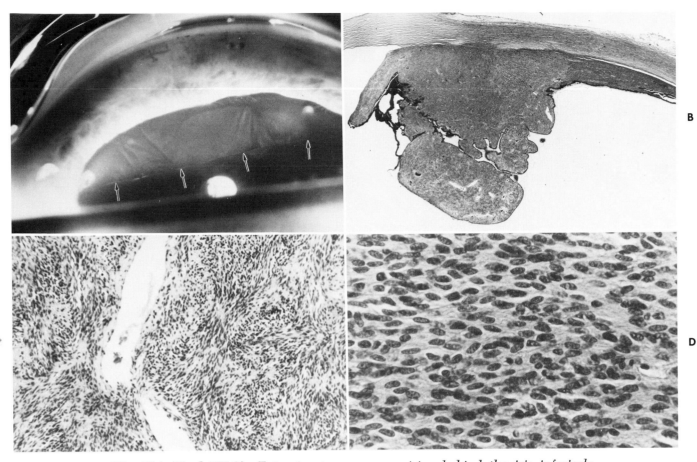

Fig. 194 (Reel XV-6). *Extensive tumor mass arising behind the iris inferiorly and invading the peripheral iris in the eye of a 27-year-old woman with a malignant melanoma of the ciliary body.* **A,** Gonioscopy reveals darkly pigmented tumor mass (arrows) between the lens posteriorly and the iris anteriorly. Inferiorly, the angle is closed due to anterior displacement of the iris against the trabecular meshwork. **B,** Low-power photomicrograph shows tumor mass closing the angle and with extension into the iris, sclera, and choroid. (H & E stain; ×40.) **C,** The tumor is of the fascicular type. (H & E stain; ×400.) **D,** The cell type is mixed but predominantly spindle cell B. (H & E stain; ×1600.)

temporally near the limbus. The cornea is clear, and the anterior chamber is of normal depth except inferiorly, where the iris is almost in contact with the cornea. The pupil is oval due to failure of the lower portion to dilate (Reel XV-6). The peripheral half of the iris from the 5 o'clock to the 7 o'clock reel XV-6 position reveals superficial neovascularization, and there is an ectropion uveae of the inferior pupillary border. The angle is closed from the 3:30 to the 8:30 position. The temporal portion of the tumor is covered by cysts and is light brown. Another large nodule of tumor between the 5 and 7 o'clock positions is dark brown and is attached to the anterior capsule of the lens. Nasally, two other nodules are visible. Gonioscopy shows that the tumor is extensive and displaces

335

FIG. 194   the iris anteriorly and the lens posteriorly (Fig. 194, A). There are some posterior subcapsular cortical lens opacities. The posterior pole is normal.

Course. Reaction to ^{32}P uptake test was strongly positive, and the left eye was enucleated. Histopathologically, a large mass of tumor was found that closed the angle and extended into the iris, sclera, and choroid (Fig. 194,B). On the surface were a number of large epithelial cysts. Microscopically, the tumor was of the fascicular type, with mixed cells but predominantly spindle cell B type (Fig. 194, C and D). The postoperative course was uneventful. Eighteen months later there were no signs of orbital recurrence or metastasis.

Malignant melanoma of the ciliary body

History. About 3 months ago this 68-year-old woman noticed some blurring of vision in her left eye. Drops given by her family physician did not help.

Findings. The vision in the right eye is 20/40 and in the left 20/50. The right eye is normal. In the left eye there is slight conjunctival injection. The cornea is clear. In the anterior chamber from the 4 o'clock to the 6 o'clock position is a dark brown mass extending out from the angle more than halfway REEL XV-7   to the pupil (Reel XV-7). Its surface is nodular, and portions are light brown. The iris adjacent to the tumor is pushed up in folds, but there does not seem to be any invasion of the iris by tumor tissue. The pupil is distorted into an oval shape. Funduscopic examination shows a large mass inside the eye directly behind the tumor mass on the iris. The fundus is otherwise normal. Intraocular tension in the right eye is 17 mm. Hg and in the left 20 mm. Hg (Schiøtz).

Course. The left eye was enucleated, and the postoperative course was uneventful. Histopathologic examination showed a massive tumor of the ciliary body that had destroyed the anterior chamber angle structures and invaded the FIG. 195   peripheral iris (Fig. 195, A). Posteriorly there was extension into the choroid, and tumor cells were found in the lumen of the intrascleral vessels (Fig. 195, B). The tumor was composed almost exclusively of classical epithelioid cells (Fig. 195, C). The patient was lost to follow-up, but subsequently it was found that she had died 7 years later of liver metastases.

Malignant melanoma of the ciliary body

History. About 6 months ago this 72-year-old woman noticed a black spot on the left eye. Soon after, she also noticed some blurring of vision and was told she had a cataract in the eye. Two weeks ago the eye became uncomfortable,

---

Fig. 195 (Reel XV-7). *Photomicrographs of a dark brown mass extending from the angle inferiorly in the left eye of a 68-year-old woman with a malignant melanoma of the ciliary body.* **A,** Low-power photomicrograph shows the massive tumor that has destroyed the anterior chamber angle and invaded the peripheral iris. (H & E stain; ×40.) **B,** Photomicrograph shows extension of tumor cells in the lumen of an intrascleral vessel. (H & E stain; ×1000.) **C,** Photomicrograph shows cell type to be almost exclusively classical epithelioid cell. (H & E stain; ×1600.)

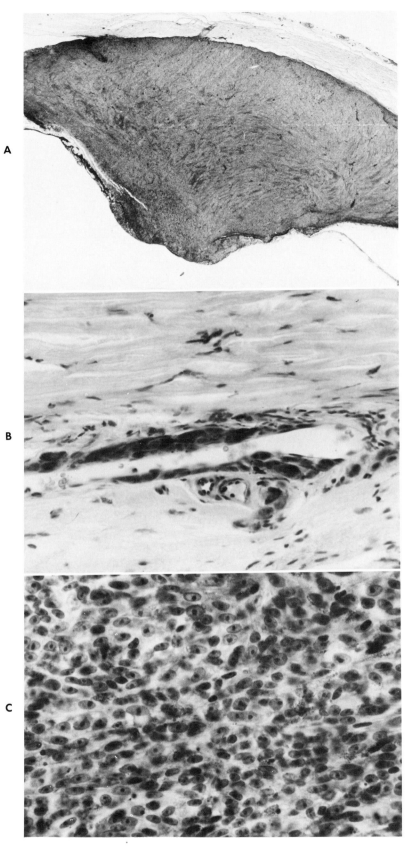

Fig. 195. For legend see opposite page.

337

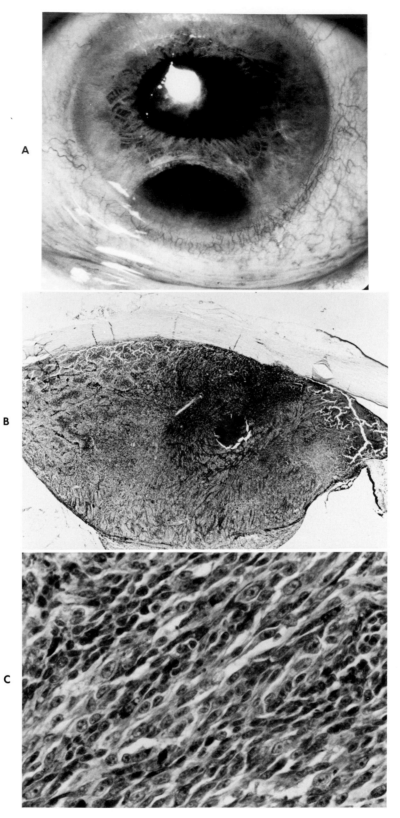

Fig. 196. For legend see opposite page.

and reaction to a ^{32}P uptake test was unequivocally positive for a tumor inferiorly.

Findings. Vision in the right eye is 20/40 and in the left accurate light projection. The right eye is normal. In the left eye there is moderate diffuse conjunctival injection. The anterior chamber is shallow, and inferiorly there is a dark brown mass from the 5 o'clock to the 7 o'clock position in contact with the cornea (Fig. 196, *A*). The iris adjacent to the tumor is pushed aside, FIG. 196 producing a number of concentric folds. The pupil is oval and displaced superiorly by tumor. There is no evidence of invasion of the iris by the tumor mass. A dense cataract does not permit even a red reflex of the fundus. Gonioscopy shows the tumor filling the angle inferiorly, but there is no sign of seeding or extension of the tumor laterally. Intraocular pressure in the right eye is 17 mm. Hg and in the left 14 mm. Hg (Schiøtz).

Course. The left eye was enucleated, and the histopathologic findings were a large, heavily pigmented malignant melanoma of the ciliary body, with extension beyond the base of the iris (Fig. 196, *B*). Microscopically, there was also extension through the sclera, and the cell type was epithelioid (Fig. 196, *C*). Postoperatively there were no complications, and 2½ years later there was no sign of metastasis. The patient was then lost to follow-up.

Malignant melanoma of the ciliary body

History. For 3 months this 64-year-old woman noticed a gradual decrease in vision in her left eye. A few days ago a black spot was noted on the eye for the first time.

Findings. Vision in the right eye is 20/25 and in the left 20/200. The right eye is normal, and the anterior segment of the left is also normal except for a black tumor mass filling the angle of the anterior chamber from the 1:30 to the 3 o'clock position (Fig. 197, *A*). This mass extends centrally about 3 mm. FIG. 197 and projects forward to come into contact with the peripheral cornea. The iris adjacent to the tumor is pushed up into folds, and the pupil is displaced nasally. Through a dilated pupil, a round, well-circumscribed dark brown mass is seen to extend to the equator. The posterior pole is normal, with nothing to account for the decreased vision.

Course. The left eye was enucleated, and the postoperative course was uneventful. The gross pathologic specimen showed a rounded tumor mass that

---

Fig. 196. *Dark brown mass involving iris inferiorly and pushing it into concentric folds in the left eye of a 72-year-old woman with a malignant melanoma of the ciliary body.* **A,** The tumor mass is in contact with a considerable portion of the cornea inferiorly, and by gonioscopy total closure of the angle but no seeding or extension of the tumor laterally can be seen. **B,** Low-power photomicrograph shows heavily pigmented malignant melanoma of the ciliary body, with extension beyond the base of the iris (extreme right). (H & E stain; ×40.) **C,** Photomicrograph shows cell type to be predominantly epithelioid. (H & E stain; ×1600.)

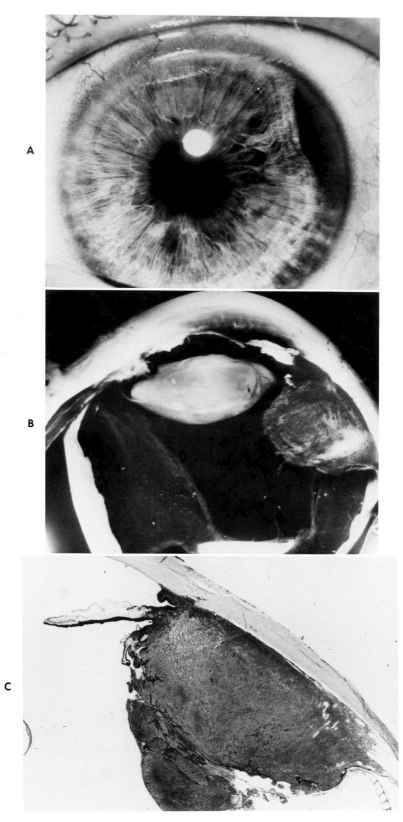

Fig. 197. For legend see opposite page.

extended well out into the vitreous cavity (Fig. 197, *B*). Histopathologically, the tumor was a malignant melanoma of the ciliary body, predominantly epithelioid cell type, with extension into the iris, angle meshwork, cornea, sclera, and choroid (Fig. 197, *C*). Two years later the Bonaccolto implant partially extruded, and the defect was repaired. Four years later the implant again became exposed and was removed. The patient was then lost to follow-up, but it was subsequently learned that she died 7 years later of lung metastases. No autopsy was performed to determine the source.

Malignant melanoma of the ciliary body with lens opacities

History. Six years ago this 52-year-old woman's left eye became red and irritable. Ocular examination revealed a mass in the iris and ciliary body with an associated cataract. The mass was thought to be a cyst of the ciliary body. Over the next 4 years she was reexamined at yearly intervals, and a slow increase in the size of the mass and a slight increase in the lens opacities were observed. A ^{32}P uptake test was performed and indicated a questionably significant difference in results from other sectors of the globe.

Findings. Vision in both eyes is 20/20. The right eye is normal. In the left eye there is a prominent forward bulge of the peripheral iris between the 4 and 5 o'clock positions and increased brown pigmentation over the bulge. With a maximally dilated pupil a small rounded mass can be seen projecting about 1 mm. beyond the pupillary margin. Adjacent to the mass are a number of concentric cortical opacities of the lower third of the lens. The remaining lens is clear. Ophthalmoscopic examination shows a brown mass extending posteriorly almost to the equator from the 4 o'clock to the 6 o'clock position. The remainder of the fundus is normal. By gonioscopic examination of the left eye the angle is seen to be completely closed from the 4 o'clock to the 6 o'clock position due to the bulge in the iris. Between the iris and lens can be seen a dark brown mass that flattens the peripheral lens adjacent to the mass (Reel XVI-1). Linear opacities of the lens cortex in this area can be also REEL XVI-1 visualized. The remainder of the angle is normal, and there is no appreciable increase in pigmentation of the trabecular meshwork. Intraocular tensions are normal in both eyes.

Course. Both excision of the tumor and enucleation were considered; but because of its very slow progression and the patient's reluctance to undergo surgery, she was followed for another year. During this time there was again a

---

Fig. 197. *Black tumor mass filling the temporal anterior chamber angle in the left eye of a 64-year-old woman with a malignant melanoma of the ciliary body.* **A,** The mass projects forward to come into contact with the peripheral cornea and pushes the iris into concentric folds. **B,** Gross pathologic specimen shows rounded tumor mass extending into the vitreous cavity. **C,** Low-power photomicrograph shows the heavily pigmented tumor mass extending into the iris, trabecular meshwork, cornea, sclera, and choroid. (H & E stain; ×40.) The cell type is predominantly epithelioid.

slight increase in the tumor's size and in the lens opacities. An iridocyclectomy was performed, and there was minimal bleeding and an uneventful postoperative course. Histopathologically, the tumor was a malignant melanoma of the ciliary body of a mixed cell type. Subsequently, some increased lens opacity occurred, and there was considerable blood in the anterior vitreous. In the next 2 months there was little absorption of the blood in the vitreous, and the vision was very poor. Enucleation was performed, and the postoperative course was uneventful. Histopathologic findings were a vitreous hemorrhage and retinal detachment but no residual tumor. Four years later there were no signs of orbital disease or metastases.

Malignant melanoma of the ciliary body

History. Three years ago this 56-year-old woman complained of blurring in her right eye, but her ophthalmologist could find no abnormalities, and the vision was normal. Blurring of vision progressed; and when recently examined, she was found to have exudates of the perimacular region.

Findings. Vision in both eyes is 20/25 with correction. In the right eye the anterior segment is normal except for a "recession" of the inferior angle seen gonioscopically. With a maximally dilated pupil a large elevated mass is seen between the 5 and 7 o'clock position. This appears to be lightly pigmented, and on its surface is the ora and pars plana region containing multiple cysts. Just below the macula are a number of subretinal exudates, and another group is seen at the equator along the inferior nasal vein. The tumor mass transilluminates partially and becomes bright green when fluorescein is given in-
REEL XVI-2 travenously (Reel XVI-2).

Course. The right eye was enucleated, and histopathologically the tumor was a malignant melanoma of the ciliary body of the spindle cell A type. Six years later the patient was in good health, with no signs of recurrence or metastasis of the tumor.

Malignant melanoma of the ciliary body

History. Recently this 85-year-old woman complained of tenderness of her right eye. A week ago she was found to have a tumor involving the iris.

Findings. The vision in the right eye is light perception nasally and in the left 20/200. In the right eye there is moderate conjunctival injection especially nasally. The cornea and anterior chamber are entirely clear. From the 12

Fig. 198. *Salmon-colored vascularized mass filling the nasal chamber angle in the right eye of an 85-year-old woman with a malignant melanoma of the ciliary body,* **A,** At the 3 o'clock position the iris is pushed into folds, but superiorly the tumor seems to be invading it. **B,** Gross pathologic specimen shows a massive tumor distorting the lens and displacing it to the side. **C,** Photomicrograph of tumor shows a mixed cell type, both spindle cell B and epithelioid. (H & E stain; ×1600.)

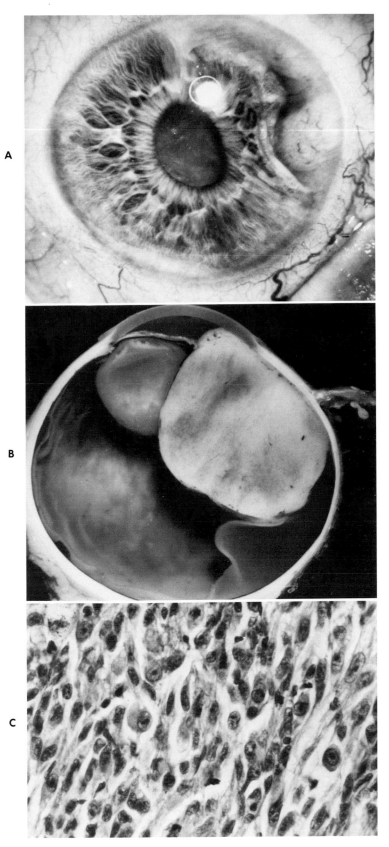

Fig. 198. For legend see opposite page.

FIG. 198 o'clock to the 4 o'clock position is a salmon-colored vascularized mass filling the angle and extending about 3 mm. centrally at the 3 o'clock position (Fig. 198, A). The iris is pushed into folds but does not appear to be invaded except at the 12 o'clock position. The pupil is displaced temporally and is ovoid. The lens cortex is diffusely opacified, and the lens appears to be distorted. In the left eye there is an immature cataract, but there are no other abnormalities. Intraocular pressure is 12 mm. Hg (Schiøtz) in the right eye and 19 mm. Hg in the left.

Course. The result of a metastatic survey was normal, but reaction to a ^{32}P uptake test was markedly positive. During the next 6 weeks there was definite enlargement of the tumor mass. The left eye was enucleated, and the gross pathologic specimen showed a massive tumor extending more than midway across the globe and displacing the lens to one side (Fig. 198, B). Histopathologically, the tumor was a malignant melanoma of the mixed cell type, both spindle cell B and epithelioid (Fig. 198, C). The postoperative course was uneventful. The patient was then lost to follow-up.

Malignant melanoma of the ciliary body

History. Two years ago this 79-year-old man noted some blurring of vision in his right eye, which progressively became worse, until 6 months ago it was reduced to bare light perception. The eye was not painful.

Findings. Vision in the right eye is inaccurate light projection and in the left 20/40. In the right eye there are a number of large, dilated blood vessels superiorly and a small area of scleral pigmentation at the 11 o'clock position FIG. 199 about 5 mm. from the limbus (Fig. 199, A). The anterior chamber is shallow superiorly, and between the 10 and 11 o'clock positions the iris is in contact with the cornea. The pupil is grossly irregular, and inferiorly there is a large posterior synechia. Projecting beyond the pupillary margin superiorly is a black tumor mass that does not transilluminate. Because of a mature cataract it is impossible to evaluate the extent of the tumor. The left eye is normal except for an incipient cataract. The intraocular pressure in both eyes is 18 mm. Hg (Schiøtz).

Course. Reaction to a ^{32}P uptake test was positive for malignancy. The right eye was enucleated, and the postoperative course was uneventful. The gross pathologic specimen showed a massive tumor of the ciliary body, with extension into the choroid (Fig. 199, B). Histopathologically, malignant melanoma cells invaded the sclera (Fig. 199, C), and the cell type was spindle cell A (Fig. 199, D). Exenteration of the orbit was considered but was not carried out due to the patient's age. A year later there was no evidence of tumor in the socket, and the vision in the left eye was further reduced due to the cataract. The patient was then lost to follow-up.

Malignant melanoma of the ciliary body with episcleral extension

History. Six weeks ago a dark spot was noted on the right eye of this 66-year-old woman. An attempt to rub it off was unsuccessful. She had no ocular symptoms.

Findings. The vision is normal in both eyes. In the right eye there is a dark

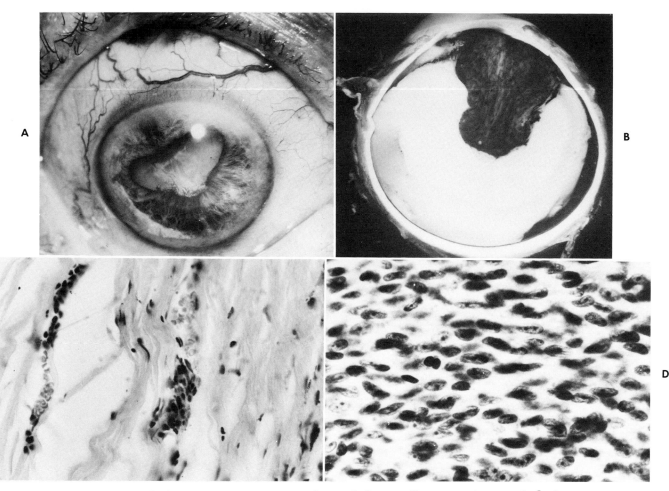

Fig. 199. *Black tumor mass projecting beyond the pupillary margin superiorly in the right eye of a 79-year-old man with a malignant melanoma of the ciliary body.* **A,** Pupil is distorted due to the tumor mass and posterior synechias. Superiorly, there are dilated episcleral and conjunctival blood vessels and a small area of dark brown scleral pigmentation. **B,** Gross pathologic specimen shows massive tumor and extension into the choroid. **C,** Photomicrograph shows tumor invading the sclera. (H & E stain; ×1000.) **D,** Photomicrograph shows spindle cell A type. (H & E stain; ×1600.)

brown, slightly elevated mass adjacent to the limbus at the 4 o'clock position (Fig. 200, *A*). The lesion is attached to the episclera, and the conjunctiva moves freely over it. With a widely dilated pupil a mass having the same color as that of the episcleral lesion is visible in the region of the ciliary body. The remaining posterior segment is normal. The left eye is normal.

FIG. 200

Course. The result of a metastatic survey was normal. Reaction to a ³²P uptake test was positive, and the right eye was enucleated. The gross pathologic specimen showed a moderately elevated tumor of the ciliary body (Fig. 200, *B*), and histopathologically the tumor was a malignant melanoma of the ciliary body with extension to the sclera. The patient was then lost to follow-up.

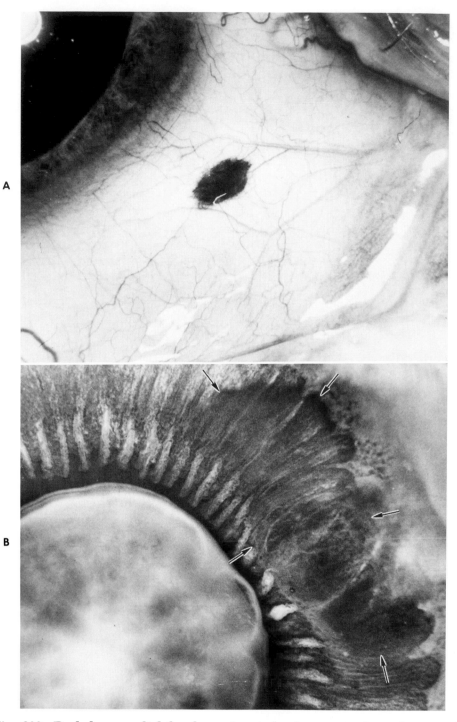

Fig. 200. *Dark brown, slightly elevated episcleral mass in the right eye of a 66-year-old woman with malignant melanoma of the ciliary body and episcleral extension.* **A,** The conjunctiva moves freely over the pigmented lesion, and with a widely dilated pupil a mass is visible in the ciliary body region. **B,** Gross pathologic specimen of the ciliary processes reveals an elevated irregular tumor mass (arrows) involving several hours of the clock. Histopathologically, the tumor is a malignant melanoma, with extension through the sclera.

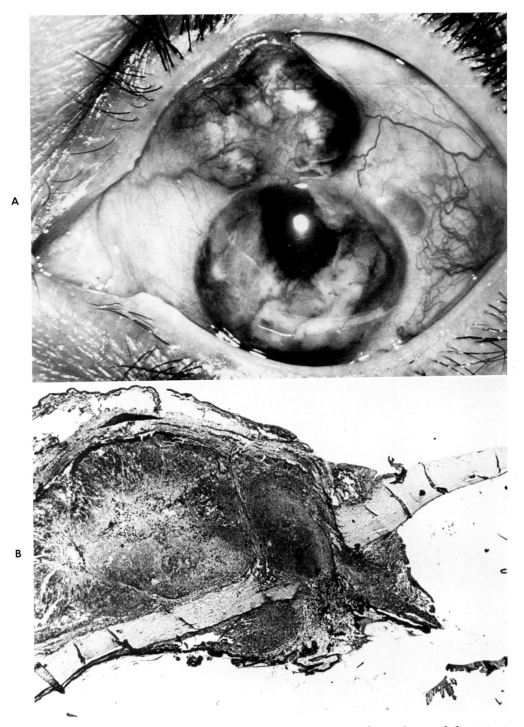

Fig. 201. *Subconjunctival elevated black mass superiorly and a nodular iris in the left eye of a 50-year-old woman with subconjunctival extension of a malignant melanoma of the ciliary body.* **A,** Filtering bleb following iridencleisis has now become solid, with tumor mass similar to that seen infiltrating the iris. **B,** Low-power photomicrograph reveals extension of tumor mass in anterior chamber through a scleral opening under the conjunctiva. (H & E stain; ×40.)

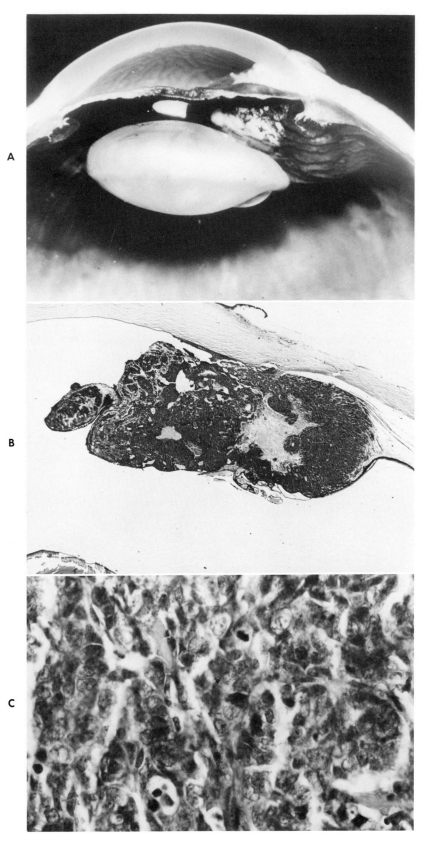

A

B

C

Fig. 202. For legend see opposite page.

Subconjunctival extension of malignant melanoma of the ciliary body

History. About 4 months ago this 50-year-old woman had an iridencleisis for what was diagnosed as unilateral glaucoma in her left eye. The eye continued to be painful, and a black mass developed under the upper lid.

Findings. Vision is 20/20 in the right eye, and the left eye is blind. The right eye is normal. In the left eye there is moderate conjunctival injection. Superiorly a black mass projects forward several millimeters and extends from the cul-de-sac down to the limbus (Fig. 201, *A*). The mass is covered by a thin FIG. 201 layer of conjunctiva. The cornea is clear, and the anterior chamber contains some blood, with a hyphema inferiorly. The depth of the anterior chamber is irregular due to the iris, which is nodular and vascularized, with a surgical coloboma superiorly. The pupil will not dilate, and visualization of the posterior segment is not possible.

Course. The left eye was enucleated. Histopathologic examination showed a malignant melanoma of the ciliary body with extensive involvement of the iris and extension of tumor tissue through a scleral opening into a "filtering bleb" (Fig. 201, *B*). Three months postoperatively several pigmented nodules appeared on the conjunctiva, and the orbit was exenterated. Six months later the orbit had filled with darkly pigmented tumor, and in another 3 months the patient died of metastases.

Malignant melanoma of the ciliary body and liver metastases

History. About 2 months ago this 55-year-old man developed blurred vision in the right eye. There was no pain in the eye, and he was apparently in good health except for some vague digestive complaints.

Findings. The vision in the right eye is 20/200 and in the left 20/20. In the right eye there are some large conjunctival vessels temporally. The cornea is clear. In the iris is a pink tumor mass from the 9 o'clock to the 11 o'clock position filling in the iris angle and pushing the iris into folds centrally (Reel XVI-3). REEL XVI-3 The pupil is ovoid due to the tumor mass. The tumor also extends inferiorly along the angle toward the 6 o'clock position. There is moderate cortical opacification and nuclear sclerosis. Only a poor view of the posterior segment can be obtained. The left eye is normal, and the intraocular tension is 19 mm. Hg (Schiøtz) in both eyes.

Fig. 202 (Reel XVI-4). *Irregular tumor mass having fingerlike projections involving the nasal angle and iris of the left eye in a 43-year-old woman with metastatic tumor of the ciliary body.* **A,** Gross pathologic specimen shows a massive ciliary body tumor, with extension through the root of the iris into the anterior chamber. The lens is slightly displaced and distorted. **B,** Low-power photomicrograph shows tumor mass, with extensive invasion of the iris, trabecular meshwork, and Schlemm's canal. (H & E stain; ×40.) **C,** Photomicrograph shows cells of the adenoid type consistent with metastatic adenocarcinoma. (H & E stain; ×1600.)

Course. A general physical examination showed the liver to be hard, firm, and irregular extending about 6 cm. below the costal margin. A liver biopsy showed malignant melanoma metastases. Because the eye was not painful, enucleation was deferred; the patient was then lost to follow-up.

Metastatic tumor of the ciliary body

History. A week ago this 43-year-old woman noticed a red spot on the left eye. There was no pain or blurring of vision, and she had no history of ocular disease or injuries. Her general health was good.

Findings. The vision in both eyes is 20/15. The right eye is normal. In the left eye there is an area of conjunctival injection extending up to the limbus from the 10 o'clock to the 11 o'clock position. At the 9 o'clock position is a small pinguecula. In the iris adjacent to the area of conjunctival injection is a tumor mass arising from the angle and extending toward the pupillary area. It has many blood vessels on its surface, which is markedly irregular due to a number of fingerlike projections on its inner surface (Reel XVI-4). The pupil is displaced temporally and is irregularly elliptical due to the tumor mass. The iris around the tumor is elevated as if tumor tissue were pushing it forward. The lens and vitreous are clear, and the fundus is normal. Intraocular pressure is 15 mm. Hg by applanation tonometry in both eyes.

REEL XVI-4

Course. Metastatic x-ray series showed multiple lesions throughout both lungs, consistent with metastasis. Moreover, further examination revealed a tumor in the left breast typical of a malignancy. Four days later the right eye was enucleated, and on the next day a mastectomy and bilateral salpingo-oophorectomy were performed. The gross pathologic specimen of the eye showed a large mass of the ciliary body distorting the lens posteriorly and extending into the anterior chamber anteriorly (Fig. 202, *A*). Histopathologically, the tumor was in the ciliary body and invaded the iris, trabecular meshwork, and Schlemm's canal (Fig. 202, *B*). Microscopically, the cells were adenoid in type consistent with metastatic adenocarcinoma (Fig. 202, *C*). A full course of fluorouracil therapy given resulted in a severe anemia and agranulocytosis, and a week later the patient died.

FIG. 202

Chapter 14

Traumatic and degenerative conditions of the ciliary body

PROLAPSE OF THE CILIARY BODY

Perforating lacerations of the sclera and occasionally of the cornea can lead to prolapse of the ciliary body. Such injuries are extremely serious in that there is often extensive hemorrhage extending into the vitreous, with profound visual loss even though permanent organization of the vitreous does not occur. Associated with the injury may be vitreous prolapse through the wound, and choroidal and retinal tissue may also be involved. Retinal detachment, if present, is difficult to treat because visualization of the area is often poor or impossible. As a general rule, the prolapsed tissue should be excised and then, despite the very poor prognosis, an attempt should be made to suture the sclera; in rare cases a good visual result can be obtained. Where retina is involved, diathermy or cryotherapy applied in several rows should be used around the edge of the perforating scleral laceration in an attempt to avoid a retinal detachment. Eyes with injuries involving the ciliary body, particularly with prolapse, are generally thought to be the most prone to sympathetic ophthalmia. Therefore, if after a week it appears that the probability of any useful vision is remote, enucleation is indicated if the vision in the other eye is good.

Blunt trauma to the globe sometimes produces an iridodialysis through which the ciliary body and occasionally vitreous will prolapse. Frequently the lens is dislocated. The complications of the dislocated lens are apparently more serious than those of the prolapsed vitreous and ciliary body. It is remarkable that often there are no untoward sequelae of such a traumatic incident. A delayed glaucoma is probably the most common. The development of a traumatic cataract is not unusual.

351

Traumatic and degenerative conditions of the ciliary body

Traumatic prolapse of the ciliary body

History. A few hours ago this 53-year-old man was struck in the left eye by the handle of his snow blower. This broke his glasses, lacerating his upper lid and sclera.

Findings. The vision in the right eye is 20/20 and in the left light perception only. The right eye is normal. The upper lid of the left eye is lacerated, and in one place there is a through-and-through hole. Superiorly, the conjunctiva and sclera appear to be lacerated with a prolapse of dark brown material around which there is much hemorrhage (Reel XVI-5). The anterior chamber contains a moderate hyphema, and the remainder of the eye cannot be examined.

REEL XVI-5

Course. An exploration of the conjunctival and scleral laceration showed that it extended about 10 mm. starting at the 11 o'clock position 4 mm. from the limbus and extending backward and temporally. Considerable ciliary body was prolapsed through the wound, and this was excised. The lid laceration was also repaired. Eleven days later the patient had no light perception in the eye, and he agreed to enucleation, which was performed. The postoperative course was uneventful, and finally the patient received a prosthesis. The result was cosmetically satisfactory.

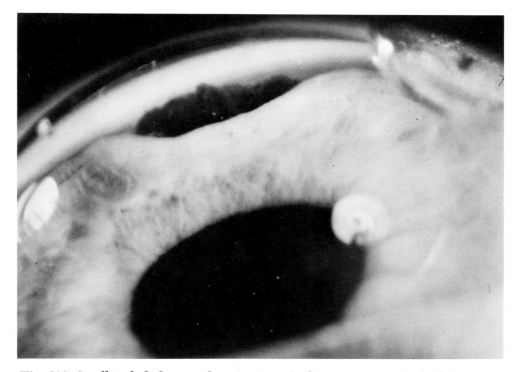

Fig. 203. *Small iridodialysis and protrusion of ciliary processes in the left eye of a 31-year-old man with a traumatic prolapse of the ciliary body into the anterior chamber. Gonioscopy shows both vitreous and iris processes protruding through the iridodialysis. Two weeks ago the patient sustained a blunt trauma to the eye.*

Prolapse of the ciliary body

Traumatic prolapse of the ciliary body into anterior chamber

History. Two weeks ago this 31-year-old man was struck in the left eye by a metal pipe. This resulted in a moderate hyphema. When it cleared, he was found to have an iridodialysis.

Findings. Vision in the right eye is 20/20 and in the left counting fingers at 1 foot. The right eye is normal. In the left there is moderate conjunctival injection. The anterior chamber is of normal depth, the pupil is ovoid, and a small iridodialysis is seen at the 2 o'clock position. There is slight posterior dislocation of the lens, and results of the fundus examination are normal. By gonioscopy vitreous can be seen protruding through the iridodialysis, and iris processes are seen to be prolapsed into the anterior chamber, some of them reaching Schwalbe's line (Fig. 203).

Course. A year and a half later the vision was still markedly reduced, and fundus examination revealed several old choroidal tears temporal to the disc, which explained the severe loss of vision. The patient was then lost to follow-up.

RECESSION OF THE IRIS ROOT
(TEAR INTO THE CILIARY BODY)

Blunt trauma to the anterior segment of the eye can result in a detachment of the ciliary body from the scleral spur and tearing of the uveal meshwork and ciliary body. The condition is commonly referred to as traumatic recession of the iris root. It may involve only a small portion of the angle, but in a more severe injury commonly it involves much if not all the circumference of the anterior chamber angle. By far the most serious complication of such an injury is the development of glaucoma, either early or late. The early type develops from a week to several years after the injury and presumably is associated with damage to the corneoscleral trabecular meshwork at the time that the ciliary body is detached from the scleral spur. Scarring and fibrosis of the trabeculum decreases its permeability to aqueous and thus reduces the facility of outflow. The late type of glaucoma may develop from several years to 40 or more years after the injury, and in some cases it has been shown to be due to secondary changes on the meshwork, with development of a cuticular membrane covering the damaged meshwork. Other cases apparently are due to scarring and sclerosis alone. As these patients become older, there is a tendency toward decreased filtration and the development of mild chronic open angle glaucoma. In the damaged eye, the facility of outflow is appreciably reduced; therefore, open angle glaucoma may develop in the damaged eye, while the undamaged eye still has a sufficient facility of outflow to remain normotensive. The most common cause of unilateral open angle glaucoma may well be traumatic recession of the iris root.

By gonioscopy the typical finding is that of an iris root that appears further posterior and wider than that in the undamaged eye. Depending on the severity and localization of the trauma, the extent of angle involvement may vary from slight to a complete 360°. The uveal meshwork is torn away and disrupted. This leaves the ciliary muscle relatively bare, as contrasted with a normal eye. Occasionally, the trabecular meshwork itself can be seen to be torn, and an iridodialysis may also be present. A subtle finding is the appearance of the scleral spur, which stands out as a white and distinct band where the uveal meshwork has been torn from it, while in the normal eye it is relatively inconspicuous behind the covering of the uveal meshwork. It is important that the ophthalmologist compare the two eyes to determine a recession of the iris root by placing gonioscopic lenses (Koeppe lenses) on both eyes simultaneously for rapid comparison. In severe injuries, the ciliary body may be torn so deeply that the angle may be three or four times the normal depth. The torn ciliary muscle is light gray and delicate appearing, sometimes resembling cotton batting. Occasionally, the tear extends through the full thickness of the muscle, and the white scleral wall is exposed, giving the appearance of a surgical cyclodialysis cleft; individual anterior ciliary arteries may be visible on the inner surface of the sclera. Peripheral anterior synechias are common adjacent to the area of angle recession and are usually associated with the hyphema that often occurs after the injury. The synechias probably have little or nothing to do with the subsequent development of glaucoma.

The treatment of a traumatic recession of the iris root is almost entirely limited to treatment of the glaucoma, which, if the injury is severe, will develop in a fairly high proportion of the cases. As would be expected, the more extensive the damage the less responsive the glaucoma is to treatment. Miotics and epinephrine are effective in some cases, but carbonic anhydrase inhibitor drugs may be necessary. Those with a late onset and presumably with a cuticular membrane are especially difficult to treat medically. A filtering procedure may be necessary. Patients who are known to have a recession of the iris root but without glaucoma should be examined periodically for the rest of their lives so that glaucoma, if it develops, will be promptly treated.

Traumatic recession of the iris root and iridodialysis

History. Three years ago this 61-year-old man was hit in the right eye with a potato thrown at him. There was almost immediate loss of vision due to a hyphema, which cleared promptly without the development of glaucoma. Traumatic mydriasis and an iridodialysis in the nasal sector became visible upon absorption of the hyphema. Three weeks ago he was again struck in the right eye with a club and sustained another hyphema. As the blood absorbed, a preretinal hemorrhage was observed. Until yesterday the tension remained in the high normal range, but then it rose to 42 mm. Hg (Schiøtz). Treatment with acetazolamide was instituted.

Findings. Vision in the right eye is 20/40 and in the left 20/30. There is moderate conjunctival injection in the right eye, with a clear cornea. The anterior chamber is abnormally deep, especially peripherally. The pupil is semidilated and irregular and reacts only minimally to light. The lens is clear, and in the fundus there are a few linear retinal hemorrhages between the disc and macula. REEL XVI-6 The left eye is normal. Gonioscopy of the right eye reveals an extensive tear into FIG. 204 the ciliary body, producing a deep cleft in some places (Reel XVI-6 and Fig. 204, A). From the 8 o'clock to the 9 o'clock position there is an iridodialysis with exposure of the ciliary processes (Fig. 204, B). Gonioscopy of the left eye reveals a normal angle containing a number of iris processes and a ciliary body band that is visible in most places. Intraocular tension is 12 mm. Hg (Schiøtz) in both eyes.

354

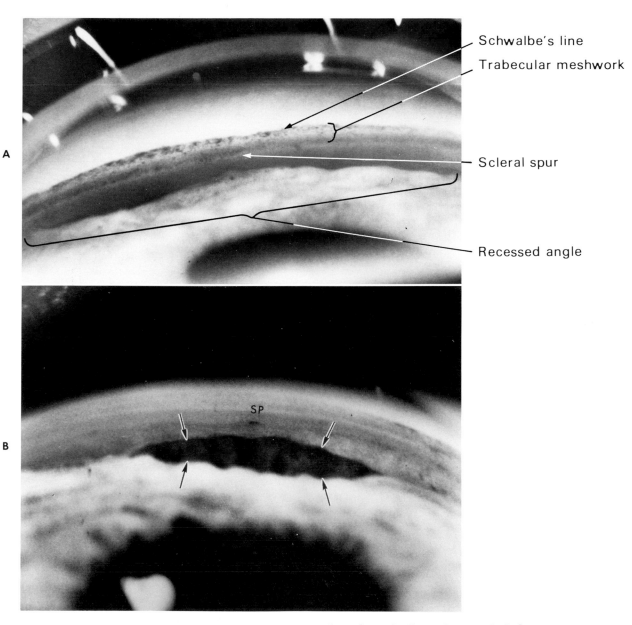

Fig. 204 (Reel XVI-6). *Extensive tear into the ciliary body and an iridodialysis in the right eye of a 61-year-old man with traumatic recession of the iris root.* **A,** Gonioscopy reveals a deep cleft in the chamber angle due to the extensive tear into the ciliary body. **B,** Gonioscopy reveals an iridodialysis (arrows) in another area, exposing the ciliary processes. The scleral spur (SP) is high, indicating the presence of a recessed iris root as well.

Course. Two months later the acetazolamide was discontinued, and the intraocular pressure did not rise. Tonography showed a borderline facility of outflow in the right eye. Four years later vision in the right eye was reduced to 20/400 because of an immature cataract, and the intraocular pressure was normal. Ten years later the vision in the right eye was markedly reduced, presumably due to a maturing cataract, and the left eye was still normal. Intraocular pressure was 16 mm. Hg (Schiøtz) in both eyes.

Traumatic recession of the iris root

History. One month ago this 12-year-old boy was struck in the left eye with a stick. This resulted in corneal abrasions, traumatic mydriasis, and macular edema. Recently he was noted to be developing a cataract.

Findings. The vision in the right eye is 20/20 and in the left 20/40. The right eye is normal. In the left eye there is a central healed corneal scar. The anterior chamber is deeper than that of the right eye, and the pupil is semidilated and slightly irregular and does not react to light. The lens is clear except for a few opacities in the anterior subcapsular region. On fundus examination the macular region appears lighter than normal, and the foveal reflex is absent, consistent with Berlin's macular edema. There is a slight iridodonesis, but the lens is not obviously dislocated. Gonioscopy of the right eye shows the angle to be fairly
FIG. 205 narrow, with the ciliary body band barely visible in some places (Fig. 205, A). In the left eye the entire 360° of the angle is about three times as wide as that of the right eye, with a "ciliary band" that is lighter than the trabecular meshwork (Fig. 205, B). In some places a diaphanous membrane can be seen deep in the angle recess, and there are a number of dark pigment clumps on the portion of the trabecular meshwork overlying Schlemm's canal. The intraocular pressure shown by applanation tonometry is 14 mm. Hg in both eyes.

Course. The patient was advised to return at 6-month intervals for repeated intraocular pressure determinations, but he was lost to follow-up.

Traumatic angle recession

History. Thirteen years ago this 31-year-old man was struck in the right eye with a baseball. The vision returned to normal, but 3 months later glaucoma and loss of vision due to a cataract were discovered in this eye. Four years later the intraocular tension was normal without medications. Three years ago the intraocular pressures were found to be elevated in both eyes. This was controlled with pilocarpine drops and acetazolamide.

Findings. Vision in the right eye is 20/300 and in the left 20/15. Both eyes appear to be normal, with miotic pupils. However, there is an immature cataract in the right eye, with marked posterior subcapsular opacities. The disc of the right eye shows slight nasal displacement of the vessels and enlargement of the central cup. In the left eye the disc is normal. By gonioscopy the right eye shows 360° recession of the iris root, with a flat iris plane. The structures of the angle are difficult to identify due to many pigmented iris processes extending well onto
FIG. 206 the trabecular meshwork (Fig. 206, A). In the left eye the angle is of normal depth and contour, but again there are numerous pigmented iris processes, some of which extended up to Schwalbe's line (Fig. 206, B). These are so numerous and extensive that they are considered to be abnormal. Visual field examination shows a relative inferior field loss in the right eye only.

Course. Without medication diurnal intraocular tension studies revealed a range between 40 and 50 mm. Hg (Schiøtz) in the right eye and 35 to 44 mm.

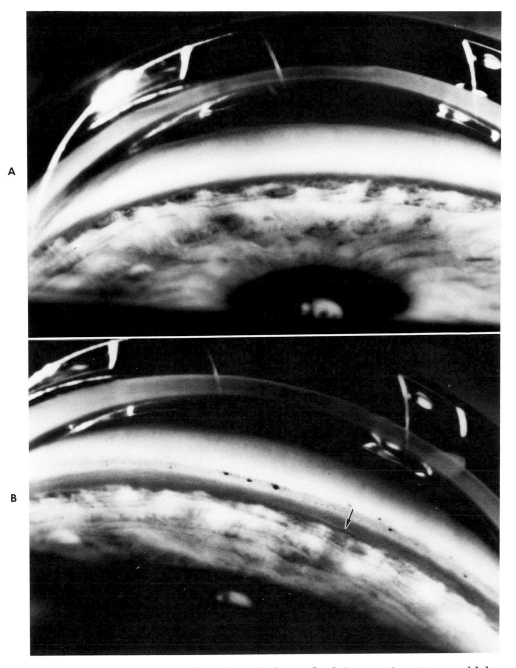

Fig. 205. *A 360° tear into the ciliary body in the left eye of a 12-year-old boy with a traumatic recession of the iris root.* **A,** Gonioscopy of the right eye reveals a fairly narrow angle. **B,** Gonioscopy of the left eye shows an angle in which the ciliary body band is wider than the trabecular meshwork. A diaphanous membrane (arrow) is occasionally visible deep in the angle recess. The left eye had been struck by a stick.

357

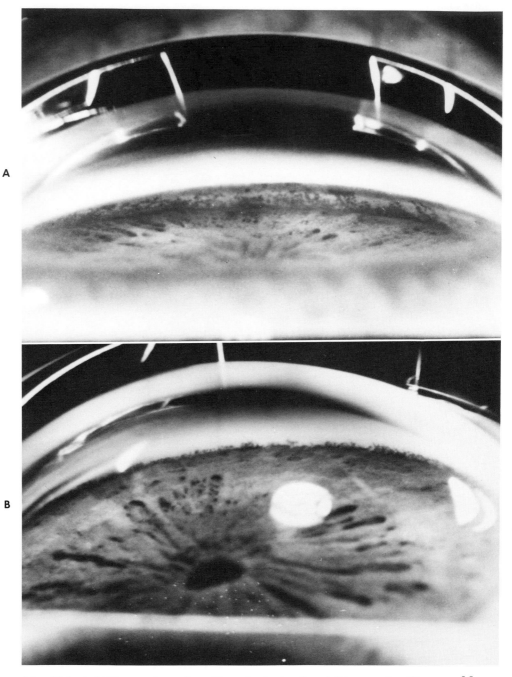

Fig. 206. *A 360° tear into the ciliary body in the right eye of a 31-year-old man with a traumatic angle recession.* **A,** Gonioscopy of the right eye reveals a flat iris plane and a wide "ciliary body band" covered by many pigmented iris processes. **B,** Gonioscopy of the left eye reveals a normal (somewhat narrow) angle containing numerous pigmented iris processes. A baseball had struck the patient's right eye.

Hg (Schiøtz) in the left. Pilocarpine (4%) drops, epinephrine (1%) drops, and ethoxzolamide (Cardrase) were instituted, resulting in reduction of the diurnal intraocular pressure range to 20 mm. Hg (Schiøtz) or lower in both eyes.

Traumatic peripheral anterior synechia and angle recession

History. Six weeks ago this 45-year-old woman was struck with a bobby pin propelled from a rubber band. Within an hour the vision was reduced to light perception only, and she was found to have an extensive traumatic hyphema. The blood gradually absorbed, without elevation of intraocular pressure or recurrent bleeding. Over the next month there was gradual improvement of vision.

Findings. Vision in the right eye is 20/80 and in the left 20/25. In the right eye the cornea is clear, and the anterior chamber is not remarkable except for an increase of depth in comparison with the left eye. The iris is atrophic and fixed by posterior synechias nasally. Iridodonesis is also present, and the pupil is semi-dilated and reacts minimally to light. The lens, vitreous, and fundus are normal through the undilated pupil. The left eye is normal. By gonioscopy most of the entire 360° of angle is about three times as wide as that of the normal left eye. In a few places there are prominent trabecular anterior synechias in sharp contrast to the excessively deep angle elsewhere (Reel XVI-7). In most places the REEL XVI-7 angle is peppered with granular brown pigment, which ends abruptly at Schwalbe's line and usually spares the scleral spur. In the left eye the ciliary body band is only partially visible, but everywhere the angle is open down to the scleral spur. There is only light pigmentation of the trabecular meshwork. The intraocular pressure in the right eye is 12 mm. Hg (Schiøtz) and in the left 20 mm. Hg (Schiøtz).

Course. Within the next few weeks there was a diffuse cortical cataractous change in the right lens, with reduction in vision so that 6 months later the vision was 20/200 with correction. At this time fundus examination showed a retinal exudate inferiorly and temporally, but no detachment. Six months later the cataract precluded all visualization of the fundus, with vision reduced to counting fingers at 10 feet. Three years later the intraocular tension was 14 mm. Hg in both eyes as shown by applanation tonometry, and tonography showed a normal facility of outflow, equal in both eyes. The patient was then lost to follow-up.

CILIARY STAPHYLOMA

Staphylomas associated with chronic glaucoma (usually absolute glaucoma) ordinarily occur anteriorly in the region of the ciliary body and therefore are commonly referred to as ciliary staphylomas. They can also be produced by injuries involving the anterior sclera. Both primary and secondary conditions that lead to thinning of the sclera anteriorly may involve the ciliary body. Their characteristics and location are variable depending on the cause and chronicity. Chronic scleritis and particularly scleral uveitis are also usually anterior in location and may result in a typical ciliary staphyloma. The region of the ciliary body represents an area of scleral weakening due to the exit of the anterior ciliary artery. Intercalary staphylomas are those arising near the limbus and are thought to result from weakening of the sclera by Schlemm's canal and the anterior ciliary vein. It is not unusual for the ciliary body to be involved in an intercalary staphyloma.

The appearance of a ciliary staphyloma is that of a bluish elevation in the area of the ciliary body due to marked thinning and ectasia of the sclera. When glaucoma results in a ciliary staphyloma, the glaucoma becomes more intractable. Treatment of the staphyloma is usually unsuccessful; however, surface diathermy and surgical buckling of the staphyloma has been successful, while the more radical procedure of scleral resection and replacement with a scleral or fascial graft may be attempted.

Ruptured ciliary staphyloma with bleb formation

History. This 85-year-old woman noted sudden painless loss of vision about 6 months ago in the left eye. More recently a dark cystic structure of the sclera developed superiorly; it was treated with cold compresses and cortisone drops.

Findings. Vision in the right eye is 20/20 with correction and in the left questionable light perception. The right eye is normal, but on the left there is an oval-shaped mass, about 8 mm. wide and 10 mm. high, protruding from the

FIG. 207   limbal region at the 12 o'clock position (Fig. 207). Covered with conjunctiva, the mass is darkly pigmented and partially transilluminates. The anterior chamber is shallow, and there is some corneal edema and early bullous keratopathy. The

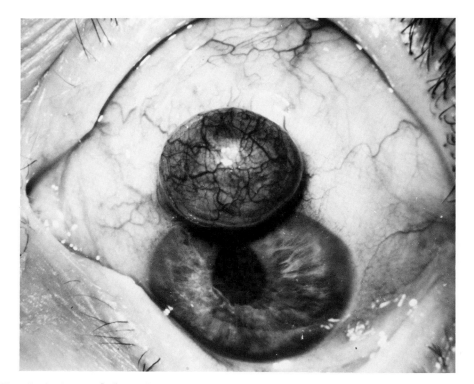

Fig. 207. *An oval-shaped mass at the limbus in the left eye of an 85-year-old woman with a ruptured ciliary staphyloma.* The mass is darkly pigmented, partially transilluminates, and is covered with conjunctiva, thus producing a bleb. The anterior chamber is shallow and the intraocular pressure markedly elevated.

pupil is distorted, as the iris is pulled up into the limbal mass. The media appear to be clear, but no fundus detail can be visualized. Intraocular tension in the right eye is 21 mm. Hg and in the left over 70 mm. Hg as shown by applanation tonometry.

Course. A ^{32}P test showed no evidence of tumor, and ultrasonography revealed no evidence of retinal detachment or intraocular mass. Intraocular tensions in the right eye were borderline, and glaucoma work-up showed the facility of the outflow to be decreased. Antiglaucomatous medication administered topically brought the patient's intraocular pressure in the right eye into the mid-teens, but in the left it remained markedly elevated. Since she was asymptomatic, no further therapy was administered to the left eye. One year later she developed streptococcal sepsis and died.

Ciliary staphylomas, interstitial keratitis, and glaucoma

History. As a child this 51-year-old woman had a severe episode of inflammation in both eyes. At age 18 she had a cataract extraction in the left eye, but her vision did not improve. Four years ago she had an episode of inflammation of her right eye, with much photophobia and some loss of vision.

Findings. The vision in the right eye is 20/100 with a high myopic astigmatic correction and in the left eye light perception only. The right cornea is dif-

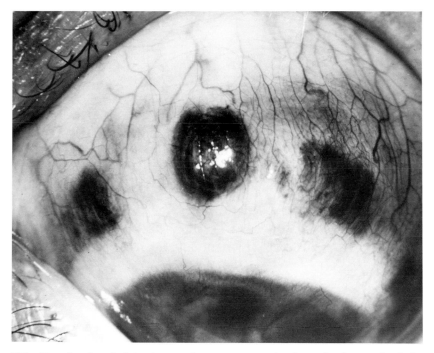

Fig. 208. *Focal scleral thinning and protrusion of ciliary body in the left eye of a 51-year-old woman with ciliary staphylomas, interstitial keratitis, and glaucoma.* The darkly pigmented areas progressively enlarged, and the eye became painful and blind.

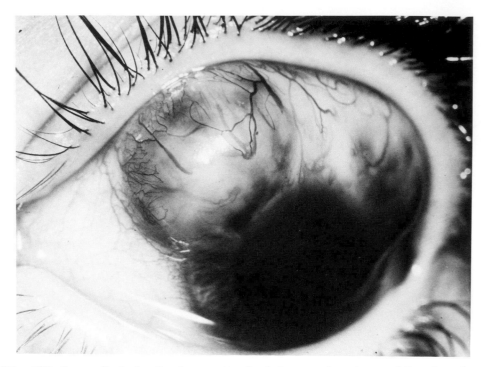

Fig. 209. *Large limbal scleral mass in the left eye of a 4-year-old girl with a traumatic ciliary staphyloma.* Recently the eye was injured, which resulted in an intraocular hemorrhage and subsequent surgical evacuation of the clot. The staphyloma occurred in an area of wound dehiscence.

fusely scarred and thinned superiorly. The anterior chamber is of normal depth. The media are difficult to visualize, and only a red reflex of the fundus can be obtained. In the left eye the cornea is markedly enlarged, and there are a number of focal ciliary staphylomas superiorly and temporally (Fig. 208). The entire cornea is vascularized and diffusely opacified. A superior coloboma of the iris is present. No details of the posterior segment of the eye can be seen.

FIG. 208

Course. Six years later the staphyloma in the left eye had increased in size, and the eye was painful. It marred the patient's appearance, and at her request the left eye was enucleated. Histopathologically, the eye showed intercalary staphylomas, with atrophy of the ciliary body, a detached retina, and absolute glaucoma. The postoperative course was uneventful, and the patient was then lost to follow-up.

Traumatic ciliary staphyloma

History. Three months ago this 4-year-old girl was struck in the left eye by a spring. This produced a small hyphema, but 2 days later there was a massive intraocular hemorrhage, which required evacuation of the clot and a peripheral iridectomy. Four days later there was a small iris prolapse through the surgical wound, and this was repaired. A week later further prolapse occurred, and another repair was done. A month later there was further wound dehiscence and evidence of ciliary body prolapse covered by conjunctiva. The intraocular pressure remained elevated, and no view of the fundus could be obtained. In another month there was further staphyloma formation, and it appeared that the eye was blind.

Findings. Apparently the vision is normal in the right eye, and there is no light perception in the left. The right eye is normal. In the left eye there is a large rounded scleral mass extending to the limbus from the 9 o'clock to the 12 o'clock position (Fig. 209). There is another similar mass at the 2 o'clock position.   FIG. 209 Both of these masses contain dark pigmented tissue. There is a surgical iridectomy superiorly, and the lens is clear, but only a dull red reflex can be obtained. Digital tension indicates that the intraocular pressure is elevated.

Course. The left eye was enucleated, and the postoperative course was uneventful. The histopathologic finding was a large intercalary staphyloma containing iris and ciliary body and secondary glaucoma.

Bibliography for part three

Cogan, D. G., and Kuwabara, T.: Tumors of the ciliary body, Int. Ophthal. Clin. **11**:27-56, Fall 1971.

Duke-Elder, S., and Perkins, E. S.: System of ophthalmology. Vol. 9, Diseases of the uveal tract, St. Louis, 1966, The C. V. Mosby Co.

Hogan, M. J., and Zimmerman, L. E.: Ophthalmic pathology, Philadelphia, 1962, W. B. Saunders Co.

Reese, A. B.: Tumors of the eye, ed. 2, New York, 1963, Paul B. Hoeber, Inc.

Scheie, H. G.: Gonioscopy in diagnosis of tumors of the iris and ciliary body, Arch. Ophthal. **51**:288-300, Mar. 1954.

Sirsat, N. V., Shriknande, S. S., and Sampat, N. B.: Medullo-epithelioma (diktyoma) of the eye, Brit. J. Ophthal. **56**:362-365, Apr. 1972.

Zimmerman, L. E.: Verhoeff's "teratoneuroma"; a critical reappraisal in light of new observations and current concepts of embryonic tumors, Trans. Amer. Ophthal. Soc. **69**:210-236, 1971.

Index

366